The Role of
Serotonin in
Psychiatric Disorders

Clinical and Experimental Psychiatry

Monograph Series of the Department of Psychiatry
Albert Einstein College of Medicine of Yeshiva University
Montefiore Medical Center
New York, N.Y.

Editor-in-Chief Herman M. van Praag, M.D., Ph.D.

Clinical and Experimental Psychiatry Monograph No. 4

The Role of Serotonin in Psychiatric Disorders

Edited by

SERENA-LYNN BROWN, M.D., Ph.D.

and

HERMAN M. VAN PRAAG, M.D., Ph.D.

Brunner/Mazel, Publishers • New York

Library of Congress Cataloging-in-Publication Data
The Role of serotonin in psychiatric disorders / edited by Serena-
Lynn Brown and Herman M. van Praag.
    p.   cm. — (Clinical and experimental psychiatry ; 4)
    Includes bibliographical reference.
    Include indexes.
    ISBN 0-87630-589-3
    1. Mental
illness—Pathophysiology.   2. Serotonin—Physiological
  effect.   3. Mental illness—Etiology.   I. Brown, Serena-Lynn.
  II. Praag, Herman M. van (Herman Meïr), 1929–   .   III. Series.
    [DNLM: 1. Mental Disorders—drug therapy.   2. Serotonin—
  therapeutic use.   W1 CL664EH v. 4 / WM 402 R745]
  RC455.4.B5R65   1990
  616.89 '07--dc20
  DNLM/DLC
  for Library of Congress   90-2285
                                                              CIP

Published by
BRUNNER/MAZEL, INC.
19 Union Square
New York, New York 10003

Manufactured in the United States of America

10 9 8 7 6 5 4 3 2 1

"To Our Fathers"

A Note on the Series

Psychiatry is in a state of flux. The excitement springs in part from internal changes, such as the development and official acceptance (at least in the U.S.A.) of an operationalized, multiaxial classification system of behavioral disorders (the DSM-III), the increasing sophistication of methods to measure abnormal human behavior and the impressive expansion of biological and psychological treatment modalities. Exciting developments are also taking place in fields relating to psychiatry; in molecular (brain) biology, genetics, brain imaging, drug development, epidemiology, experimental psychology, to mention only a few striking examples.

More generally speaking, psychiatry is moving, still relatively slowly, but irresistibly, from a more philosophical, contemplative orientation, to that of an empirical science. From the fifties on, biological psychiatry has been a major catalyst of that process. It provided the mother discipline with a third cornerstone, i.e., neurobiology, the other two being psychology and medical sociology. In addition, it forced the profession into the direction of standardization of diagnoses and of assessment of abnormal behavior. Biological psychiatry provided psychiatry not only with a new basic science and with new treatment modalities, but also with the tools, the methodology and the mentality to operate within the confines of an empirical science, the only framework in which a medical discipline can survive.

In other fields of psychiatry, too, one discerns a gradual trend towards scientification. Psychological treatment techniques are standardized and manuals developed to make these skills more easily transferrable. Methods registering treatment outcome—traditionally used in the behavioral/cognitive field—are now more and more requested and, hence, developed for dynamic forms of psychotherapy as well. Social and community psychiatry, until the sixties more firmly rooted in humanitarian ideals and social awareness than in empirical studies, profited greatly from its liaison with the social sciences and the expansion of psychiatric epidemiology.

Let there be no misunderstanding. Empiricism does *not imply* that it is

vii

only the measurable that counts. Psychiatry would be mutilated if it would neglect that what is not yet capturable in numbers and probably never will be. It *does imply* that what is measurable should be measured. Progress in psychiatry is dependent on ideas and on experiment. Their linkage is inseparable.

This monograph series, published under the auspices of the Department of Psychiatry of the Albert Einstein College of Medicine/Montefiore Medical Center, is meant to keep track of important developments in our profession, to summarize what has been achieved in particular fields, and to bring together the viewpoints obtained from disparate vantage points—in short, to capture some of the excitement ongoing in modern psychiatry, both in its clinical and experimental dimensions. Our Department hosts the Series, but naturally welcomes contributions from others.

Bernie Mazel is not only the publisher of this series, but it was he who generated the idea—an ambitious plan which, however, we all feel is worthy of pursuit. The edifice of psychiatry is impressive, but still somewhat flawed in its foundations. May this Series contribute to consolidation of its infrastructure.

—HERMAN M. VAN PRAAG, M.D., PH.D.
Silverman Professor and Chairman
Department of Psychiatry
Albert Einstein College of Medicine
Montefiore Medical Center
Bronx, New York

Contents

ix

Contributors

Alan Apter, M.D., Director, Adolescent Unit, Geha Hospital, Petah-Tikva, Israel; Senior Lecturer, Sackler School of Medicine, Tel Aviv Medical Center, Tel Aviv, Israel; formerly Research Fellow in Psychopharmacology and Biological Psychiatry, Department of Psychiatry, Albert Einstein College of Medicine/Montefiore Medical Center, Bronx, New York

Gregory M. Asnis, M.D., Professor of Psychiatry and Director of the Affective Disorders Program, Department of Psychiatry, Albert Einstein College of Medicine of Yeshiva University/Montefiore Medical Center, Bronx, New York

Avraham Bleich, M.D., Colonel and Head, Mental Health Department, Israel Defense Force; Lecturer, Sackler School of Medicine, Tel Aviv Medical Center, Tel Aviv, Israel; formerly Research Fellow in Psychopharmacology and Biological Psychiatry, Department of Psychiatry, Albert Einstein College of Medicine/Montefiore Medical Center, Bronx, New York

Harry A. Brandt, M.D., Professor and Director, Eating Disorder Program, Department of Psychiatry, University of Maryland School of Medicine, Baltimore, Maryland

Timothy D. Brewerton, M.D., Associate Professor, Department of Psychiatry and Behavioral Sciences, Medical University of South Carolina, Charleston, South Carolina

Serena-Lynn Brown, M.D., Ph.D., Assistant Professor and Director, Psychopharmacology Clinic, Department of Psychiatry, Albert Einstein College of Medicine/Montefiore Medical Center, Bronx, New York

Dennis S. Charney, M.D., Professor, Department of Psychiatry, Yale University School of Medicine, New Haven, Connecticut; Chief, Psychiatry Service, West Haven Veterans Administration Medical Center, West Haven, Connecticut

Pedro Delgado, M.D., Assistant Professor of Psychiatry, Department of

Psychiatry, Yale University School of Medicine, New Haven, Connecticut; Chief, Outpatient Psychiatry, West Haven Veterans Administration Medical Center, West Haven, Connecticut

Jill M. Harkavy Friedman, Ph.D., Assistant Professor and Coordinator, Anxiety and Depression Clinic, Department of Psychiatry, Albert Einstein College of Medicine/Montefiore Medical Center, Bronx, New York

George R. Heninger, M.D., Professor of Psychiatry and Director, Abraham Ribicoff Research Facilities, Department of Psychiatry, Yale University School of Medicine, New Haven, Connecticut

David C. Jimerson, M.D., Associate Professor of Psychiatry and Director of Research, Department of Psychiatry, Harvard Medical School and Beth Israel Hospital, Boston, Massachusetts

Rene S. Kahn, M.D., Chief Resident, Department of Psychiatry, Mount Sinai School of Medicine, New York, New York; formerly Research Fellow in Psychopharmacology and Biological Psychiatry, Department of Psychiatry, Albert Einstein College of Medicine/Montefiore Medical Center, Bronx, New York

Oren Kalus, M.D., Research Fellow in Psychopharmacology and Biological Psychiatry, Department of Psychiatry, Albert Einstein College of Medicine/Montefiore Medical Center, Bronx, New York

Martin L. Korn, M.D., Assistant Professor and Deputy Director, Psychopharmacology Clinic, Albert Einstein College of Medicine/Montefiore Medical Center, Bronx, New York

Michael D. Lesem, M.D., Assistant Professor and Chief, Adult Psychiatric Services, Department of Psychiatry, Harris County Psychiatric Center, University of Texas Medical School at Houston, Houston, Texas

Herbert Y. Meltzer, M.D., Douglas D. Bond Professor of Psychiatry, Department of Psychiatry, Case Western Reserve University School of Medicine, Cleveland, Ohio

Dennis L. Murphy, M.D., Chief, Laboratory of Clinical Science, National Institute of Mental Health, Bethesda, Maryland

J. Frank Nash, Ph.D., Assistant Professor of Psychiatry, Department of Psychiatry, Case Western Reserve University School of Medicine, Cleveland, Ohio

Demitri F. Papolos, M.D., Assistant Professor and Chief, Inpatient Service, Department of Psychiatry, Albert Einstein College of Medicine/Montefiore Medical Center, Bronx, New York

Stephen J. Peroutka, M.D., Ph.D., Assistant Professor of Neurology, Department of Neurology, Stanford University Medical Center, Stanford, California

Lawrence H. Price, M.D., Associate Professor of Psychiatry and Director, Clinical Neuroscience Research Unit, Department of Psychiatry, Yale University School of Medicine, New Haven, Connecticut

Andrew J. Sleight, Ph.D., Postdoctoral Fellow, Department of Neurology, Stanford University Medical Center, Stanford, California

Herman M. van Praag, M.D., Ph.D., Professor and Chairman, Department of Psychiatry, Albert Einstein College of Medicine/Montefiore Medical Center, Bronx, New York

Scott Wetzler, Ph.D., Assistant Professor of Psychiatry and Head, Clinical Assessment Program, Division of Psychology, Department of Psychiatry, Albert Einstein College of Medicine/Montefiore Medical Center, Bronx, New York

Joseph Zohar, M.D., Associate Professor of Psychiatry and Director, Anxiety Clinic, Beer-Sheva Mental Health Center and Ben Gurion University, Beer-Sheva, Israel

Rachel C. Zohar-Kadouch, M.D., Outpatient Psychiatric Clinic, Sorocca Medical Center, Beer-Sheva, Israel

The Role of
Serotonin in
Psychiatric Disorders

1

Introduction
Why Study Serotonin in Clinical Psychiatric Research?

SERENA-LYNN BROWN
HERMAN M. VAN PRAAG

Over the past several decades, the field of biological psychiatry has emerged as a major new subspecialty of general psychiatry. A number of discoveries, including the specificity of certain classes of medications for the treatment of different psychiatric disorders and the elucidation of possible biological markers in several major psychiatric illnesses, have spurred the growth of research in this area. Several areas of intensive study have involved an examination of the role of the monoaminergic neurotransmitters—in particular, serotonin (5-hydroxytryptamine, or 5-HT) and norepinephrine (NE)—in the mood and anxiety disorders, schizophrenia, and other forms of psychiatric dysfunction. Now, with the development of more specific 5-HTergic medications and the completion of clinical trials suggesting the efficacy of these drugs in treating a variety of psychiatric illnesses, interest in 5-HT in biological psychiatry has again burgeoned.

It is the purpose of this volume to provide the reader with an understanding of the knowledge to date on the role of 5-HT in the major psychiatric disorders, and to address the clinical relevance of data derived from research in this area. Each of the eight chapters in this volume that cover specific psychiatric diagnoses or psychopathological dimensions provides a concise review of the literature to date in the field, proposes a particular role for 5-HTergic dysfunction, and suggests the clinical importance of understanding such disorders in this manner. Three chapters that are not addressed to specific psychiatric diagnoses per se have been included to cover topics that might be of special importance to clinicians who seek to understand the biological underpinnings of such disorders. These chapters have been placed at the beginning of the book, since they synthesize material that will be helpful in reading the more clinically relevant chapters.

Chapter 2 provides a solid grounding for understanding the process of identification and characterization of 5-HT receptors. Possible functional correlates of 5-HT receptors in the central nervous system are discussed, and the potential clinical relevance and significance of each 5-HT receptor subtype are postulated.

The receptor sensitivity hypothesis of antidepressant action is reviewed in Chapter 3, with emphasis on more recent data concerning the role of 5-HT in the mechanism of action of antidepressant treatments. This chapter also suggests the importance of the 5-HT receptor sensitivity or neuronal enhancement hypothesis, since it is the only working model of antidepressant action that has generated a novel treatment modality that has proved effective (i.e., lithium augmentation of other psychotropic medication).

More clinical in nature, Chapter 4 reviews the neuroendocrine challenge paradigm, a research probe that is thought to provide a "window" on central monoamine function, enabling investigators to study receptor function in vivo. This technique has been utilized by a number of researchers to collect data on 5-HTergic function in many of the psychiatric disorders discussed in this volume. This chapter provides the basic principles and rationale for the use of such a technique, reviews data supporting the role of 5-HT in the secretion of specific hormones studied in these tests, and discusses results of neuroendocrine challenge investigations involving 5-HTergic challenge agents in normal individuals and psychiatric patients.

The clinician or scientist reading Chapters 5–13 can essentially follow much of the history of how researchers in biological psychiatry developed an understanding of the role of 5-HTergic dysfunctions in psychiatric disorders. Initially, several decades ago, the "monoamine hypothesis of depression" was proposed, suggesting that monoamines, particularly NE and 5-HT, are deficient in depression. Thus, the tricyclic antidepressants and the monoamine oxidase inhibitors were seen to exert their therapeutic actions by increasing synaptic availability of these neurotransmitters, either through blockade of presynaptic uptake or through inhibiting monoamine degradation.

Over the next 25 years, research into the biology of depression proliferated. Convincing evidence emerged that 5-HT dysfunction is related to depression. However, data were disparate and difficult to compress into a unifying "5-HT theory" of depression, since one set of data seemed to support a "5-HT hypofunction" theory of depression and another a "5-HT hyperfunction" theory.

Because of this, in Chapter 5, which reviews the literature in the field of 5-HT and depression, a different way of viewing these findings is proposed that succeeds in uniting them in a comprehensible way. In line with our belief that the specificity of 5-HT dysfunctions may be better related to certain psychopathological phenomena rather than to depression per se, we have suggested that such 5-HT dysfunction may be related to suicidality in depression, to suicidality in general, and, finally, to dysregulation of aggression, possibly as a consequence of impulse control disorder, rather than to depression itself as a single diagnostic or nosological entity.

Evidence emerging over the past few years has suggested a dysregulation of 5-HT function in anxiety. Initially, a number of 5-HT-potentiating agents were shown to be effective in the treatment of panic disorder. As detailed in Chapter 6, because patients tend to show an initial deterioration followed by rapid improvement over a several-week treatment period with these drugs, our group has suggested that such data provide evidence for hypersensitivity of postsynaptic 5-HT receptors in panic disorder, with treatment involving a compensatory downregulation of these receptors. Recent neuroendocrine challenge study data described in Chapter 6 have provided more evidence supporting this hypothesis.

Chapter 7 examines recent evidence, from several lines of study, that implicates 5-HTergic dysfunction as having a major role in obsessive compulsive disorder. Again, drugs that are 5-HT reuptake inhibitors have been shown to possess clinical efficacy in the treatment of this disorder, whereas, strikingly, drugs that block NE reuptake appear to be ineffective in such treatment. This chapter reports on neuroendocrine challenge data that are consistent with the hypothesis that an increase in central 5-HT receptor sensitivity may also be associated with specific psychopathological characteristics of this disorder.

Although biological research on schizophrenia has been dominated by the "dopamine hypothesis" over the past few decades, recent data have suggested an important role for 5-HT in this disorder as well. As reviewed in Chapter 8, certain neuroleptics (e.g., chlorpromazine, thioridazine, and clozapine) have a high affinity for 5-HTergic, as well as dopaminergic, receptors. In addition, as it has become increasingly evident that treatment of schizophrenia with neuroleptics is only partially effective in diminishing the psychotic, productive symptoms, and hardly affects negative symptoms, new data on more selective 5-HT antagonists have provided promising indications for the treatment of both positive and negative symptomatology. Ongoing research on biological markers in schizophrenia has repeatedly demonstrated a dysregulation of 5-HT parameters in schizophrenia although, as with depression, some of these results are contradictory and difficult to integrate into a unifying theory at this time.

As the methodology for measuring in vivo 5-HTergic parameters has grown, such measurements have been made in an increasing number of psy-

chiatric disorders and, where 5-HTergic dysfunctions have been demonstrated, this has led to new modes of psychopharmacological treatment.
Chapter 9 reviews research to date on 5-HTergic findings in the childhood
psychiatric disorders. Studies suggesting abnormally enhanced 5-HTergic
metabolism in infantile autism, childhood anorexia nervosa, and the more
pervasive disorders of childhood are discussed, and the few studies examining 5-HTergic variables in enuresis, Tourette's syndrome, Klein-Levine syndrome, Lesch-Nyhan syndrome, childhood depression, and childhood
obsessive compulsive disorder are summarized. It is again proposed that the
ubiquitous nature of the involvement of 5-HTergic mechanisms in childhood psychopathology may suggest that the specificity of the 5-HT disturbance may be more closely related to psychopathological dimensions such
as anxiety, aggression, and impulsivity, which cut across diagnoses, and
that in the more pervasive childhood psychiatric disorders, 5-HT mechanisms may be more vulnerable to disruption by abnormalities in developmental processes in general.

Chapter 10 discusses evidence suggesting that 5-HT dysregulation may
play a major role in the etiology of the eating disorders, particularly bulimia nervosa. Serotonergic neuroendocrine challenge study results from
bulimic patients and matched normal controls are presented, demonstrating
both blunting of hormonal response to 5-HTergic challenge and greater
headache response to such challenge in bulimics (regardless of the presence
of concurrent anorexia nervosa or major depression) as compared with
control subjects. It is proposed that such results provide evidence for altered postsynaptic 5-HT receptor sensitivity in bulimia nervosa, possibly
associated with dysfunctional presynaptic parameters as well. A pathophysiological association among bulimia, major depression, and migraine, mediated by 5-HT, is postulated, and the evidence for such a relationship is
discussed.

With the advent of the diagnosis of "seasonal affective disorder," there
has been a resurgence of interest in the relationships among circadian
rhythms, seasonality, and the affective disorders. Chapter 11 describes the
role of melatonin in the regulation of biological rhythms, and the critical
relationship between 5-HT and melatonin. Data are reviewed that suggest
an abnormal melatonin function in patients with affective disorder. It is hypothesized that specific disturbances in 5-HT function in the pineal-raphe-
suprachiasmatic nucleus system may determine an abnormality in
photoperiodic regulation that may be involved in the pathogenesis of at
least some types of affective disorder.

Over the past decade, a number of researchers have demonstrated a high
correlation between decreased 5-HT metabolism and a history of suicide attempts, especially those with a violent component, across psychiatric diag-

noses. As other research in the area of outwardly directed aggression has consistently demonstrated a negative correlation between 5-HT metabolism and violence among a variety of subject populations, Chapter 12 again suggests that the psychopathological correlate of such decreased 5-HT function might involve dysregulation of aggression, irrespective of psychiatric diagnosis.

Finally, Chapter 13 is both a review and a look toward the future, spelling out more clearly the belief that the functional approach to psychopathology provides the best means of studying, and ultimately understanding, psychiatric illnesses. The chapter briefly reviews the data on 5-HT and psychiatric dysfunction, and proposes that decreased central 5-HT metabolism may be more closely related to psychopathological dysfunctions, such as aggression dysregulation and anxiety, than to discrete nosological categories, such as major depression. After reviewing the role of dopamine in the facilitation of goal-directed behavior and of NE in pleasure and its opposite (anhedonia), we propose a dimensional monoamine hypothesis of psychopathological dysfunction. This theory suggests that disorders of drive, mood, and hedonic function seen in a number of psychiatric disorders, such as major depression, cannot be viewed as merely arising from dysfunction in one monoamine system, but rather as the result of specific abnormalities originating in all three of these mutually interconnected neurotransmitter systems. We believe that only by looking at psychiatric illness dimensionally, rather than nosologically, and by examining the interactions and interconnections between neurotransmitter systems, rather than concentrating solely on one system, can one answer the major questions in biological psychiatry today.

We hope that this volume will be of help both to active scientific researchers and to clinicians seeking to understand possible biological dysfunction in the disorders that they treat on a daily basis. Knowledge in this area is growing and changing every day. What is known today may be disproved tomorrow, while answers that are lacking today may be found in the very near future. However, we have attempted to present in this volume an up-to-date compendium of what is known in the field of serotonin and the psychiatric disorders. We hope that our suggestions concerning a dimensional versus a nosological approach to psychopathology, and an interaction among the serotonergic, dopaminergic, and noradrenergic neurotransmitter systems along such axes, will be helpful in conceptualizing a number of psychiatric problems and in making sense of the extensive, and sometimes confusing, body of data on the efficacy of different medications in the various psychiatric disorders.

2

Central Serotonin Receptors
Functional Correlates
and Clinical Relevance

STEPHEN J. PEROUTKA
ANDREW J. SLEIGHT

In the 30 years since the differentiation of M and D receptors (Gaddum & Picarelli, 1957), it has become clear that multiple 5-hydroxytryptamine (5-HT) receptors exist. Moreover, since the introduction of radioligand binding techniques in the 1970s, the identification of 5-HT receptor subtypes has proliferated at a brisk rate. This trend has been disturbing to many investigators in the field, despite the fact that radioligand studies have been remarkably accurate in their ability to identify binding sites that, eventually, prove to be 5-HT receptors. At the present time, a state of equilibrium has been achieved in which most of the 5-HT binding sites have been successfully correlated with various physiological, biochemical, and behavioral effects of 5-HT. Future studies are likely to identify even more 5-HT binding-site subtypes and, ultimately, receptors.

The identification and characterization of these 5-HT receptor subtypes have a number of clinical implications. For example, neuropsychiatric disorders such as anxiety, depression, and hallucinosis have been specifically linked to specific 5-HT receptor subtypes in the central nervous system (CNS). (See Table 2-1.) This chapter will summarize data concerning the pharmacological characteristics and possible functional correlates of central 5-HT receptors, and discuss the potential clinical significance of each 5-HT receptor subtype.

This work was supported in part by the John A. and George L. Hartford Foundation, the McKnight Foundation, the Alfred P. Sloan Foundation, and NIH Grants NS12151-13 and NS 23560-02.

TABLE 2-1
Summary of Clinical Indications for 5-HT Receptor Agent

Disease	*Possible 5-HT Receptor(s) Involved*
Anxiety	5-HT$_{1A}$, 5-HT$_2$, 5-HT$_3$
Depression	5-HT$_{1A}$, 5-HT$_2$, uptake system
Obsessive compulsive disorder	Uptake system
Migraine (acute)	5-HT$_{1D}$
Migraine (prophylactic)	5-HT$_2$
Appetite suppression	5-HT$_{1A}$, 5-HT$_{1C}$, uptake system

CHARACTERIZATION OF 5-HT BINDING-SITE SUBTYPES

In 1979, radioligand binding techniques were used to differentiate two distinct subtypes of 5-HT receptors in the CNS (Peroutka & Snyder, 1979). One class of sites, designated 5-HT$_1$ receptors, displayed nanomolar affinity for 5-HT and could be labeled with ^{3}H-5-HT. More recently, 5-HT$_1$ sites have been demonstrated to comprise at least four subtypes: 5-HT$_{1A}$, 5-HT$_{1B}$, 5-HT$_{1C}$, and 5-HT$_{1D}$ sites. The 5-HT$_2$ binding site, by contrast, displays micromolar affinity for 5-HT and was labeled with ^{3}H-spiperone (Leysen et al., 1978). A third major class of 5-HT receptors, 5-HT$_3$ sites, was defined more recently and was characterized in the CNS (Kilpatrick et al., 1987). At present, cDNA clones have been identified for the 5-HT$_{1A}$ (Fargin et al., 1988), the 5-HT$_{1C}$ (Julius et al., 1988), and the 5-HT$_2$ receptors (Prichett et al., 1988).

5-HT$_{1A}$ RECEPTORS

The 5-HT$_{1A}$ binding site was first identified by David Nelson and colleagues and was defined as specific ^{3}H-5-HT binding in brain membranes that was sensitive to nanomolar concentrations of spiperone (Pedigo et al., 1981). Subsequently, the 5-HT$_{1A}$ binding site was more selectively labeled with ^{3}H-8-hydroxy-2-(di-n-propylamino)-tetralin (8-OH-DPAT) (Gozlan et al., 1983; Hoyer et al., 1985; Peroutka, 1986) and other radioligands. (See Table 2-2.) Regardless of which radioligand is used to label the site, it displays high and selective affinity for 8-OH-DPAT, 5-methoxydimethyltryptamine, ipsapirone, and buspirone. The 5-HT$_{1A}$ site is densely present in the CA1 region and dentate gyrus of the hippocampus and in the raphe nuclei (Pazos & Palacios, 1985; Hoyer et al., 1986). Because of the large number of agents that display potent and selective affinity for the 5-HT$_{1A}$ site, multiple correlations have been established between the pharmacological characteristics of this binding site and specific physiological effects (Peroutka, 1987). (See Table 2-2.)

TABLE 2-2
Characteristics of $5\text{-}HT_{1A}$, $5\text{-}HT_{1B}$, $5\text{-}HT_{1C}$

	$5\text{-}HT_{1A}$	$5\text{-}HT_{1B}$	$5\text{-}HT_{1C}$	$5\text{-}HT_{1D}$	$5\text{-}HT_2$	$5\text{-}HT_3$
Radiolabeled by	^{3}H-5-HT ^{3}H-8-OH-DPAT ^{3}H-Ipsapirone ^{3}H-WB 4101 ^{3}H-Buspirone ^{3}H-PAPP ^{3}H-Spiroxatrine	^{3}H-5-HT ^{125}I-CYP (Rat and mouse only)	^{3}H-5-HT ^{3}H-Mesulergine ^{125}I-LSD ^{125}I-DOI ^{3}H-SCH 23390	^{3}H-5-HT	^{3}H-Spiperone ^{3}H-Mesulergine ^{125}I-LSD ^{3}H-Ketanserin ^{3}H-Mianserin ^{125}I-Methyl-LSD ^{3}H-DOB	^{3}H-GR 65360 ^{3}H-Quipazine ^{3}H-Zacopride ^{3}H-BRL 43694 ^{3}H-ICS 205-930 ^{3}H-QICS 205-930
High-density regions	Raphe nuclei Hippocampus	Substantia nigra Globus pallidus	Choroid plexus	Basal ganglia	Layer IV Cortex	Peripheral neurons Entorhinal cortex
Potent pharmacological agents (i.e., <10 nM)	5-CT 8-OH-DPAT 5-HT RU 24969 d-LSD	RU 24969 5-CT 5-HT	Mesulergine Metergoline Methysergide	5-CT 5-HT Metergoline	Spiperone Mesulergine Methysergide Metergoline Mianserin	GR 65360 ICS 205-930 BRL 43694
Second messenger	Inhibition of adenylate cyclase	?	PI turnover	Inhibition of adenylate cyclase	PI turnover	?
Membrane effects	Hyperpolarization (K$^+$ channel)	?	Depolarization (Cl$^-$ channel)	?	Depolarization	Depolarization (Ca^{2+} channel)
Functional correlates	Basilar artery Thermoregulation Hypotension Sexual behavior 5-HT syndrome Food intake	"Autoreceptor"	Food intake	?	Vascular contractions Platelet-shape changes Rat forepaw edema Tryptamine seizures Head twitches Back-muscle contractions	Transmitter release Bezold-Jarisch reflex

Inhibition of Adenylate Cyclase Activity

Serotonergic modulation of adenylate cyclase, for example, has been linked to the 5-HT$_{1A}$ site. Guanosine 5'-triphosphate (GTP) and guanosine 5'-diphosphate (GDP), but not guanylic acid (GMP), inhibit the binding of ^{3}H-8-OH-DPAT to brain membranes (Hall et al., 1985; Schlegel & Peroutka, 1986). In addition, guanine nucleotides significantly reduce agonist potencies for ^{3}H-8-OH-DPAT binding sites, whereas antagonist potencies are not affected by nucleotides. 5-HT also inhibits forskolin-stimulated adenylate cyclase in rat and guinea pig hippocampal membranes (De Vivo & Maayani, 1986; Bockaert et al., 1987).

The pharmacological data derived from this system appear to be consistent with a single, homogeneous population of receptors. 8-OH-DPAT and d-LSD are similar to 5-HT in their ability to inhibit cyclase activity. Buspirone, on the other hand, is only a partial agonist in this system (De Vivo & Maayani, 1986). By contrast, spiperone, (-) pindolol, and (-) propranolol are competitive antagonists at this receptor, whereas ketanserin has no effect on 5-HT–induced inhibition of the cyclase activity (Oksenberg & Peroutka, 1988). The 5-HT$_{1A}$ receptor also appears to mediate inhibition of vasoactive intestinal peptide-stimulated cyclic adenosine monophosphate formation in purified striatal and cortical cultured neurons (Weiss et al., 1986). Thus, the 5-HT$_{1A}$ receptor seems to be negatively coupled to an adenylate cyclase in certain brain regions.

Hyperpolarization of Neuronal Membranes

Neurophysiological analyses have also benefited from the recent development and characterization of 5-HT$_{1A}$ selective agents. For example, such studies have clearly demonstrated that the 5-HT$_{1A}$ receptor mediates inhibition of raphe nuclei. Buspirone, a 5-HT$_{1A}$ selective agent, causes complete inhibition of dorsal raphe neuronal firing in the rat (VanderMaelen et al., 1986) and mouse (Trulson & Arasteh, 1986). Other 5-HT$_{1A}$ selective agents, such as ipsapirone, 8-OH-DPAT, and 5-CT, were also found to mimic the effect of 5-HT on raphe cell firing (VanderMaelen et al., 1986). (-)Propranolol, a beta-adrenergic agent that also displays high affinity for the 5-HT$_{1A}$ receptor, reversibly blocks the inhibitory effects of ipsapirone and 8-OH-DPAT on raphe cell inhibition (Sprouse & Aghajanian, 1987). The hippocampus is a second anatomical structure containing a high concentration of 5-HT$_{1A}$ sites that has been used to study 5-HT$_{1A}$ receptor function (Pazos & Palacios, 1985). The 5-HT$_{1A}$ selective agonists directly inhibit CA1 pyramidal cells (Andrade & Nicoll, 1987).

Other Systems

Contractions of the canine basilar artery induced by 5-HT have been proposed to be a functional correlate of the 5-HT$_{1A}$ receptor (Taylor et al.,

1986; Peroutka et al., 1986). Specific components of the 5-HT behavioral syndrome have also been linked to activation of 5-HT_{1A} receptors (Tricklebank, 1985; Smith & Peroutka, 1986). It has been suggested, as well, that stimulation of central 5-HT_{1A} receptors gives rise to an increase in food intake (hyperphagia) in rats (Dourish et al., 1985a), and that this is a model for somatodendritic autoreceptor stimulation (Hutson et al., 1986).

This effect, however, can be seen only under specific conditions. For example, if rats are deprived of food before the experiment, the 5-HT_{1A} agonist 8-OH-DPAT causes a decrease in food intake (Dourish et al., 1985b). In addition, studies in male rats have shown that 5-HT_{1A} selective agonists facilitate seminal emissions and ejaculations (Kwong et al., 1986). The hypotensive potencies of 8-OH-DPAT and RU 24969 in pentobarbitone-anesthetized rats suggest that the 5-HT_{1A} site may mediate these effects (Doods et al., 1985). Finally, the thermoregulatory effects of 8-OH-DPAT and RU 24969 also appear to be mediated by the 5-HT_{1A} receptor (Tricklebank et al., 1986; Gudelsky et al., 1986).

Clinical Relevance

Recent clinical investigations have focused on the ability of 5-HT_{1A} selective agents to act as human anxiolytics. Buspirone is the first pharmacological agent in this class of drugs to be approved for human use. (See Table 2-3.) Ipsapirone, gepirone, and SM-3997 are also 5-HT_{1A} selective agents that are in various stages of clinical or preclinical development. Each of these drugs displays a relatively selective interaction with 5-HT_{1A} receptor binding sites in brain membranes. In addition, these agents are also similar in that they appear to be "partial agonists" in biochemical assays. For example, buspirone, in comparison with 5-HT, has only a moderate effect on the inhibition of forskolin-stimulated adenylate cyclase activity (De Vivo & Maayani, 1986) and causes only a modest contraction of the canine basilar artery (Peroutka et al., 1986). The clinical efficacy of these agents in the treatment of human anxiety disorders suggests that the 5-HT_{1A} receptor plays a significant role in anxiogenesis.

The 5-HT_{1A} agonist 8-OH-DPAT has also been shown to possess antidepressant properties in some animal models of depression (Kennett et al., 1987). In addition, buspirone, gepirone, and ipsapirone have demonstrated clinical efficacy in the treatment of depression, which suggests that the 5-HT_{1A} receptor may play a role in this disorder. If rats are treated chronically with antidepressants, a reduction in the number of 5-HT_{1A} binding sites can be seen (Palfreyman et al., 1986), as well as a downregulation of the 5-HT_{1A} mediated inhibition of forskolin-stimulated adenylate cyclase activity (Sleight et al., 1988).

TABLE 2-3
Clinical Status of 5-HT Receptor Subtype Selective Drugs

	Company	*Clinical Indication*	*Status*
5-HT$_{1A}$ agents			
Buspirone	Mead Johnson	Anxiety	Marketed
Ipsapirone	Troponwerke	Anxiety	Phase II
Gepirone	Mead Johnson	Anxiety; depression	Phase III
SM 3997	Pfizer	Anxiety	Phase II
5-HT$_2$ agents			
Cyproheptadine	MS&D	Appetite stimulant; dumping syndrome	Marketed
Pizotifen	Sandoz	Migraine prophylaxis	Marketed
Mianserin	Organon	Depression	Marketed
Methysergide	Sandoz	Migraine prophylaxis	Marketed
Ketanserin	Janssen	Hypertension	Marketed
Ritanserin	Janssen	Anxiety; schizophrenia	Phase II
Altanserin	Janssen	Anxiety; depression	Phase II
Nefazodone	Mead Johnson	Depression	Phase II
5-HT$_3$ agents			
BRL 24924	Beecham	GI motility disturbances	Phase III
ICS 205-930	Sandoz	Migraine: emesis; GI disturbances	Phase II
GR38032F	Glaxo	Emesis; anxiety; schizophrenia	Phase II
BRL 43694	Beecham	Migraine; emesis	Phase I

5-HT$_{1B}$ RECEPTORS

The 5-HT$_{1B}$ receptor has been directly labeled in rat brain with ^{125}I-cyano-pindolol (Hoyer et al., 1985). The 5-HT$_{1B}$ site has high affinity for 5-HT and RU 24969 and relatively low affinity for d-LSD and 8-OH-DPAT. The highest densities of 5-HT$_{1B}$ sites in rat brain are found in the globus pallidus, dorsal subiculum, and substantia nigra (Pazos & Palacios, 1985). Interestingly, the 5-HT$_{1B}$ site, as defined by radioligand binding studies, appears to be species specific. The 5-HT$_{1B}$ site is present in rat and mouse brain, but not in guinea pig, cow, chicken, turtle, frog, or human brain membranes (Hoyer et al., 1986; Heuring et al., 1986).

To date, functional correlates of this site have been limited to studies of the serotonin "autoreceptor." Briefly, 5-HT autoreceptors are studied in synaptosomal or slice preparations in which depolarization-evoked release of stored ^{3}H-5-HT is measured by superfusion techniques. The release of ^{3}H-5-HT can be inhibited by 5-HT and related agonists, presumably through a presynaptic autoreceptor. Engel et al. (1986) have convincingly demonstrated that in rat brain synaptosomes, the effects of 5-HT and other agents are mediated by the 5-HT$_{1B}$ receptor. No significant correlation was observed between drug potencies at the 5-HT autoreceptor and drug affinities for 5-HT$_{1C}$ or 5-HT$_2$ binding sites. However, a significant correlation was obtained between drug affinities for 5-HT$_{1B}$ sites and the rat 5-HT autoreceptor. As a result, the 5-HT$_{1B}$ binding site appears to be the receptor that mediates release of 5-HT from nerve terminals in rat brain.

A similar conclusion was reached from an analysis of 5-HT and related drug effects on the release of ^{3}H-5-HT induced by depolarization of rat cerebellum synaptosomes (Raiteri et al., 1986). By contrast, the 5-HT heteroreceptor mediating release of endogenous glutamate induced by depolarization of rat cerebellum synaptosomes did not conform to the previously described pharmacological characteristics of 5-HT$_{1A}$, 5-HT$_{1B}$, 5-HT$_{1C}$, and 5-HT$_2$ binding sites.

Clinical Relevance

The major issue concerning the 5-HT$_{1B}$ receptor is its apparent absence in human brain membranes (Heuring et al., 1986; Hoyer et al., 1986), a finding that has been confirmed by two independent laboratories. At the same time, it should be noted that a number of drugs, such as mCPP, have been described as being "5-HT$_{1B}$ selective." Clinically, mCPP displays unique neuropsychiatric effects in humans. However, it is an extremely nonselective pharmacological agent, since it also displays a similar affinity for a number of neurotransmitter receptors in humans (Hamik & Peroutka, 1989). Therefore, it is difficult to attribute the neuropsychiatric effects of mCPP to its interactions with a specific 5-HT receptor subtype. Moreover, its interactions with the 5-HT$_{1B}$ receptor in rat brain appear to be irrelevant to its clinical effects, since the 5-HT$_{1B}$ site does not appear to exist in human brain.

5-HT$_{1C}$ RECEPTORS

The 5-HT$_{1C}$ site was first discovered as a result of the autoradiographic analysis of 5-HT binding site subtypes. The 5-HT$_{1C}$ site was characterized initially in membranes from pig choroid plexus and cortex (Pazos et al., 1984, 1985; Hoyer et al., 1985). The site was labeled by both ^{3}H-5-HT and ^{3}H-mesulergine. Independently, Yagaloff and Hartig (1985) labeled the site with ^{125}I-LSD in the rat choroid plexus. The 5-HT$_{1C}$ site has high affinity for 5-HT, methysergide, and mianserin, and relatively low affinity for RU 24969. These pharmacological characteristics are also shared by the putative 5-HT$_{1C}$ site identified in rat cortex (Hoyer et al., 1985; Peroutka, 1986).

The recent work of Sanders-Bush and colleagues has convincingly demonstrated that 5-HT stimulation of phosphatidylinositol hydrolysis is mediated by the 5-HT$_{1C}$ site in choroid plexus membranes (Conn et al., 1986). Drug effects on 5-HT–stimulated phosphatidylinositol hydrolysis in choroid plexus were compared with drug potencies at ^{125}I-LSD binding sites in the same tissue. Mianserin and ketanserin were found to be potent antagonists of 5-HT–induced changes, whereas spiperone was more than an order of magnitude less potent in this system. The authors concluded that the 5-HT$_{1C}$ site in choroid plexus is functionally linked to the phosphatidylinositol second messenger system.

It has also been suggested that the 5-HT$_{1C}$ receptor may be involved in the regulation of food intake, since the administration of mCPP to rats causes a decrease in food intake. This effect cannot be explained merely by the affinity of mCPP for 5-HT$_{1B}$ receptors; thus, it may be mediated by 5-HT$_{1C}$ receptors.

Clinical Relevance

Although 5-HT$_{1C}$ receptors have been identified in other parts of the brain, it is clear that they are located predominantly in the choroid plexus. Therefore, it has been proposed that they may modulate the production and/or absorption of cerebrospinal fluid. Clearly, this receptor may have an important role in this function, but at present, pharmacological agents that are selective for the 5-HT$_{1C}$ receptor do not exist. Thus it is not yet possible to determine whether the 5-HT$_{1C}$ receptor plays a role in human neuropsychiatric disorders.

5-HT$_{1D}$ RECEPTORS

A fourth subtype of 5-HT$_1$ sites labeled by ^{3}H-5-HT recently was identified in bovine brain membranes (Heuring & Peroutka, 1987). The 5-HT$_{1A}$ selective agents such as 8-OH-DPAT, ipsapirone, and buspirone display micromolar affinities for these sites. RU 24969 and (–) pindolol are approximately two orders of magnitude less potent at these sites than at 5-HT$_{1B}$ sites that have been identified in rat brain. Agents that display nanomolar potencies for 5-HT$_{1C}$ sites, such as mianserin and mesulergine, are two to three orders of magnitude less potent at ^{3}H-5-HT–labeled 5-HT$_{1D}$ binding sites in bovine caudate. In addition, both 5-HT$_2$ and 5-HT$_3$ selective agents are essentially inactive at these binding sites. These ^{3}H-5-HT sites display nanomolar affinity for 5-carboxyamidotryptamine (5-CT), 5-methoxytryptamine, metergoline, and 5-HT.

Regional studies demonstrate that this class of sites is most dense in the basal ganglia, but exists in all regions of bovine brain. Sumatriptan is an extremely potent and selective 5-HT$_{1D}$ agent (Peroutka & McCarthy, 1989) and is a potent agonist at 5-HT receptors, mediating the contraction of cerebral blood vessels (Feniuk et al., 1987). The 5-HT_{1D} binding site also appears to modulate the inhibition of adenylate cyclase activity in the cow substantia nigra (Hoyer & Schoeffter, 1988) and can therefore be considered a 5-HT "receptor."

Clinical Relevance

The 5-HT_{1D} receptor is unique in many respects. First of all, it is the densest 5-HT receptor subtype in human brain. Its high density in the basal ganglia suggests that it may play an important role in many neuropsychiatric conditions. Sumatriptan has now been shown to be extremely effective in the acute treatment of migraine (Doenicke et al., 1988). This effect may be mediated by the 5-HT_{1D} receptors present in cerebral blood vessels, since the drug shows little affinity for other neurotransmitter binding sites.

5-HT_2 RECEPTORS

Because of the availability of a large number of potent and selective antagonists, the 5-HT_2 class of binding sites has been extensively analyzed. ^{3}H-spiperone, ^{3}H-LSD, ^{3}H-mianserin, ^{3}H-ketanserin, ^{3}H-mesulergine, ^{125}I-LSD and N_1-methyl-2-^{125}I-LSD can be used to label the 5-HT_2 binding site (Leysen et al., 1978; Leysen et al., 1984). Classical serotonergic antagonists have high affinity for this site, while 5-HT and related tryptamines are markedly less potent. The highest level of 5-HT_2 binding is in the cerebral cortex and caudate, with all other brain regions having substantially fewer binding sites (Pazos et al., 1985).

Phosphatidylinositol Turnover

The 5-HT–induced phosphoinositide hydrolysis seen in rat cerebral cortex appears to be a result of 5-HT_2 receptor activation (Sanders-Bush & Conn, 1987); 5-HT stimulates phosphoinositide turnover with an EC_{50} of 1 μM. The response to 5-HT is blocked by nanomolar concentrations of ketanserin and other 5-HT_2 antagonists. Furthermore, tricyclic antidepressants decrease both 5-HT_2 binding sites and 5-HT–induced phosphoinositide turnover (Kendall & Nahorski, 1985). In addition, the rat thoracic aorta, cultured bovine aortic smooth muscle cells, and platelets are three additional systems in which 5-HT appears to modulate phosphoinositide turnover via a receptor that is similar to the 5-HT_2 binding site.

Depolarization of Neuronal Membranes

At the present time, two specific neurophysiological effects of 5-HT have been attributed to activation of the 5-HT_2 receptor (Aghajanian et al., 1987). In the facial motor nucleus, 5-HT facilitates the excitatory effects of glutamate. This effect is antagonized by selective 5-HT$_2$ antagonists such as methysergide, cyproheptadine, and cinanserin (McCall & Aghajanian, 1980). Similar data were derived from intracellular studies of this brain-stem nucleus (VanderMaelen & Aghajanian, 1980). Thus, 5-HT causes a slow depolarization of facial motor neuron membranes and an increased input resistance, which leads to increased excitability of the cell. The membrane effects of 5-HT are blocked by methysergide (VanderMaelen & Aghajanian, 1980). These data suggest that 5-HT$_2$ receptors mediate 5-HT–induced excitation of facial motor neurons.

More recently, Davies et al. (1987) demonstrated that 5-HT causes a slow depolarization of 68% of cortical neurons, which is associated with a decreased conductance. The response displayed some voltage dependency and was easily desensitized by repeated applications of 5-HT. The selective 5-HT$_2$ receptor antagonists ritanserin and cinanserin blocked the depolarizing effects of 5-HT. Therefore, the effects of 5-HT on cortical pyramidal neurons share many similarities with the depolarizing effects of 5-HT in the facial motor nucleus, and also appear to be mediated by 5-HT$_2$ receptors.

Other Systems

In contrast to 5-HT–induced contractions of the canine basilar artery, 5-HT–induced contractions of many other vascular tissues are mediated by 5-HT$_2$ receptors (Peroutka, 1984). A number of behavioral effects of 5-HT have also been attributed to 5-HT$_2$ receptors. For example, drug antagonism of the "head-shake" or "head-twitch component" of the 5-HT behavioral syndrome has clearly been related to a blockade of 5-HT$_2$ receptors (Peroutka et al., 1981; Leysen et al., 1984). Likewise, tryptamine-induced seizure activity can be prevented by selective 5-HT$_2$ antagonists (Leysen et al., 1978). Behavioral studies of the discriminative cue properties of 5-HT agonists have concluded that this behavioral response may be mediated by 5-HT$_2$ receptors (Glennon et al., 1983).

Another behavioral correlate of 5-HT$_2$ receptor activation is the back-muscle contractions seen following intrathecally administered 2,5-dimethoxy-alpha, 4-dimethyl-benzene ethamine hydrochloride (DOM), a selective 5-HT$_2$ agonist. This effect appears to be mediated by spinal 5-HT$_2$ receptors, since intrathecally administered 5,7-dihydroxytryptamine causes a marked increase in the number of back-muscle contractions (Marsden et al., 1989).

Antagonism of 5-HT–induced forepaw edema in the rat by 22 antagonists correlates with drug affinity for 5-HT$_2$ sites labeled by ^{3}H-spiperone (Ortmann et al., 1982). Similarly, drug antagonism of tracheal smooth-muscle contraction, in vivo bronchoconstriction, and contraction of guinea pig ileum is consistent with mediation by 5-HT$_2$ sites (Leysen et al., 1984).

The 5-HT$_2$ receptors have also been implicated in the regulation of aldosterone production (Matsuoka et al., 1985). The 5-HT induction of platelet shape changes and aggregation may also be mediated by 5-HT$_2$ receptors (Leysen et al., 1984).

5-HT$_2$ Receptors and Hallucinosis

Glennon and associates have hypothesized that hallucinogens act as agonists at the 5-HT$_2$ receptor in the CNS (Glennon, 1987). This theory is based largely on the observation that d-LSD and other hallucinogens produce similar stimulus effects in drug-discrimination studies and that specific 5-HT$_2$ antagonists are able to block these discriminative cue effects (Glennon, 1987). However, recent studies in Stanford's laboratory indicate that nanomolar concentrations of d-LSD act as an antagonist of 5-HT$_2$ receptors in rat cortex (Pierce & Peroutka, 1988). This conclusion was based on two major observations. First, GTP fails to alter the ability of d-LSD to compete for 5-HT$_2$ receptors, a finding that suggests a lack of agonist activity at this site (Battaglia et al., 1984). Second, nanomolar concentrations of d-LSD significantly inhibit the effects of micromolar 5-HT on PI turnover in the rat cortex, a biochemical system mediated by 5-HT$_2$ receptors (Sanders-Bush & Conn, 1987; Kendall & Nahorski, 1985).

The ability of d-LSD to antagonize 5-HT$_2$–mediated effects of 5-HT has also been reported in many other systems. For example, the guinea pig trachea contracts in response to micromolar concentrations of 5-HT (Heller & Baraban, 1987). The ability of 5-HT antagonists to block this effect correlates significantly with drug affinities for the 5-HT$_2$ binding site (Van Nueten et al., 1982; Cohen et al., 1985). DOB acts as a partial agonist in this system by producing approximately 50% of the maximal contraction induced by 5-HT (Heller & Baraban, 1987). By contrast, nanomolar concentrations of d-LSD display no agonist effects in this system, and yet are able to antagonize the effect of micromolar 5-HT. These data are analogous to the PI turnover data described in a recent report (Pierce & Peroutka, 1988), and further confirm and the ability of d-LSD to antagonize 5-HT–mediated effects via the 5-HT$_2$ receptor.

The rat uterus is a second example of smooth muscle in which 5-HT–induced contractions appear to be mediated by 5-HT$_2$ receptors (Millar et al., 1982; Cohen et al., 1985). Once again, d-LSD acts as an antagonist in this system, with a pA$_2$ value of approximately 8.5 (Gaddum et al., 1955; Cerletti & Doepfner, 1958; Hashimoto et al., 1977). In rats, 5-HT–induced paw edema has also been linked to the 5-HT$_2$ receptor (Ortmann et al., 1982). The effect of 5-HT in this model system is also antagonized by d-LSD, as well (Doepfner & Cerletti, 1958). In summary, although 5-HT$_2$ receptors may play an important role in the mechanism of action of hallucinogenic agents, these observations suggest that hallucinogenic drug activity is not derived from direct activation of 5-HT$_2$ receptors.

Clinical Relevance

Owing primarily to the large number of selective 5-HT$_2$ antagonists, the 5-HT$_2$ receptor has been implicated in a number of neuropsychiatric conditions. For example, antidepressants selectively downregulate the density of 5-HT$_2$ receptors (Peroutka & Snyder, 1980a; 1980b). A number of 5-HT$_2$ antagonists are also used in the prophylactic treatment of migraine. In addition, more recent data have suggested that drugs that interact with both the dopamine D$_2$ and the 5-HT$_2$ receptor may have unique antipsychotic effects. However, a specific clinical role for 5-HT$_2$ receptor selective agents in neuropsychiatric diseases has not yet been identified. (See Table 2-2).

5-HT$_3$ RECEPTORS

In addition, 5-HT has a number of potent effects in the peripheral nervous system, which are not affected by 5-HT$_1$ and/or 5-HT$_2$ selective drugs such as 8-OH-DPAT and ketanserin. However, unlike 5-HT effects in the CNS, effects of 5-HT in the periphery can often be blocked with such drugs as MDL 72222, (−)cocaine, metoclopramide, and ICS 205-930 (Richardson & Engel, 1986; Richardson et al., 1985). Because the receptors that mediate these effects have an extremely distinct pharmacology that does not appear to coincide with the 5-HT$_1$ and 5-HT$_2$ classes of receptors, they have been designated 5-HT$_3$ receptors (Richardson & Engel, 1986; Bradley et al., 1986).

It is also clear that heterogeneity exists within the 5-HT$_3$ class of receptors. At least three distinct subtypes of 5-HT$_3$ sites have been hypothesized (Richardson & Engel, 1986), since the potency of selective 5-HT$_3$ antagonists is significantly different in different physiological systems. For example, MDL 72222 has a pA$_2$ of 9.1 against 5-HT–induced effects on postganglionic sympathetic and parasympathetic neurons in the rabbit heart, but is inactive against putative 5-HT$_3$ receptors in the guinea pig ileum (Richardson & Engel, 1986). The development of more selective and varied pharmacological agents should further define the pharmacological characteristics and functional correlates of 5-HT$_3$ receptors and their probable subtypes.

At present, the identification and characterization of 5-HT$_3$ receptors in the CNS are an active area of research. Indeed, Kilpatrick et al. (1987) recently reported that ^{3}H-GR 65630 labels an apparent 5-HT$_3$ recognition site in rat brain membranes. The site appears to coincide with peripheral 5-HT$_3$ receptors, since it displays high (i.e., nanomolar) affinity for such drugs as

GR 65360, ICS 205-930, BRL 43694, and MDL 72222. More recently, the Stanford laboratory used ³H-quipazine to label an apparent 5-HT₃ membrane recognition site in rat brain membranes. Various other investigators are also attempting to identify 5-HT₃ receptors in the CNS.

Clinical Relevance

The 5-HT₃ antagonists appear to be potent antiemetics and may have novel effects on gastrointestinal motility. Clinically, the drugs may also have antimigraine properties that extend beyond their antiemetic effects. In addition, 5-HT₃ drugs have been hypothesized as possessing anxiolytic or antipsychotic properties. However, the clinical data remain preliminary. More extensive studies are in progress to determine accurately the clinical utility of 5-HT₃ agents in neuropsychiatric illnesses.

OTHER 5-HT RECEPTOR SUBTYPES

The existence of a variety of other 5-HT receptor subtypes has been hypothesized, as well. In general, the feature that distinguishes the following sites from the foregoing receptors is that they have only been identified in a single laboratory. If their presence can be confirmed by other, independent investigators, then it is likely that each of the sites will be added to the growing list of 5-HT receptor subtypes.

The fact that 5,7-dihydroxytryptamine–induced lesions of the raphe system cause a loss of ³H-8-OH-DPAT binding in the striatum but not hippocampus has led Michel Hamon and colleagues to hypothesize that ³H-8-OH-DPAT also labels a presynaptic 5-HT autoreceptor (Gozlan et al., 1983). In addition, the putative hallucinogen ³H-DOB has been reported to label an apparent 5-HT₂ recognition site (Lyon et al., 1987). Studies are in progress to determine more clearly the possible relevance of this site to 5-HT₂ sites labeled by ³H-antagonists. Finally, Gershon and colleagues have reported that a site designated 5-HT₁ₚ exists in gut membranes (Mawe et al., 1986). This site can be labeled by ³H-5-HT and displays a pharmacological profile that is distinct from all other known 5-HT₁ binding site subtypes. Moreover, the pharmacological characteristics of this site correlate with the physiological effects of 5-HT in the gut (Mawe et al., 1986).

FUTURE TRENDS

In this chapter, evidence has been provided from a variety of molecular, biochemical, and physiological studies to suggest that a number of 5-HT receptors exist. At present, the differentiation of 5-HT receptors into 5-HT₁ₐ, 5-HT₁ᵦ, 5-HT₁c, 5-HT₁ᴅ, 5-HT₂, and 5-HT₃ subtypes appears to be the most relevant classification system. Future pharmacological progress most likely will continue to depend on the development of highly potent and selective agonists and antagonists for each 5-HT receptor subtype.

A more important trend involves the advances that are currently being made in molecular biology. To date, although a 5-HT receptor sequence has not been identified, rapid progress in this area is likely to yield detailed structural data on the 5-HT_{1A}, 5-HT_{1C}, and 5-HT_3 receptors in the very near future. Once determined, the classification system based on the radioligand binding studies may need to be revised. Indeed, DNA cloning of the 5-HT_{1A}, 5-HT_{1C}, and 5-HT_2 receptors has shown that the 5-HT_{1C} receptor is more related to the 5-HT_2 receptor than the 5-HT_1 receptor (Fargin et al., 1988; Julius et al., 1988; Prichett et al., 1988).

REFERENCES

Aghajanian, G. K., Sprouse, J. S., & Rasmussen, K. (1987). Physiology of the midbrain serotonin system. In H. Meltzer (Ed.), *Psychopharmacology: The third generation of progress* (pp. 141–149). New York: Raven Press.

Andrade, R., & Nicoll, R. (1987). Novel anxiolytics discriminate between postsynaptic serotonin receptors mediating different physiological responses on single neurons of the rat hippocampus. *Naunyn-Schmiedeberg's Arch. Pharmacol., 336,* 5–10.

Battaglia, G., Shannon, M., & Titeler, M. (1984). Guanyl nucleotide and divalent cation regulation of cortical S_2 serotonin receptors. *J. Neurochem., 43,* 1213–1219.

Bockaert, J., Dumuis, A., Bouhelal, R., Sebben, M., & Cory, R. N. (1987). Piperazine derivatives including the putative anxiolytic drugs, buspirone and ipsapirone, are agonists at 5-HT_{1A} receptors negatively coupled with adenylate cyclase in hippocampal neurons. *Arch. Pharmacol., 335,* 588–592.

Bradley, P. B., Engel, G., Feniuk, W., Fozard, J. R., Humphrey, P. P. A., Middlemiss, D. N., Mylecharane, E. J., Richardson, B. P., & Saxena, P. R. (1986). Proposals for the classification and nomenclature of functional receptors for 5-hydroxytryptamine. *Neuropharmacol., 25,* 563–576.

Cerletti, A., & Doepfner, W. (1958). Comparative study on the serotonin antagonism of amide derivatives of lysergic acid and of ergot alkaloids. *J. Pharmacol., 122,* 124–136.

Cohen, M. L., Schenck, K. W., Colbert, W., & Wittenauer, L. (1985). Role of 5-HT_2 receptors in serotonin-induced contractions of nonvascular smooth muscle. *J. Pharmacol. Exp. Ther., 232,* 770–774.

Conn, P. J., Sanders-Bush, E., Hoffman, B. J., & Hartig, P. R. (1986). A unique serotonin receptor in choroid plexus is linked to phosphatidlyinositol turnover. *Proc. Nat. Acad. Sci., 83,* 4086–4088.

Davies, M. F., Deisz, R. A., Prince, D. A., & Peroutka, S. J. (1987). Two distinct effects of 5-hydroxytryptamine on cortical neurons. *Brain Res., 423,* 347–352.

De Vivo, M., & Maayani, S. (1986). Characterization of the 5-hydroxytryptamine$_{1A}$

receptor-mediated inhibition of forskolin-stimulated adenylate cyclase activity in guinea pig and rat hippocampal membranes. *J. Pharmacol. Exp. Ther., 238,* 248–253.

Doenicke, A., Brand, J., & Perrin, V. L. (1988). Possible benefit of GR 43175, a novel 5-HT$_1$-like receptor agonist, for the acute treatment of severe migraine. *Lancet, I,* 1309–1311.

Doepfner, W., & Cerletti, A. (1958). Comparison of lysergic acid derivatives and antihistamines as inhibitors of the edema provoked in the rat's paw by serotonin. *Int. Arch. Allergy, 12,* 89–97.

Doods, H. N., Kalkman, H. O., De Jonge, A., Thoolen, M., Wilffert, B., Timmermans, P., & Van Zwieten, P. A. (1985). Differential selectivities of RU 24969 and 8-OH-DPAT for the purported 5-HT$_{1A}$ and 5-HT$_{1B}$ binding sites. Correlation between 5-HT$_{1A}$ affinity and hypotensive activity. *Eur. J. Pharmacol., 112,* 363–370.

Dourish, C. T., Hutson, P. H., & Curzon, G. (1985a). Low doses of the putative serotonin agonist 8-hydroxy-2-(di-n-propylamino) tetralin (8-OH-DPAT) elicit feeding in the rat. *Psychopharmacology, 86,* 197–204.

Dourish, C. T., Hutson, P. H., & Curzon, G. (1985b). Characteristics of feeding induced by the serotonin agonist 8-hydroxy-2-(di-n-propylamino) tetralin (8-OH-DPAT). *Brain Res. Bull., 15,* 377–384.

Engel, G., Gothert, M., Hoyer, D., Schlicker, E., & Hillenbrand, K. (1986). Identity of inhibitory presynaptic 5-Hydroxytryptamine premises 5-HT premises autoreceptors in the rat brain cortex with 5-HT binding sites. *NAaunyn-Schmiedeberg's Arch. of Pharmacol., 332,* 1–7.

Fargin, A., Raymond, J. R., Lohse, M. J., Kobilka, B. K., Caron, M. G., & Lefkowitz, R. J. (1988). The genomic clone G-21 which resembles a beta-adrenergic receptor sequence encodes the 5-HT$_{1A}$ receptor. *Nature, 335,* 358–360.

Feniuk, W., Humphrey, P. P. A., & Perren, M. J. (1987). Selective vasoconstrictor action of GR 43175 on arteriovenous anasomoses (AVAs) in the anaesthetized cat. *Br. J. Pharmacol., 92,* 756.

Gaddum, J. H., Khan, A., Hathway, D. E., & Stephens, F. F. (1955). Quantitative studies of antagonists for 5-hydroxytryptamine. *Quart. J. Exp. Physiol., 40,* 49–74.

Gaddum, J. H., & Picarelli, Z. P. (1957). Two kinds of tryptamine receptor. *Br. J. Pharmacol. Chemother., 12,* 323–328.

Glennon, R. A. (1987). Psychoactive phenylisopropylamines. In H. Meltzer (Ed.), *Psychopharmacology: The third generation of progress* (pp. 1627–1639). New York: Raven Press.

Glennon, R. A., Young, R., & Rosecrans, J. A. (1983). Antagonism of the effects of the hallucinogen DOM and the purported 5-HT agonist quipazine by 5-HT$_2$ antagonists. *Eur. J. Pharmacol., 91,* 189–196.

Gozlan, H., El Mestikawy, S., Pichat, L., Glowinski, J., & Hamon, M. (1983). Identification of presynaptic serotonin autoreceptors using a new ligand: ^{3}H-PAT. *Nature, 305,* 140–142.

Gudelsky, G. A., Koenig, J. I., & Meltzer, H. Y. (1986). Thermoregulatory responses to serotonin (5-HT) receptor stimulation in the rat. *Neuropharmacol., 25,* 1307–1313.

Hall, M. D., El Mestikawy, S., Emerit, M. B., Pichat, L., Hamon, M., & Gozlan, H. (1985). [³H]8-hydroxy-2-(Di-n-Propyl-amino) tetralin binding to pre- and postsynaptic 5-hydroxytryptamine sites in various regions of the rat brain. *J. Neurochem., 44*, 1685-1696.

Hamik, A., & Peroutka, S. J. (1989). 1-(m-Chlorophenyl)piperazine (mCPP) interactions with neurotransmitter receptors in human brain. *Biol. Psychiat., 25*, 569-575.

Hashimoto, H., Hayashi, M., Nakahara, Y., Niwaguchi, T., & Ishii, H. (1977). Actions of D-lysergic acid diethylamide (LSD) and its derivatives on 5-hydroxytryptamine receptors in the isolated uterine smooth muscle of the rat. *Eur. J. Pharmacol., 45*, 341-348.

Heller, W. A., & Baraban, J. M. (1987). Potent agonist activity of DOB at 5-HT₂ receptors in guinea pig trachea. *Eur. J. Pharmacol., 138*, 115-117.

Heuring, R. E., & Peroutka, S. J. (1987). Characterization of a novel ³H-5-HT binding site subtype in bovine brain membranes. *J. Neurosci., 7*, 894-903.

Heuring, R. E., Schlegel, J. R., & Peroutka, S. J. (1986). Species variations in 5-HT₁B and 5-HT₁C binding sites defined by RU 24969 competition studies. *Eur. J. Pharmacol., 122*, 279-282.

Hoyer, D., Engel, G., & Kalkman, H. O. (1985). Molecular pharmacology of 5-HT₁ and 5-HT₂ recognition sites in rat and pig brain membranes: Radioligand binding studies with [³H]5-HT, [³H]8-OH-DPAT, (-)[¹²⁵I]iodocyanopindolol, [³H]mesulergine and [³H]ketanserin. *Eur. J. Pharmacol., 118*, 13-23.

Hoyer, D., Pazos, A., Probst, A., & Palacios, J. M. (1986). Serotonin receptors in the human brain: I. Characterization and autoradiographic localization of 5-HT₁A recognition sites. Apparent absence of 5-HT₁B recognition sites. *Brain Res., 376*, 85-96.

Hoyer, D., & Schoeffter, P. (1988). 5-HT₁D Receptor-mediated inhibition of forskolin-stimulated adenylate cyclase activity in calf substantia nigra. *Eur. J. Pharmacol., 147*, 145-147.

Hutson, P. H., Dourish, C. T., & Curzon, G. (1986). Neurochemical and behavioral evidence for the modulation of the hyperphagic action of 8-OH-DPAT by 5-HT cell body autoreceptors. *Eur. J. Pharmacol., 129*, 347-352.

Julius, J., MacDermott, A. B., Axel, R., & Jessell, T. M. (1988). Molecular characterization of a functional cDNA encoding the serotonin 1c receptor. *Science, 241*, 558-564.

Kendall, D. A., & Nahorski, S. R. (1985). 5-Hydroxytryptamine-stimulated inositol phospholipid hydrolysis in rat cerebral cortex slices: Pharmacological characterization and effects of antidepressants. *J. Pharmacol. Exp. Ther., 233*, 473-479.

Kennett, G. A., Dourish, C. T., & Curzon, G. (1987). Antidepressant-like action of 5-HT₁A agonists and conventional antidepressants in an animal model of depression. *Eur. J. Pharmacol., 134*, 265-274.

Kilpatrick, G. J., Jones, B. J., & Tyers, M. B. (1987). The identification distribution of 5-HT₃ receptors in rat brain using radioligand binding. *Nature, 330*, 746-748.

Kwong, L. L., Smith, E. R., Davidson, J. M., & Peroutka, S. J. (1986). Differential

24   *The Role of Serotonin in Psychiatric Disorders*

interactions of "prosexual" drugs with 5-hydroxytryptamine$_{1A}$ and alpha$_2$-adrenergic receptors. *Behav. Neurosci., 100,* 664–668.

Leysen, J. E., de Chaffoy de Courcelles, D. C., De Clerck, F., Niemegeers, J. E., & Van Nueten, J. M. (1984). Serotonin-S$_2$ receptor binding sites and functional correlates. *Neuropharmacology, 23,* 1493–1501.

Leysen, J. E., Niemegeers, C. J. E., Tollenaere, J. P., & Laduron, P. M. (1978). Serotonergic component of neuroleptic receptors. *Nature, 272,* 163–166.

Lyon, R. A., Davis, K. H., & Titeler, M. (1987). ^{3}H-DOB (4-bromo-2,5-dimethoxyphenylisopropylamine) labels a guanyl nucleotide-sensitive state of cortical 5-HT$_2$ receptors. *J. Pharmacol. Exp. Ther., 31,* 194–199.

Marsden, C. A., Sleight, A. J., Fone, K. C. F., Johnson, J. V., Crespi, F., Martin, K. F., Garrett, J. C., & Bennett, G. W. (1989). Functional identification of 5-HT receptor subtypes. *Comp. Biochem. Physiol.,* (A)*93,* 107–114.

Matsuoka, H., Ishii, M., Goto, A., & Sugimoto, T. (1985). Role of serotonin type 2 receptors in regulation of aldosterone production. *Am. Physiol. Soc., 234,* 1843–1849.

Mawe, G. M., Branchek, T. A., & Gershon, M. D. (1986). Peripheral neural serotonin receptors: Identification and characterization with specific antagonists and agonists. *Proc. Nat. Acad. Sci., 83,* 9799–9803.

McCall, R. B., & Aghajanian, G. K. (1980). Pharmacological characterization of serotonin receptors in the facial motor nucleus: A microiontophoretic study. *Eur. J. Pharmacol., 65,* 175–183.

Millar, J. A., Facoory, B. D., & Laverty, R. (1982). Mechanism of action of ketanserin. *Lancet, i,* 1154.

Oksenberg, D., & Peroutka, S. J. (1988). Antagonism of 5-HT$_{1A}$ receptor-mediated modulation of adenylate cyclase activity by pindolol and propranolol isomers. *Biochem. Pharmacol., 37,* 3429–3433.

Ortmann, R., Bischoff, S., Radeke, E., Buech, O., & Delini-Stula, A. (1982). Correlations between different measures of anti-serotonin activity of drugs. *Naunyn-Schmiedeberg's Arch. Pharmacol., 321,* 265–270.

Palfreyman, M. G., Mir, A. K., Kubina, M., Middlemiss, D. N., Richards, M., Tricklebank, M. D., & Fozard, J. R. (1986). Monoamine receptor sensitivity changes following chronic administration of MDL 72394 a site directed inhibitor of monoamine oxidase. *Eur. J. Pharmacol., 106,* 539–546.

Pazos, A., Cortes, R., & Palacios, J. M. (1985). Quantitative autoradiographic mapping of serotonin receptors in the rat brain. II. Serotonin-2 receptors. *Brain Res., 346,* 231–249.

Pazos, A., Hoyer, D., & Palacios, J. M. (1984). Mesulergine, a selective serotonin-2 ligand in the rat cortex, does not label these receptors in porcine and human cortex: Evidence for species differences in brain serotonin-2 receptors. *Eur. J. Pharmacol., 106,* 531–538.

Pazos, A., & Palacios, J. M. (1985). Quantitative autoradiographic mapping of serotonin receptors in the rat brain. I. Serotonin-1 receptors. *Brain Res., 346,* 205–230.

Pedigo, N. W., Yamamura, H. I., & Nelson, D. L. (1981). Discrimination of multiple [^{3}H]5-hydroxytryptamine binding sites by the neuroleptic spiperone in rat brain. *J. Neurochem., 36,* 220–226.

Peroutka, S. J. (1984). Vascular serotonin receptors: Correlation with 5-HT$_1$ and 5-HT$_2$ binding sites. *Biochem. Pharmacol., 33,* 2349–2353.

Peroutka, S. J. (1986). Pharmacological differentiation and characterization of 5-HT$_{1A}$, 5-HT$_{1B}$ and 5-HT$_{1C}$ binding sites in rat frontal cortex. *J. Neurochem., 47,* 529–540.

Peroutka, S. J. (1987). Serotonin receptors. In H. Meltzer (Ed.), *Psychopharmacology: The third generation of progress* (pp. 303–311). New York: Raven Press.

Peroutka, S. J., Huang, S., E. Allen, G. S. (1986). Canine basilar artery contractions mediated by 5-hydroxytryptamine$_{1A}$ receptors. *J. Pharmacol. Exp. Ther., 237,* 901–906.

Peroutka, S. J., Lebovitz, R. M., & Snyder, S. H. (1981). Two distinct central serotonin receptors with different physiological functions. *Science, 212,* 827–829.

Peroutka, S. J., & McCarthy, B. G. (1989). Sumatriptan (GR 43175) interacts selectively with 5-HT$_{1B}$ and 5-HT$_{1D}$ binding sites. *Eur. J. Pharmacol., 163,* 133–136.

Peroutka, S. J., & Snyder, S. H. (1979). Multiple serotonin receptors: Differential binding of ³H-serotonin, ³H-lysergic acid diethylamide and ³H-spiroperidol. *Mol. Pharmacol., 16,* 687–699.

Peroutka, S. J., & Snyder, S. H. (1980a). Long-term antidepressant treatment decreases spiroperidol-labeled serotonin receptor binding. *Science, 210,* 88–90.

Peroutka, S. J., & Snyder, S. H. (1980b). Regulation of serotonin$_2$ (5-HT$_2$) receptors labeled with ³H-spiroperidol by chronic treatment with the antidepressant amitriptyline. *J. Pharmacol. Exp. Ther., 215,* 582–587.

Pierce, P. A., & Peroutka, S. J. (1988). Antagonism of 5-HT$_2$-mediated phosphatidylinositol turnover by d-lysergic acid diethylamide. *J. Pharmacol. Exp. Ther., 247,* 918–925.

Prichett, D. B., Bach, A. W. J., Wozny, M., Taleb, O., Dal Toso, R., Shih, J. C., & Seeberg, P. H. (1988). Structure and functional expression of cloned rat serotonin 5-HT$_2$ receptor. *EMBO J., 7,* 4135–4140.

Raiteri, M., Maura, G., Bonanno, G., & Pittaluga, A. (1986). Differential pharmacology and function of two 5-HT$_1$ receptors modulating transmitter release in cerebellum. *J. Pharmacol. Exp. Ther., 237,* 644–648.

Richardson, B. P., & Engel, G. (1986). The pharmacology and function of 5-HT$_3$ receptors. *Trends Neurosci., 7,* 424–428.

Richardson, B. P., Engel, G., Donatsch, P., & Stadler, P. A. (1985). Identification of serotonin M-receptor subtypes and their specific blockade by a new class of drugs. *Nature, 336,* 126–131.

Sanders-Bush, E., & Conn, P. J. (1987). Neurochemistry of serotonin neuronal systems: Consequences of serotonin receptor activation. In H. Meltzer (Ed.), *Psychopharmacology: The third generation of progress* (pp. 95–103). New York: Raven Press.

Schlegel, J. R., & Peroutka, S. J. (1986). Nucleotide interactions with 5-HT$_{1A}$ binding sites directly labeled by [³H]-8-hydroxy-2-(DI-n-propylamino)tetralin ([³H]-8-OH-DPAT). *Biochem. Pharmacol., 35,* 1943–1949.

Sleight, A. J., Marsden, C. A., Palfreyman, M. G., Mir, A. K., & Lovenberg, W. (1988). Chronic MAO A and MAO B inhibition decreases the 5-HT$_{1A}$ receptor mediated inhibition of forskolin-stimulated adenylate cyclase. *Eur. J. Pharmacol., 154,* 255–261.

Smith, L. M., & Peroutka, S. J. (1986). Differential effects of 5-hydroxytryptamine$_{1A}$ selective drugs on the 5-HT behavioral syndrome. *Pharmacol. Biochem. Behav., 24,* 1513–1519.

Sprouse, J. S., & Aghajanian, G. K. (1987). Electrophysiological responses of serotonergic dorsal raphe neurons to 5-HT$_{1A}$ and 5-HT$_{1B}$ agonists. *Synapse, 1,* 3–9.

Taylor, E. W., Duckles, S. P., & Nelson, D. L. (1986). Dissociation constants of serotonin agonists in the canine basilar artery correlate to K_i values at the 5-HT$_{1A}$ binding site. *J. Pharmacol. Exp. Ther., 236,* 118–125.

Tricklebank, M. D. (1985). The behavioral response to 5-HT receptor agonists and subtypes of the central 5-HT receptor. *Trends Pharmacol. Sci., 6,* 403–407.

Tricklebank, M. D., Middlemiss, D. N., & Neill, J. (1986). Pharmacological analysis of the behavioral and thermoregulatory effects of the putative 5-HT$_1$ receptor agonist, RU 24969, in the rat. *Neuropharmacology, 25,* 877–886.

Trulson, M. E., & Arasteh, K. (1986). Buspirone decreases the activity of 5-hydroxytryptamine-containing dorsal raphe neurons in-vitro. *J. Pharm. Pharmacol., 38,* 380–382.

VanderMaelen, C. P., & Aghajanian, G. K. (1980). Intracellular studies showing modulation of facial motoneuron excitability by serotonin. *Nature, 287,* 346–347.

VanderMaelen, C. P., Matheson, G. K., Wilderman, R. C., & Patterson, L. A. (1986). Inhibition of serotonergic dorsal raphe neurons by systemic and iontophoretic administration of buspirone, a non-benzodiazepine anxiolytic drug. *Eur. J. Pharmacol., 129,* 123–130.

Van Nueten, J. M., Leysen, J. E., Vanhoutte, P. M., & Janssen, P. A. J. (1982). Serotonergic responses in vascular and non-vascular tissues. *Arch. Int. Pharmacodyn., 256,* 331–334.

Weiss, S., Sebben, M., Kemp, D., & Bockaert, J. (1986). Serotonin 5-HT$_1$ receptors mediate inhibition of cyclic AMP production in neurons. *Eur. J. Pharmacol., 120,* 227–230.

Yagaloff, K. A., & Hartig, P. R. (1985). ^{125}I-LSD binds to a novel serotonergic site on rat choroid plexus epithelial cells. *J. Neurosci., 5,* 3178–3183.

3

The Receptor Sensitivity Hypothesis of Antidepressant Action
A Review of Antidepressant Effects on Serotonin Function

DENNIS S. CHARNEY
PEDRO L. DELGADO
LAWRENCE H. PRICE
GEORGE R. HENINGER

On the basis of data from a variety of techniques, including neurotransmitter receptor binding, single-unit electrophysiology studies, measurement of brain second-messenger function, and behavioral paradigms involving pharmacological stimulation of behavior using drugs that bind to specific neurotransmitter receptors, the original biogenic amine hypothesis of antidepressant action involving alterations in monoamine metabolism has been modified. The evidence from these investigations suggested that the ability of long-term antidepressant treatment to reduce beta-adrenergic receptor sensitivity, while enhancing the responses of serotonergic and alpha$_1$-adrenergic receptor stimulation, is related to the therapeutic mechanism of action of antidepressant treatments.

The receptor sensitivity hypothesis suggesting that modulation of receptor sensitivity may be a mechanism of action common to tricyclic antidepressants, atypical antidepressants, monoamine oxidase (MAO) inhibitors, and electroconvulsive therapy, initially inspired a great deal of enthusiasm. It was believed that if information from preclinical studies identifying receptor sensitivity changes following antidepressant treatment were applied to clinical research strategies in depressed patients, new insights into the pathophysiology of depressive illness and the development of improved and more specific therapeutic agents would result.

The purpose of this chapter is to review the current status of the receptor sensitivity hypothesis of antidepressant action in relation to effects on serotonin function. Since an enormous literature exists regarding this hypothesis, only findings that have emerged since our 1981 comprehensive review (Charney, Menkes, & Heninger, 1981) will be discussed. An attempt will be made to synthesize the findings and draw conclusions, especially in relation to the following.

1. Do the data support the hypothesis that a specific alteration in serotonin neuronal transmission following long-term antidepressant treatment can account for the mechanism of action of all, or even most, antidepressant treatments?

2. If a common mechanism of action of antidepressant treatment related to serotonin function has not been identified, what aspects of the effects of long-term antidepressant treatment on serotonin neuronal activity are most relevant?

3. Has the serotonin receptor sensitivity hypothesis of antidepressant action led to new discoveries regarding the etiology and treatment of major depression that support a receptor dysfunction in this disorder?

4. What new strategies should be employed to further the knowledge of the role of serotonin function in the mechanism of action of antidepressant drugs and the etiology of major depression in order to facilitate the development of new treatments?

ANTIDEPRESSANT EFFECTS ON
SECOND MESSENGER FUNCTION

Serotonin-Sensitive Adenylate Cyclase Activity

A 5-HT–activated adenylate cyclase system has been identified in mammalian tissue. Depending on the experimental conditions, there is evidence that 5-HT_1 receptor sites are positively or negatively linked to adenylate cyclase (Conn & Sanders-Bush, 1987). Recently, it has been reported that 5-HT inhibits forskolin-stimulated adenylate cyclase in hippocampal preparations. This inhibitory action has pharmacological properties consistent with a 5-HT_{1A} site (DeVivo & Maayani, 1985, 1986). As far as we know, the effects of long-term antidepressant treatment on this 5-HT-receptor–mediated response have not been examined.

Lithium has been shown to increase hippocampal 5-HT–stimulated cyclic adenosine monophosphate accumulation after chronic (three weeks) but not subacute (five days) treatment. Lithium produced a facilitation of 5-HT-sensitive adenylate cyclase activity despite a decrease in the density of

5-HT$_1$ receptors and no effect on receptor-adenylate cyclase coupling (Hotta & Yamawaki, 1986).

The Phosphatidylinositol System

An important mechanism for signal transduction is the phosphatidylinositol cycle. This cycle is a major second-messenger system mediating actions of numerous hormones and neurotransmitters, including norepinephrine (NE), serotonin, acetylcholine, histamine, and several peptides (Abdel-Latif, 1986). Serotonin has been shown to stimulate phosphatidylinositol hydrolysis in mammalian brain (Berridge, Downes, & Hanley, 1982). It is generally accepted that activation of 5-HT$_2$ receptors mediates 5-HT–stimulated phosphoinositide hydrolysis in the cerebral cortex. In subcortical regions, 5-HT stimulates a phosphoinositide hydrolysis by mechanisms other than the 5-HT$_2$ receptor (Conn & Sanders-Bush, 1985, 1986). The 5-HT$_{1C}$ receptor has been suggested to be linked to phosphoinositide hydrolysis in the choroid plexus (Conn & Sanders-Bush, 1986, 1987).

Chronic but not acute treatment with imipramine, desipramine, and iprindol, but not zimelidine, reduces the stimulation of ^{3}H-inositol phosphates by 5-HT in cerebral cortex (Kendall & Nahorski, 1985; Godfrey et al., 1988). These results suggest that some antidepressant drugs may reduce brain 5-HT$_2$ receptor function.

Lithium has been shown to have important actions on phosphoinositol hydrolysis. It is a potent inhibitor of inositol-1-phosphatase, but at concentrations considerably higher than required clinically (Berridge, Downes, & Hanley, 1982). A recent investigation using therapeutic concentrations of lithium demonstrated that it reduced the actions on tracheal muscle relaxation of muscarinic, cholinergic, and histamine H$_1$ receptor stimulation. These effects are probably mediated by lithium's interference with the phosphatidylinositol cycle. It has been speculated that such effects of lithium could involve numerous neurotransmitters and peptides, account for the mood-stabilizing therapeutic properties of lithium, and provide a rational design for new antidepressant antimanic agents (Menkes et al., 1986).

The ability of lithium to alter protein phosphorylation has been studied. Lithium increases the phosphorylation of a 64-kDa membrane protein in cortex and hippocampus. This phosphorylation is not dependent on exogenous calcium or calcium/calmodulin (Klein et al., 1987). The nature of this protein and its possible significance in the therapeutic action of lithium remain to be established.

SEROTONIN RECEPTOR BINDING STUDIES

Chronic antidepressant treatment has inconsistent effects (Charney, Menkes, & Heninger, 1981; Sugrue, 1983; Green & Nutt, 1985) and long-term lithium administration produces a reduction in ^{3}H-5-HT binding (Hotta & Yamawaki, 1986; Treiser & Kellar, 1980; Treiser et al., 1981). Recent investigations involving radioligands such as spiperone and ritanserin, which label 5-HT$_2$ receptors, have observed that these receptors are decreased in density by many, but not all, antidepressant drugs.* (See Table 3-1.) Chronic lithium administration reduces the density of 5-HT$_2$ receptors in hippocampus but not in frontal cortex (Goodwin et al., 1986). For many of these drugs, the reduction in 5-HT$_2$ density appears to require long-term drug administration; however, an important exception is mianserin, which has this effect after a few doses (Blackshear, Martin, & Sanders-Bush, 1986; Blackshear, Friedman, & Sanders-Bush, 1983; Holmeste & Tang, 1983; Gandolfi, Barbaccia, & Costa, 1985).

Several important questions have arisen regarding the relevance of the observed 5-HT$_2$ binding decrements to the therapeutic action of antidepressants. At first glance, it would appear to be difficult to reconcile the decrease in 5-HT$_2$ receptors after antidepressant drug administration with the physiological supersensitivity to serotonin that has been observed in a variety of brain areas following such treatment. However, a reciprocal relationship between 5-HT$_1$ and 5-HT$_2$ receptors has been observed with 5-HT$_2$ receptors having an inhibitory effect on responses to 5-HT in prefrontal cortex (Lakoski & Aghajanian, 1985). In addition, electroconvulsive therapy (ECT) increases 5-HT$_2$ receptor density, an effect opposite to that of antidepressant drugs (Kellar et al., 1981; Vetulani, Lebrecht, & Pile, 1981; Kellar & Bergstrom, 1983; Green, Johnson, & Nimgaonkar, 1983; Green, Heal, & Goodwin, 1986).

The mechanism by which long-term treatment with many antidepressants reduces 5-HT$_2$ receptor density has not been definitively established. The downregulation of 5-HT$_2$ receptors does not require intact 5-HT nerve terminals (Scott & Crews, 1986). In addition, the 5-HT$_2$ receptor recognition site does not respond predictably to in vivo manipulations. For example, increased 5-HT$_2$ receptor density does not develop after denervation (Quik & Azmita, 1983), and, paradoxically, chronic 5-HT$_2$ receptor antagonist administration decreases the density of the 5-HT$_2$ receptor binding site (Blackshear, Friedman, & Sanders-Bush, 1983; Leysen et al., 1986). The ability of many antidepressant drugs acutely to antagonize 5-HT receptors may relate to the decrease in 5-HT$_2$ receptor density with long-term treatment (Wander et al., 1986).

---

*Hyttel, Overo, & Arnt, 1984; Peroutka & Snyder, 1980; Kellar et al., 1981; Vetulani, Lebrecht, & Pilc, 1981; Kendall et al., 1982; Kellar & Bergstrom, 1983; Green, Johnson, & Nimgaonkar, 1983; Stolz, Marsden, & Middlemiss, 1983; Fuxe et al., 1983; Goodwin, Green, & Johnson, 1984; Blackshear, Martinn, & Sanders-Bush, 1986; Green, Heal, & Goodwin, 1986.

TABLE 3-1
The Effects of Chronic Antidepressant Administration on Serotonin Receptor Function*

Antidepressant Category	Receptor Binding			Neurophysiological Sensitivity		Behavioral Sensitivity		
	$5\text{-}HT_1$	$5\text{-}HT_2$	IMI	$5\text{-}HT$ Autoreceptor	$5\text{-}HT$ Postsynaptic	$5\text{-}HT_1$	$5\text{-}HT_{1A}$ Autoreceptor	$5\text{-}HT_2$
NE reuptake inhibitors	0↓	→	↓0	0	↑	→	→	↑0
Mixed NE and 5-HT reuptake inhibitors	0	→	↓0	0	↑	→	→	↑↓0
5-HT reuptake inhibitors	0	↑0	↑	→	0	→	→	↓0
MAO inhibitors	→	→	↑0	→	0	→	→	→
Atypical antidepressants:								
Trazodone	0	→	—	—	—	—	—	0↑
Bupropion	—	0	0	—	—	—	—	0↓
Mianserin	0	→	0	—	↑	—	→	—
Nomifensine	—	0	—	—	—	—	—	—
Maprotiline	—	0	—	—	↑	—	—	—
ECT	0	↑	↓0	—	↑	↓↑	→	→

*The specific techniques used to evaluate serotonin receptor subtypes are described in the text. ↑, Increase; ↓, decrease; 0, no change; —, not tested; averaged over different brain regions and different drugs; mixed results are indicated by more than one symbol.

It is likely that antidepressants produce a complex interactive effect on serotonin and noradrenergic neuronal function. For example, recent studies indicate that serotonin neurons may regulate beta-adrenergic receptor number and function in the brain (Nimgaonkar et al., 1985; Asakura et al., 1987; Janowsky et al., 1982; Stockmeier, Martino, & Kellar, 1985). An intact serotonergic neuronal input is corequired for the downregulation of cortical beta-adrenergic receptors by tricyclic antidepressants and ECT (Asakura et al., 1987; Janowsky et al., 1982; Manier et al., 1987; Dumbrille-Ross & Tang, 1983).

Antidepressant Binding Sites

There is now substantial evidence that several ligands of different structures, including ^{3}H-imipramine, ^{3}H-paroxetine, and ^{3}H-indalpine, bind with high affinity to a recognition site associated with the 5-HT transporter complex. This recognition site mediates the inhibition of the Na^+-dependent uptake of 5-HT. The available evidence suggests that the binding site labeled by ^{3}H-imipramine is not identical to the transporter recognition site for 5-HT, but, rather, an allosteric coupling exists between the two sites. Consequently, the ^{3}H-imipramine recognition site may represent a novel type of presynaptic receptor, whose function it is to modulate 5-HT uptake, and it may play a role in the mode of action of antidepressants (Langer et al., 1986).

The effects of antidepressant treatment on ^{3}H-imipramine binding have been variable. Tricyclic antidepressants decrease the number of brain ^{3}H-imipramine recognition sites in some, but not all, studies[†]. Haloperidol and lithium also reduce ^{3}H-imipramine site density (Plenge & Mellerup, 1982; Hrdina, 1984). Iprindol and mianserin do not alter ^{3}H-imipramine binding site density (Kinnier, Chuang, & Costa, 1980; Hrdina, 1984) and zimelidine and deprenyl increase ^{3}H-imipramine binding (Gentsch, Lichtsteine, & Feer, 1984; Severson & Anderson, 1986). (See Table 3-1.)

NEUROPHYSIOLOGICAL STUDIES OF SEROTONIN FUNCTION

Previous single-unit electrophysiological investigations have consistently identified enhanced serotonergic and alpha$_1$-adrenergic responsiveness in various postsynaptic brain regions following chronic antidepressant administration. There is also electrophysiological evidence favoring beta-adrenergic subsensitivity, but this has not been studied as extensively (Charney, Menkes, & Heninger, 1981).

[†]Langer et al., 1986; Barbaccia et al., 1983; Kinnier, Chuang, & Costa, 1980; Raisman, Briley, & Langer, 1980; Plenge & Mellerup, 1982; Hrdina, 1984; Gentsch, Lichtsteine, & Feer, 1984; Severson & Anderson, 1986.

Most of the recent electrophysiological work has involved the evaluation of drugs with specific and potent effects on serotonin reuptake and MAO inhibitors on serotonergic neurotransmission.[‡] (See Table 3-1.) These experiments, which have been conducted primarily by deMontigny and associates, measured the responsiveness of hippocampal pyramidal cells to iontophoretic application of serotonin as a reflection of postsynaptic serotonin function and the activity of the hippocampal pyramidal neurons in electrical stimulation of the ventral medial ascending serotonin pathway to obtain a measure of net serotonin neurotransmission. They also evaluated the responsiveness to lysergic acid diethylamide (LSD) of serotonin neurons of the dorsal raphe nucleus, to assess serotonin autoreceptor function (Blier & deMontigny, 1983; Blier, deMontigny, & Tardif, 1984; Chaput, deMontigny, & Blier, 1986). These investigations have demonstrated that chronic treatment with serotonin reuptake inhibitors, such as zimelidine, indalpine, and citalopram, increased serotonergic transmission by inducing a desensitization of the serotonin autoreceptor without altering postsynaptic serotonin sensitivity (Blier & deMontigny, 1983; Blier, deMontigny, & Tardif, 1984; Chaput, deMontigny, & Blier, 1986). In contrast, antidepressant drugs such as imipramine, desipramine, and iprindol induce postsynaptic serotonin receptor supersensitivity, but do not change autoreceptor function (deMontigny & Aghajanian, 1978). The explanation for this observation may be that tricyclic drugs are rapidly demethylated into their secondary forms, which are weak serotonin uptake inhibitors. These results suggest that sustained blockade of serotonin reuptake is probably required for desensitization of the autoreceptor. In these studies, the responsiveness of hippocampal pyramidal neurons to NE was not modified by any of the antidepressant drugs investigated.

New data indicate that prolonged inhibition of MAO-A, but not MAO-B, results in enhanced serotonin neurotransmission (Blier & deMontigny, 1985; Blier, deMontigny, & Azzaro, 1986a). Short-term administration of MAO-A inhibitors reduces dorsal raphe firing rate and results in complete recovery with long-term treatment. This is probably due to autoreceptor desensitization, because the ability of LSD to decrease dorsal raphe activity is reduced with chronic MAO-A inhibitor administration. The depression of firing rate of hippocampal pyramidal neurons induced by stimulation of the ventral medial serotonin pathway is increased by phenelzine and clorgy-

---

[‡]Blier & deMontigny, 1983; Blier, deMontigny, & Tardif, 1984; deMontigny, Blier, & Chaput, 1984; deMontigny, 1984; Turmel & deMontigny, 1984; Blier & deMontigny, 1985; Blier & deMontigny, 1985; Blier, deMontigny, & Azzaro, 1986a; Blier, deMontigny, & Azzaro, 1986b; Chaput, deMontigny, & Blier, 1986; Olpe & Schellenberg, 1981; Rowan & Anwyl, 1985; deMontigny & Aghajanian, 1978.

line, but not deprenyl, which suggests that the former two drugs enhance net serotonin transmission.

The MAO inhibitors also produce an immediate decrease in locus coeruleus firing rate. This effect, although maximal at two days, persists with long-term administration, in contrast to the recovery that occurs in serotonin neuronal firing rate. The effect of stimulation of the dorsal noradrenergic bundle is not modified by treatment with MAO inhibitors (Blier & deMontigny, 1985). A decrease in activity of noradrenergic neurons, coupled with unchanged efficacy of the noradrenergic neuronal stimulation, indicated that MAO inhibition results in a net decrease of noradrenergic neurotransmission. Since serotonin, but not norepinephrine, neurons progressively recover their normal firing rate during sustained MAO inhibition, an enhancement of serotonin neurotransmission, rather than a reduction in noradrenergic transmission, appears more likely to be related to the delayed antidepressant effects of the MAO inhibitors.

Lithium and Serotonin Neuronal Activity

A series of investigations suggests that short-term (48 hours) lithium administration enhances the serotonergic neurotransmission via actions on presynaptic serotonin neuronal function (Treiser et al., 1981; Blier & deMontigny, 1985; Grahame-Smith & Green, 1974; Sangdee & Franz, 1980). The response of hippocampal pyramidal neurons to electrical stimulation of the ventral medial serotonin pathway is increased twofold by short-term lithium treatment. Pretreatment with 5-7-DHT abolishes this enhancement. Neurophysiological studies of the dorsal raphe nucleus indicate that lithium alters neither the number of active neurons nor their mean firing rate (Blier & deMontigny, 1985). Short-term lithium potentiates the tryptophan-tranylcypromine–induced serotonin syndrome (Grahame-Smith & Green, 1974) and the depressant effects of tryptophan on transmission between bulbospinal pathways and sympathetic preganglionic neurons (Sangdee & Franz, 1980). In rhesus monkeys, the prolactin rise following intravenous tryptophan, but not m-chlorophenyl piperazine (mCPP), is enhanced by short-term lithium administration (Heninger, Charney, & Smith, 1986).

Three possible mechanisms have been suggested as accounting for the enhancing effect of lithium on 5-HT neuronal function: (1) increased uptake of tryptophan by serotonin neurons, (2) decreased reuptake of serotonin, or (3) enhanced release of serotonin from terminals.

The first possibility is unlikely because the increase in tryptophan reuptake induced by lithium does not take place in all brain regions, and in particular, not in the hippocampus (Swann et al., 1981). The second possibility is also unlikely because acute blockade of serotonin reuptake by serotonin reuptake inhibitors fails to augment the effectiveness of electrical stimulation of serotonin neurons (Blier & deMontigny, 1983; Blier, deMontigny, & Tardif, 1984; Chaput, deMontigny, & Blier, 1986). The third possibility is more likely and is supported by the finding that basal, as well as potassium-stimulated release of serotonin, is increased in the hippocampus by lithium treatment (Treiser et al., 1981). It has been proposed that lithium might augment serotonin release through its action on phosphoinositol metabolism (Berridge, Downes, & Hanley, 1982; Menkes et al., 1986).

EFFECTS OF LONG-TERM ANTIDEPRESSANT TREATMENT ON BEHAVIORAL MODELS

The importance of behavioral models of receptor function is that they allow an assessment of the overall integrated functioning of specific neuronal systems. The authors' previous review concluded that the results of behavioral studies were consistent with the hypothesis that long-term antidepressant treatment enhanced postsynaptic alpha-adrenergic and serotonergic receptor function (Charney, Menkes, & Heninger, 1981). The findings were qualified by the observation that the behavioral potentiation of NE and serotonin function in several of the studies occurred only more than 24 hours after the last antidepressant treatment. This observation raised questions regarding the applicability of the findings to clinical situations.

Behavioral Models of Serotonin Function

Behavioral studies conducted over the past five years indicate that it can no longer be simply stated that 5-HT receptor function is enhanced by long-term antidepressant treatment (Willner, 1985). (See Table 3-1.) It has been established that the various behavioral models utilized to assess serotonin function depend on the functions of specific serotonin receptor subtypes. For example, it has been suggested that the serotonin-agonist–induced head-twitch response is related to the function of the 5-HT_2 receptor, whereas effects on 5-HT_1 receptors may relate more to the development of the serotonin syndrome (Lucki, Nobler, & Frazer, 1984; Leysen, 1984).

The results of studies evaluating the head-twitch response to serotonin agonists following long-term antidepressant treatment are not uniform. Most of the significant findings were observed 24 or more hours after the last antidepressant dose, when drug levels are low. The 5-methoxy-DMT–induced increase in the head-twitch response is reduced by chronic treatment with imipramine and amitriptyline one and 18 hours after the last dose. However, 24 and 48 hours after the last dose, both imipramine and amitriptyline, as well as trazadone, iprindol, and desipramine, increase the head-twitch response. Chronic mianserin does not change the 5-methoxy-DMT head-twitch response (Friedman, Cooper, & Dallob, 1983). Tranylcypromine, zimelidine, and mianserin have been reported to decrease the head-twitch response to 5-methoxy-DMT one and 24 hours after the last dose. Repeated ECT produces an increase in the 5-methoxy-DMT–induced head-twitch response 48 hours after the last treatment (Goodwin, Green, & Johnson, 1984; Wielosz, 1985). The 5-HTP-induced head-twitch response is enhanced 18 hours after the final ECT and desipramine dose (Green, 1983). The head-twitch response to quipazine is reduced at two hours but unchanged at 72 hours after the final amitriptyline dose. Fluvoxamine and citalopram have no effect on the quipazine-induced head-twitch response (Pawlowski & Melzacka, 1986).

Few recent studies have been conducted to evaluate the effects of longterm antidepressant treatment on the serotonin syndrome. The MAO inhibitors reduce the effects of 5-methoxy-DMT or LSD in eliciting the serotonin syndrome 24 hours after the last dose (Lucki & Frazer, 1982). Amitriptyline and imipramine reduce the 5-methoxy-DMT–induced serotonin syndrome at less than two hours (Stolz, Marsden, & Middlemiss, 1983; Stolz & Marsden, 1982), have no effect at 12-24 hours (Lucki & Frazer, 1982), and increase the response 48 hours or more after the last dose (Stolz, Marsden, & Middlemiss, 1983; Stolz & Marsden, 1982). Long-term chlorimipramine and fluoxetine reduce the 5-methoxy-DMT response at two and 48 hours after the final treatment (Stolz, Marsden, & Middlemiss, 1983).

Long-term desipramine, tranylcypromine, and zimelidine treatment 24 hours after the last dose and repeated ECT attenuate the serotonin syndrome induced by the 5-HT$_{1A}$ receptor agonist 8-OH-DPAT in the rat (Goodwin, De Souza, & Green, 1987). In contrast, lithium administration for 14 days enhances the serotonin syndrome produced by 8-OH-DPAT, probably via a postsynaptic mechanism (Goodwin et al., 1986). Long-term clorgyline treatment has been shown to block the effects of mCPP on food intake, sedation, and induction of limb movements. The effects of mCPP may also be mediated via actions on 5-HT$_{1B}$ receptors (Goodwin, De Souza, & Green, 1985). Chronic lithium administration does not modify the locomotor responses to the putative 5-HT$_{1B}$ receptor agonist RU24969 (Goodwin et al., 1986).

Behavioral studies are now being conducted that purport to assess presynaptic 5-HT$_{1A}$ receptor function following long-term antidepressant treatment. The effect of 8-OH-DPAT on rectal temperature is reduced by a spectrum of antidepressants, such as amitriptyline, desipramine, zimelidine, mianserin, and tranylcypromine, and by ECT (Goodwin, De Souza, & Green, 1985, 1987; Gudelsky et al., 1986). These effects were seen during drug treatment (one hour after last treatment) and withdrawal (42 hours after final treatment) and only developed fully after long-term administration (Goodwin, De Souza, & Green, 1987). Long-term lithium administration also reduces the hypothermic response to 8-OH-DPAT 18 hours after the last dose (Goodwin et al., 1986).

CLINICAL STUDIES OF SEROTONIN FUNCTION AND THE MECHANISMS OF ACTION OF ANTIDEPRESSANT TREATMENTS

Effects on Serotonin Turnover

At the time of the 1981 review, several studies had investigated the effect of antidepressant treatments on cerebrospinal fluid (CSF) 5-HIAA levels. Amitriptyline, imipramine, chlorimipramine, and zimelidine reduced CSF 5-HIAA. Nortriptyline and phenelzine produced smaller decreases in CSF 5-HIAA that tended toward significance, and ECT had no consistent effects. The alterations in CSF 5-HIAA by antidepressant treatments were not related to treatment response and no consistent relationship was identified between pretreatment CSF 5-HIAA levels and subsequent therapeutic responses to amitriptyline, chlorimipramine, and imipramine (Charney, Menkes, & Heninger, 1981). More recently, a National Institute of Mental Health collaborative study of the biology of depressive disorders reported that in unipolar patients, low CSF 5-HIAA and high urinary metanephrine were associated with therapeutic responses to imipramine, but not amitriptyline (Bowden et al., 1985, 1987).

Since 1981, relatively few studies have been conducted to evaluate the effects of antidepressants on serotonin turnover, which perhaps reflects the generally disappointing results of previous investigations. Mianserin produces either no change or a decrease in MHPG levels and no change in CSF 5-HIAA or HVA. Amitriptyline and imipramine reduce CSF MHPG and 5-HIAA without altering CSF HVA, and ECT increases CSF 5-HIAA and not HVA levels (Asberg & Wagner, 1986). As before, most antidepressant studies of alterations of monoamine metabolites have not shown these to be related to clinical outcome (Veith et al., 1983; Sharma, Venkitasubramanian, & Agnihotri, 1986).

Assessment of Serotonin Receptor Function

Many of the studies designed to evaluate monoamine receptor function using pharmacological probes have evaluated serotonergic function. (See Table 3-2.) A series of studies has determined the effect of a variety of antidepressant drugs on the ability of intravenous tryptophan to increase prolactin.[§] Extensive evidence reviewed elsewhere indicates that the prolactin response to tryptophan can be used as a reflection of serotonergic function

---

[§]Charney, Heninger, & Sternberg, 1984; Charig et al., 1986; Cowen, 1987; Price, Charney, & Heninger, 1985; Price, Charney, and Heninger (in press); Price et al., 1987; Price et al. (submitted); Cowen et al., 1986; Anderson & Cowen, 1986; Glue et al., 1986.

TABLE 3-2
Clinical Investigations of Antidepressant Effects on Serotonin
Receptor Function in Depressed Patients*

Antidepressant Category	TRP→↑ PRL	5-HTP→↑ CORT	IMI Binding
NE reuptake inhibitors	↑	↓	0
Mixed NE and 5-HT reuptake inhibitors	↑	↓	0
5-HT reuptake inhibitors	↑	—	↑
MAOI	↑	↑	—
Atypical antidepressants:			
Trazodone	0	—	—
Bupropion	0	—	—
Mianserin	0	—	—
Nomifensine	—	—	—
Maprotiline	—	—	0
ECT	—	—	0

*Unless otherwise noted, the specific techniques used to evaluate monoamine receptor subtypes are described in the text. AMP, Amphetamine; CORT, cortisol; TRP, tryptophan; PRL, prolactin; IMI, imipramine; APO, apomorphine; GH, growth hormone; BROMO, bromocriptine. ↑, Increase; ↓, decrease; 0, no change; —, not tested; averaged over different brain regions and different drugs; mixed results are indicated by more than one symbol.

(Charney, Heninger, & Sternberg, 1984), perhaps involving the 5-HT$_1$ receptor (Glue et al., 1986; Heninger, Charney, & Smith, 1987). It has been observed in depressed patients that, in rank order, fluvoxamine > amitriptyline > tranylcypromine > desipramine significantly increase the prolactin response to tryptophan (Charney, Heninger, & Sternberg, 1984; Price, Charney, & Heninger, 1985; Price et al., 1987; Price et al., 1988). In healthy subjects, desipramine and chlorimipramine increase the prolactin response to tryptophan, perhaps to a greater degree than in patients (Cowen et al., 1986; Anderson & Cowen, 1986).

The potentiation of the tryptophan-prolactin response, however, is not universal among antidepressants because in depressed patients, trazodone and buproprion do not enhance the tryptophan-induced increase in prolactin (Price, Charney, & Heninger, in press; Charney, Price, & Heninger, unpublished data). The inability of trazodone to increase the prolactin response to tryptophan probably relates to the postsynaptic serotonin antagonist properties of trazodone.

In a related observation, the amitriptyline-induced enhancement of the prolactin response to tryptophan is further increased after abrupt discontinuation of amitriptyline in the context of little clinical change. This finding has been explained by the ability of amitriptyline to produce serotonin receptor supersensitivity because of its postsynaptic serotonin receptor antagonist properties. The functional consequences of the serotonin receptor supersensitivity are most manifest when the drug antagonism is removed following amitriptyline discontinuation (Charney, Heninger, & Sternberg, 1984). These results suggest that not all antidepressant drugs provide a robust enhancement of serotonin function, and that there is no linear relationship between an enhancement of serotonin function and therapeutic responsiveness.

Several investigations suggest that lithium enhances serotonin function in healthy subjects and depressed patients. The prolactin response to tryptophan is enhanced by lithium treatment in healthy subjects and depressed patients (Price et al., 1987; Glue et al., 1986), as is the fenfluramine-induced increase in prolactin secretion in depressed bipolar patients (Slater et al., 1976). Fenfluramine has little effect on cortisol secretion in healthy subjects and in unmedicated euthymic manic-depressive patients. However, in 11 manic-depressive patients treated with lithium, fenfluramine induced an increase in cortisol (Muhlbauer & Muller-Oerlinghausen, 1985).

Another paradigm used to evaluate serotonin function is the cortisol increase following 5-HTP administration. Depressed patients receiving imipramine, desipramine, or nortriptyline exhibited a decreased cortisol response to 5-HTP compared with the drug-free condition (Meltzer et al., 1984). These findings clearly contrast with the enhancement of serotonin function identified by the tryptophan infusion test. This may be due to the possibility that 5-HTP–induced increases in cortisol are related to effects on the 5-HT$_2$ receptors, whereas tryptophan neuroendocrine actions appear to occur via 5-HT$_1$ receptor stimulation (Heninger, Charney, & Smith, 1987). In addition, 5-HTP may have peripheral effects at the level of the adrenal gland (Van de Kar et al., 1985), and actions on catecholamine as well as indoleamine function (Ng et al., 1972; Fuxe et al., 1971).

Most, but not all, investigations have reported a decrease in platelet imipramine binding in drug-free, severely depressed patients (Langer et al., 1986). A decrease in the density of ^{3}H-imipramine in postmortem brains of depressed patients has been reported by two groups (Stanley, Virgillio, & Gershon, 1982; Perry et al., 1983). These results suggest that the possible existence of an endogenous "imipramine-like" substance may be relevant to the etiology of mood disorders and the mechanism of antidepressant drugs (Langer et al., 1986; Barbaccia & Costa, 1984). In general, antidepressant treatments do not consistently change the density or affinity of platelet imipramine receptors in depressed patients in relation to clinical improvement, which suggests that any disturbance in the serotonin transporter site may be a trait disorder (Asberg & Wagner, 1986; Asarch, Shih, & Kulcsar, 1980; Raisman et al., 1981; Suranyi-Cadotte, 1985; Langer et al., 1986; Wagner et al., 1987).

THERAPEUTIC STUDIES RELEVANT TO THE SEROTONIN RECEPTOR SENSITIVITY HYPOTHESIS

The addition of lithium treatment to ongoing antidepressant administration in patients who were either refractory or only partially responsive to treatment was based on the hypothesis that an enhancement of serotonin function was critical to therapeutic efficacy. The original open study by de-Montigny et al. (1981) and a double-blind placebo-controlled study by Heninger, Charney, and Sternberg (1983) have now been replicated by numerous investigations and have established lithium augmentation as a routine clinical treatment.** The earlier studies by Shopsin and colleagues demonstrating that parachlorophenylalanine, which decreases 5-HT synthesis, induces a recurrence of depressive symptoms in recovered depressed patients receiving antidepressant treatment, also support an important role for 5-HT in antidepressant action (Shopsin et al., 1975, 1976).

Recent work by Delgado and colleagues has utilized another strategy to evaluate the relationship between alterations in serotonin function produced by antidepressant medications and therapeutic efficacy (Delgado et al., 1988). (See Table 3-3.) Taking advantage of the known dependence of brain serotonin on plasma levels of tryptophan, they used a modified version of the tryptophan-free amino acid drink method described by Young et al. (1985) for rapidly lowering plasma tryptophan. This new method involves a 24-hour, low-tryptophan diet, followed the next morning by a tryptophan-free, 16-amino-acid drink. The ingestion of a tryptophan-free amino-acid drink induces hepatic protein synthesis and thereby depletes plasma tryptophan as it is incorporated into newly synthesized protein. With this strategy, a rapid and profound depletion of plasma tryptophan of over 90% has been achieved and the therapeutic effects of a variety of antidepressants temporarily reversed during the tryptophan-depleted state (Delgado et al., 1988). It is inferred that the reversal of antidepressant action in depression by this method is related to the expected decrease in brain serotonin availability, which supports an important role for serotonin function in the maintenance of antidepressant efficacy (Delgado et al., 1988).

**deMontigny et al.,1983; Nelson & Byck, 1982; Price, Conwell, & Nelson,1983; Birkhimer et al., 1983; Joyce, Hewland, & Jones, 1983; Louie & Meltzer, 1984; deMontigny, Elie, & Caille, 1985; Joyce, 1985; Schrader & Levien, 1985; Roy & Pickar, 1985; Nelson & Mazure, 1986; Kushnir, 1986; Price, Charney, & Heninger, 1986.

TABLE 3-3
Therapeutic Studies Relevant to Serotonin Receptor Sensitivity
Hypotheses of Antidepressant Action

Hypothesis and Therapeutic Approach	*Results and Implications*
Serotonin neurotransmission potentiation	
1. PCPA reversal of antidepressant action	Consistent with the serotonin neurotransmission potentiation hypothesis of antidepressant action, PCPA, a tryptophan hydroxylase inhibitor that reduces serotonin synthesis, and over 90 percent depletion of plasma tryptophan by a 17-amino-acid drink, both reverse the therapeutic effects of antidepressants.
2. Dietary depletion of tryptophan reversal of antidepressant action	
3. Lithium augmentation of antidepressant action	In numerous investigations, lithium has been demonstrated to augment the therapeutic effects of a spectrum of antidepressant drugs in treatment-fractory depressed patients. This treatment was developed and based on the serotonin neurotransmission potentiation hypothesis of antidepressant action.

DO ANTIDEPRESSANT EFFECTS ON SEROTONIN FUNCTION REPRESENT A COMMON MECHANISM OF ACTION?

Neurophysiological studies have consistently indicated that a spectrum of antidepressant drugs increase serotonergic neurotransmission. This increase appears to take place through at least two separate mechanisms. Specific and potent serotonin reuptake inhibitors and MAO inhibitors produce a decreased sensitivity of the serotonin autoreceptor, whereas various other antidepressant treatments, including atypical drugs, produce postsynaptic receptor supersensitivity by an undetermined mechanism.

The increase in serotonin neurotransmission observed in neurophysiological studies has not been associated with an increase in the density of serotonin receptors. In contrast, $5\text{-}HT_2$ receptors, labeled by radioligands such as ^3H-ketanserin, are reduced by long-term administration of many, but not all, antidepressant treatments.

The discrepant neurophysiological and binding studies must be considered in the context of serotonin receptor subtypes that have been evaluated by these methods and the functional interaction between $5\text{-}HT_1$ and $5\text{-}HT_2$ receptors. Although radioligand binding studies provide evidence for the existence of distinct $5\text{-}HT_1$ and $5\text{-}HT_2$ binding sites, the range of functional properties of these receptors remains to be established. The $5\text{-}HT_1$ receptor subtypes can be differentiated physiologically in the dorsal raphe nucleus, where 5-HT$_{1A}$, but not 5-HT$_{1B}$, ligands mimic the inhibitory action of 5-HT. It is this receptor that becomes subsensitive after long-term treatment with 5-HT reuptake inhibitors and MAO inhibitors (Aghajanian, Sprouse, & Rasmussen, 1988; Sprouse & Aghajanian, 1987). Radioligand binding studies have not specifically evaluated changes in the density of somatodendritic autoreceptors with antidepressant treatment.

In contrast to the dorsal raphe where 5-HT$_{1A}$ ligands are full agonists, in the hippocampus these compounds behave as partial agonists or antagonists (Sprouse & Aghajanian, 1987). Neurophysiological investigations indicate that hippocampal 5-HT receptors become supersensitive after prolonged treatment with tricyclic antidepressants, atypical antidepressants, and ECT. Radioligand binding studies have not specifically assessed changes in postsynaptic 5-HT$_{1A}$ receptors following antidepressant treatment.

Studies in human brain have shown a high concentration of 5-HT$_2$ sites throughout the cerebral cortex, with the exception of pre- and postcentral gyri (Sprouse & Aghajanian, 1987). Neurophysiological studies indicate that in brain areas where both 5-HT$_1$ and 5-HT$_2$ receptors exist, the 5-HT$_2$ receptor opposes inhibitory and enhances excitatory effects produced by activation of the 5-HT$_1$ receptor (Aghajanian, Sprouse, & Rasmussen, 1987; Aghajanian, Sprouse, & Rasmussen, 1988). For example, in the prefrontal cortex, 5-HT receptor activation works in opposition to the depressant effects of 5-HT on cell firing, whereas in the facial motor nucleus, 5-HT$_2$ receptors enhance a facilitatory action of 5-HT on cell firing. Therefore, in prefrontal cerebral cortex, the antidepressant-induced decrease in 5-HT$_2$ receptors may be associated with a potentiation of the depressant effects of 5-HT on cell firing.

The apparent discordance between the neurophysiological findings and the findings using behavioral models of serotonin function may be related to several factors. First, many of the behavioral paradigms measure the function of 5-HT$_2$ receptors, which are distinct from the 5-HT$_1$ receptors that have been studied neurophysiologically. In addition, the behaviors assessed are primarily mediated in the brain stem and spinal cord and not the forebrain, which is most relevant to antidepressant properties and on which many of the neurophysiological studies have been conducted. As with adrenergic receptor systems, it is essential that behavioral paradigms be developed that are capable of evaluating the function of brain regions (cortex, limbic forebrain) most likely to be involved in antidepressant actions.

It is important to emphasize that of the different receptor sensitivity hypotheses, it is only the serotonin neuronal enhancement hypothesis that has led to a new, effective treatment approach. Unique to the discovery of new treatments of major psychiatric disorders, the original studies of lithium augmentation were based on a clearly defined preclinical hypothesis of psychotropic drug mechanism (i.e., potentiation of serotonin function). Although the demonstrated efficacy of lithium augmentation was consistent with the preclinical prediction, direct clinical demonstration of the mechanism of this action is currently lacking.

The recent observations of Price, Charney, & Heninger (1986) indicate that the rapid antidepressant effects of lithium augmentation (less than seven days) are less common than originally suggested, and that up to three weeks of lithium administration may be required to obtain therapeutic responses. These findings suggest that the acute effect of lithium on the increase of presynaptic serotonin release may not be the primary therapeutic mechanism, and that its effect on the regulation of serotonin neurotransmission, and perhaps other neuronal systems mediated by the phosphoinosital cycle, must be considered. This may explain why the addition of serotonin precursors, tryptophan, 5-HTP, and fenfluramine, to antidepressant regimens in treatment-refractory patients has been disappointing therapeutically.

IMPLICATIONS FOR THE MONOAMINE HYPOTHESIS OF DEPRESSIVE ILLNESS

At present, no satisfactory animal model of endogenous depression exists, and in clinical studies of depressed patients, it has been difficult to directly evaluate brain function in vivo. For these reasons, investigations in laboratory animals designed to identify the therapeutic mechanism of antidepressant drugs have also been used to gain insights into the pathophysiology of depression. One problem with this approach is that it assumes a direct relationship between the mode of action of antidepressant treatment and the etiological disturbance. Although this may be true, there is little empirical evidence suggesting that such an association must exist. In fact, there are many examples in medicine indicating that a specific link between drug mechanism and illness pathophysiology is not necessary for drug efficacy. For example, antihypertension or antiarrhythmic drugs may have therapeutic effects without affecting the primary pathophysiological disturbance.

The biological markers reflective of monoamine function for which depressed-patient/healthy-subject differences have been most commonly reported (including decreased platelet imipramine binding, blunted clonidine-induced growth hormone increases, and decreased prolactin rise following administration of tryptophan) have not been consistently altered by antidepressant treatment. Several, but not all, recent investigations have reported increased beta-receptor and 5-HT$_2$ receptor density in postmortem brain tissue of suicide victims.*** These findings are consistent with hypotheses suggesting that decreases in beta-adrenergic and 5-HT$_2$ receptor density relate to antidepressant action.

The inability to identify a common mechanism of action of antidepressant treatments suggests that depression is probably biologically heterogeneous and not associated with a single dysfunction (e.g., serotonin). Therefore, in clinical studies, a greater emphasis is needed on defining neurobiological subtypes of depressive illness. Depressive subtypes can be identified using biological tests, such as the responses to specific pharmacological challenges and brain imaging of receptor density and function. In addition, more studies are needed to determine whether depressed patients can be categorized by their responses to specific antidepressant treatments. Previous investigations with this strategy either used drugs that were nonspecific with regard to neurochemical profile (Beckmann & Goodwin, 1975) or studied small sample sizes (Potter et al., 1981; Aberg-Wistedt, 1982; d'Elia et al., 1981; Emrich et al., 1987).

Another critical focus that remains a target for future studies is the possibility that in mood disorders, neuronal systems that link serotonin and noradrenergic neurons are dysfunctional. Important interactions between noradrenergic and serotonin systems are not surprising when considered in the context that they are both distributed throughout the brain via ascending and descending pathways, particularly limbic structures and the sensory areas of the cortex. Therefore, it has been hypothesized that these aminergic systems are functionally linked in the assessment of sensory information, including mood, cognitive, and somatic sensory processing.

Antidepressant treatments may work at many different sites that indirectly affect the neuronal loops that coordinate interactions between these two long-axon monoaminergic systems (Costa, Ravizza, & Barbaccia, 1986). The challenge inherent in this theory is to find out which neurotransmitters and neuropeptides modulate the neuronal loop operating in this coordinating fashion. The reciprocal regulation of adrenergic receptors (α_1, α_2, β) and serotonergic receptors (5-HT$_1$, 5-HT$_2$) may be an important mechanism for the homeostatic control of brain noradrenergic and serotonergic activity.†† The effects induced by long-term administration of antidepressants on the relative functional sensitivity of the various receptor systems may correct a disorder of noradrenergic and serotonergic regulation in mood disorders.

This hypothesis is consistent with the observation that specific and po-

***Mann et al., 1986; Arango et al., 1987; Zanko & Biegon, 1983; Meyerson et al., 1982; Crow et al., 1984.
††Cowen et al., 1982; Dumbrille-Ross & Tang, 1983; Tricklebank, Forler, & Fozard, 1984; Rappaport, Sturtz, & Guicheney, 1985; Handley & Singh, 1986; Heal et al., 1986.

tent 5-HT (fluoxetine, fluvoxamine) and NE (desipramine) reuptake inhibitors appear to be equally effective antidepressant treatments across a broad spectrum of depressed patients. A noradrenergic dysregulation hypothesis of depression has been advanced by Siever and Davis (1985).

IDENTIFICATION OF NOVEL TREATMENTS WITH EFFECTS ON SEROTONIN NEURONS

A potentially therapeutically useful area of exploration may be determination of the antidepressant effects of drugs with specific actions on serotonin receptor subtypes. A recent study using behavioral adaptation to restraint as a behavioral analogue of depression suggested that 5-HT_{1A} agonists may possess antidepressant effects (Kennett, Dourish, & Curzon, 1987). It has not been established whether this effect occurs via stimulation of pre- or postsynaptic 5-HT_{1A} receptors. A recent neurophysiological investigation has found that chronic administration of the 5-HT_{1A} agonist gepirone results in 5-HT_{1A} autoreceptor subsensitivity, an action also observed with some other antidepressants (Blier & deMontigny, 1987). Therefore, a careful evaluation of the antidepressant properties of 5-HT_{1A} agonists such as buspirone and gepirone appears warranted.

Alternatively, it would be of interest to test the therapeutic effectiveness of 5-HT_{1A} receptor antagonists as they become available. Analogous to the effects of alpha$_2$-receptor antagonists on NE turnover, these drugs should increase presynaptic 5-HT release. Continued assessment of the antidepressant properties of 5-HT_2 receptor antagonists, such as ritanserin, will also be important;[‡‡] it will allow evaluation of the clinical relevance of the downregulation of 5-HT_2 receptors induced by many antidepressants. Based on the effects of 5-HT_{1A} and 5-HT_2 antagonists, a combination of these drugs with classical antidepressants in treatment-refractory patients will provide further data regarding the role of the potentiation of serotonin neurotransmission in the therapeutic mechanisms of antidepressant drugs. (See Table 3-4.)

Although progress toward the development of new, more efficacious antidepressant treatments has been slow, there is reason for optimism. Recent methodological advances in basic neuroscience have resulted in the rapid compilation of new neurotransmitters and receptor systems, improved peptide-discovery methods, and increased understanding of receptor-generated regulatory phenomena from the initial recognition site through second and third messenger systems. This knowledge, in conjunction with the rapid ad-

---

[§§]Data on file, Janssen Pharmaceutica, N. V. B-2340 Beerse, Belgium.

TABLE 3-4
Novel Therapeutic Approaches for the Treatment of Depression
Based on Effects on Serotonin Function

Therapeutic Approach	Neurobiological Actions and Rationale
Serotonin receptor subtypes	
1. 5-HT$_{1A}$ receptor antagonists	Enhance serotonin neuronal firing and turnover. Useful test of serotonin neurotransmission hypothesis of antidepressant action. Such drugs are not available clinically.
2. 5-HT$_{1A}$ receptor agonists	Preclinical neurophysiological and behavioral investigations suggest potential for antidepressant action. Buspirone and more specific 5-HT$_{1A}$ agonists are available for antidepressant testing.
3. 5-HT$_2$ receptor antagonists	Will allow evaluation of the clinical relevance of downregulation of 5-HT$_2$ receptors by antidepressants. Ritanserin is available for antidepressant testing.

vances in molecular biology, may lead to a new generation of centrally active compounds with the potential for antidepressant efficacy.

REFERENCES

Abdel-Latif, A. A. (1986). Calcium-mobilizing receptors, polyphosphoinositides, and the generation of second messengers. *Pharmacol. Rev., 38,* 227–272.

Aberg-Wistedt, A. (1982). A double-blind study of zimelidine, a serotonin uptake inhibitor, and desipramine, a noradrenaline uptake inhibitor, in endogenous depression. I. Clinical findings. *Acta Psychiatr. Scand., 66,* 50–65.

Aghajanian, G. K., Sprouse, J. S., & Rasmussen, K. (1987). Physiology of the midbrain serotonin system. In H. Meltzer (Ed.), *Psychopharmacology: A third generation of progress* (pp. 141–149). New York: Raven Press.

Aghajanian, G. K., Sprouse, J. S., & Rasmussen, K. (1988). Electrophysiology of central serotonin receptor subtypes. In E. Sanders-Bush (Ed.), *The serotonin receptors* (pp. 225–252). Clifton, New Jersey: Humana Press.

Anderson, I. M., & Cowen, P. J. (1986). Clomipramine enhances prolactin and growth hormone responses to L-tryptophan. *Psychopharmacology, 89,* 131–133.

Arango, V., Ernsberger, P., Tierney, H., Stanley, M., Reis, D. J. & Mann, J. J. (1987). Quantitative autoradiography demonstrates increased 5-HT$_2$ receptors in the frontal cortex of suicide victims. *Soc. Neuroscience Abstr., 66*(10), 216.

Asakura, M., Tsukamoto, T., Kubota, H., Imafuku, J., Ino, M., Nishizaki, J., Sato, A., Shinbo, K., & Hasegawa, K. (1987). Role of serotonin in the regulation of β-adrenoceptors by antidepressants. *Eur. J. Pharmacol., 141,* 95–100.

Asarch, K. B., Shih, J. C., & Kulcsar, A. (1980). Decreased ³H-imipramine binding in depressed males and females. *Commun. Psychopharmacol., 4,* 425–432.

Asberg, M., & Wagner, A. (1986). Biochemical effects of antidepressant treatment-studies of monoamine metabolites in cerebrospinal fluid and platelet ³H-imipramine binding. In R. Porter, G. Bock, and S. Clark (Eds.), *Antidepressants and receptor function* (pp. 57–76). New York: Wiley.

Barbaccia, M. L., Brunello, N., Chuang, D-M., & Costa, E. (1983). On the mode of action of imipramine: Relationship between serotonergic axon terminal function and down-regulation of β-adrenergic receptors. *Neuropharmacology, 22,* 373–383.

Barbaccia, M. L., & Costa, E. (1984). Autocoids for drug receptors: A new approach in drug development. *NY Acad. Sci., 430,* 103–114.

Beckmann, M., & Goodwin, F. K. (1975). Antidepressant response to tricyclics and urinary MHPG in unipolar patients. Clinical response to imipramine and amitriptyline. *Arch. Gen. Psychiatry, 32,* 17–21.

Berridge, M. J., Downes, C. P., & Hanley, M. R. (1982). Lithium amplifies agonist-dependent phosphatidylinositol responses in brain and salivary glands. *Biochem. J., 206,* 587–595.

Birkhimer, L. J., Alderman, A. A., Schmitt, C. E., & Ednie, K. J. (1983). Combined trazodone-lithium therapy for refractory depression. *Am. J. Psychiatry, 140,* 1382–1383.

Blackshear, M. A., Friedman, R. L., & Sanders-Bush, E. (1983). Acute and chronic effects of serotonin antagonists on serotonin binding sites. *Naunyn-Schmiedeberg's Arch. Pharmacol., 324,* 125–129.

Blackshear, M. A., Martin, L. I., & Sanders-Bush, E. (1986). Adaptive changes in the 5-HT₂ binding site after chronic administration of agonists and antagonists. *Neuropharmacology, 25,* 1267–1271.

Blier, P., & deMontigny, C. (1983). Electrophysiological investigations on the effect of repeated zimelidine administration on serotonergic neurotransmission in the rat. *Soc. Neurosci., 3,* 1270–1278.

Blier, P., & deMontigny, C. (1985). Serotonergic but not noradrenergic neurons in rat central nervous system adapt to long-term treatment with monoamine oxidase inhibitors. *Neuroscience, 16,* 949–955.

Blier, P., & deMontigny, C. (1985). Short-term lithium administration enhances serotonergic neural transmission: Electrophysiological evidence in the rat CNS. *Eur. J. Pharmacol., 113,* 69–77.

Blier, P., & deMontigny, C. (1987). Modification of 5-HT neuron properties by sustained administration of the 5-HT₁ₐ agonist gepirone: Electrophysiological studies in the rat brain. *Synapse, 1,* 470–480.

Blier, P., deMontigny, C., & Azzaro, A. J. (1986a). Effect of repeated amiflamine administration on serotonergic and noradrenergic neurotransmission: Electrophysiological studies in the rat CNS. *Naunyn-Schmiedeberg's Arch. Pharmacol., 334,* 253–260.

Blier, P., deMontigny, C., & Azzaro, A. J. (1986b). Modification of serotonergic and noradrenergic neurotransmissions by repeated administration of monoamine oxidase inhibitors: Electrophysiological studies in the rat central nervous system. *J. Pharmacol. Exp. Ther., 237,* 987–994.

Blier, P., deMontigny, C., & Tardif, D. (1984). Effects of the two antidepressant drugs mianserin and indalpine on the serotonergic system: Single-cell studies in the rat. *Psychopharmacology, 84,* 242–249.

Bowden, C. L., Koslow, S. H., Hanin, I., Maas, J. W., Davis, J. M., & Robins, E. (1985). Effects of amitriptyline and imipramine treatment on brain amine neurotransmitter metabolites in cerebrospinal fluid. *Clin. Pharmacol. Ther., 37,* 316–324.

Bowden, C. L., Koslow, S., Maas, J. W., Davis, J., Garver, D. L., & Hanin, I. (1987). Changes in urinary catecholamines and their metabolites in depressed patients treated with amitriptyline or imipramine. *J. Psychiatr. Res., 21,* 111–128.

Chaput, Y., deMontigny, C., & Blier, P. (1986). Effects of a selective 5-HT reuptake blocker, citalopram, on the sensitivity of 5-HT autoreceptors: Electrophysiological study in the rat brain. *Naunyn-Schmiedeberg's Arch. Pharmacol., 333,* 342–348.

Charig, E. M., Anderson, I. M., Robinson, J. M., Nutt, D. M., & Cowen, P. J. (1986). L-tryptophan and prolactin release: Evidence for interaction between $5HT_1$, and $5HT_2$ receptors. *Human Psychopharm., 1,* 93–97.

Charney, D. S., Heninger, G. R., & Sternberg, D. E. (1984). Serotonin function and mechanism of action of antidepressant treatment: Effects of amitriptyline and desipramine. *Arch. Gen. Psychiatry, 41,* 359–365.

Charney, D. S., Menkes, D. B., & Heninger, G. R. (1981). Receptor sensitivity and the mechanism of action of antidepressant treatment. *Arch. Gen. Psychiatry, 38,* 1160–1180.

Cohen, R. M., Aulakh, C. S., & Murphy, D. L. (1983). Long-term clorgyline treatment antagonizes the eating and motor function responses to MCPP. *Eur. J. Pharmacol., 94,* 175–179.

Conn, P. J., Janowsky, A., & Sanders-Bush, E. (1986). Denervation supersensitivity of 5HT-1C receptors in rat choroid plexus. *Brain Res., 400,* 396–398.

Conn, P. J., & Sanders-Bush, E. (1985). Serotonin-stimulated phosphoinositide turnover: Mediation by the S_2 binding site in rat cerebral cortex but not in subcortical regions. *J. Pharmacol. Exp. Ther., 234,* 195–203.

Conn, P. J., & Sanders-Bush, E. (1986). Regulation of serotonin-stimulated phosphoinositide hydrolysis: Relation to the serotonin 5HT-2 binding site. *J. Neurosci., 6,* 3669–3675.

Conn, P. J., & Sanders-Bush, E. (1987). Central serotonin receptors: Effector systems, physiological roles and regulation. *Psychopharmacology, 92,* 267–277.

Costa, E., Ravizza, L., & Barbaccia, M. L. (1986). Evaluation of current theories on the mode of action of antidepressants. In G. Bartholini, K. G. Lloyd, and P. L. Morselli (Eds.), *Mode of action of antidepressants* (pp. 9–21). New York: Raven Press.

Cowen, P. J. (1987). Psychotropic drugs and human 5-HT neuroendocrinology. *TIPS, 8,* 105–108.

Cowen, P. J., Geaney, D. P., Schachter, M., Green, A. R., & Elliott, J. M. (1986). Desipramine treatment in normal subjects: Effects on neuroendocrine responses to tryptophan and on platelet serotonin (5-HT)-related receptors. *Arch. Gen. Psychiatry, 43,* 61–67.

Cowen, P. J., Grahame-Smith, D. G., Green, A. R., & Heal, D. J. (1982). β-adrenoceptor agonists enhance 5-hydroxytryptamine-mediated behavioural responses. *Br. J. Pharmacol., 76,* 265–270.

Crow, T. J., Cross, A. J., Copper, S. J., Deakin, J. F. W., Ferrier, I. N., Johnson, J. A., Joseph, M. H., Owen, F., Poulter, M., Lofthouse, R., Corsellis, J. A. N., Chambers, D. R., Blessed, G., Perry, E. K., Perry, R. H., & Tomlinson, B. E. (1984). Neurotransmitter receptors and monoamine metabolites in the brains of patients with Alzheimer type dementia and depression and suicides. *Neuropharmacology, 23,* 1561–1569.

Delgado, P. L., Charney, D. S., Price, L. H., Aghajanian, G. K., Landis, H., & Heninger, G. R., May (1988). Tryptophan depletion alters mood in depression. *Amer. Psychiatric Assoc. New Research Abstracts,* NR164.

d'Elia, G., Hallstrom, T., Nystrom, C., & Ottosson, J.-O. (1981). Zimelidine vs. maprotiline in depressed outpatients. A preliminary report. *Acta Psychiatr. Scand., 63*(Suppl)290, 225–235.

deMontigny, C. (1984). Electroconvulsive shock treatments enhance responsiveness of forebrain neurons to serotonin. *J. Pharmacol. Exp. Ther., 228,* 230–234.

deMontigny, C., & Aghajanian, G. K. (1978). Tricyclic antidepressants: Long-term treatment increases responsivity of rat forebrain neurons to serotonin. *Science, 202,* 1303–1306.

deMontigny, C., Blier, P., & Chaput, Y. (1984). Electrophysiologically-identified serotonin receptors in the rat CNS: Effect of antidepressant treatment. *Neuropharmacology, 23,* 1511–1520.

deMontigny, C., Cournoyer, G., Morissette, R., Langlois, R., & Caille, G. (1983). Lithium carbonate addition in tricyclic antidepressant-resistant depression: Correlations with the neurobiologic actions of tricyclic antidepressant drugs and lithium ion on the serotonin system. *Arch. Gen. Psychiatry, 40,* 1327–1334.

deMontigny, C., Elie, R., & Caille, G. (1985). Rapid response to the addition of lithium in iprindole-resistant unipolar depression: A pilot study. *Am. J. Psychiatry, 142,* 220–223.

deMontigny, C., Grunberg, F., Mayer, A., & Deschenes, J. P. (1981). Lithium induces rapid relief of depression in tricyclic antidepressant drug nonresponders. *Br. J. Psychiatry, 138,* 252–256.

De Vivo, M., & Maayani, S. (1986). Characterization of the 5-hydroxytryptamine$_{1A}$ receptor-mediated inhibition of forskolin-stimulated adenylate cyclase activity in guinea pig and rat hippocampal membranes. *J. Pharmacol. Exp. Ther., 238,* 248–253.

De Vivo, M., & Maayani, S. (1985). Inhibition of forskolin-stimulated adenylate cyclase activity by 5-HT receptor agonists. *Eur. J. Pharmacol., 119,* 231–234.

Dumbrille-Ross, A., & Tang, S. W. (1983). Noradrenergic and serotonergic input necessary for imipramine-induced changes in beta but not S$_2$ receptor densities. *Psychiatr. Res., 9,* 207–215.

Emrich, H. M., Berger, M., Riemann, D., & von Zerssen, D. (1987). Serotonin reuptake inhibition vs. norepinephrine reuptake inhibition: A double-blind differential-therapeutic study with fluvoxamine and oxaprotiline in endogenous and neurotic depressives. *Pharmacopsychiat., 20,* 60–63.

Friedman, E., Cooper, T. B., & Dallob, A. (1983). Effects of chronic antidepressant treatment on serotonin receptor activity in mice. *Eur. J. Pharmacol., 89,* 69–76.

Fuxe, K., Butcher, L. L., & Engel, J. (1971). D,L-5-hydroxytryptophan-induced changes in central monoamine neurons after peripheral decarboxylase inhibition. *J. Pharm. Pharmacol., 23,* 420–424.

Fuxe, K., Ogren, S. O., Agnati, L. F., Benfenati, F., Fredholm, B., Andersson, K., Zini, L., & Eneroth, P. (1983). Chronic antidepressant treatment and central 5-HT synapses. *Neuropharmacology, 22,* 389–400.

Gandolfi, O., Barbaccia, M. L., & Costa, E. (1985). Different effects of serotonin antagonists on ^{3}H-mianserin and ^{3}H-ketanserin recognition sites. *Life Sci., 36,* 713–721.

Gentsch, C., Lichtsteine, M., & Feer, H. (1984). ^{3}H-Imipramine and ^{3}H-cyanoimipramine binding in rat brain tissue: Effect of long-term antidepressant administration. *J. Neural. Transm., 59,* 257–264.

Glue, P. W., Cowen, P. J., Nutt, D. J., Kolakowska, T., & Grahame-Smith, D. G. (1986). The effect of lithium on 5-HT-mediated neuroendocrine responses and platelet 5-HT receptors. *Psychopharmacology, 90,* 398–402.

Godfrey, P. P., McClue, S. J., Young, M. M., & Heal, D. J. (1988). 5-Hydroxytryptamine-stimulated inositol phospholipid hydrolysis in the mouse cortex has pharmacological characteristics compatible with mediation via 5-HT$_2$ receptors but this response does not reflect altered 5-HT$_2$ function after 5,7-dihydroxytryptamine lesioning or repeated antidepressant treatments. *J. Neurochem., 50,* 730–738.

Goodwin, G. M., De Souza, R. J., & Green, A. R. (1985). Presynaptic serotonin receptor-mediated response in mice attenuated by antidepressant drugs and electroconvulsive shock. *Nature, 317,* 531–533.

Goodwin, G. M., De Souza, R. J., & Green, A. R. (1987). Attenuation by electroconvulsive shock and antidepressant drugs of the 5-HT$_{1A}$ receptor-mediated hypothermia and serotonin syndrome produced by 8-OH-DPAT in the rat. *Psychopharmacology, 91,* 500–505.

Goodwin, G. M., De Souza, R. J., Wood, A. J., & Green, A. R. (1986). Lithium decreases 5-HT$_{1A}$ and 5-HT$_2$ receptor and α_2-adrenoceptor mediated function in mice. *Psychopharmacology, 90,* 482–487.

Goodwin, G. M., De Souza, R. J., Wood, A. J., & Green, A. R. (1986). The enhancement by lithium of the 5-HT$_{1A}$ mediated serotonin syndrome produced by 8-OH-DPAT in the rat: Evidence for a post-synaptic mechanism. *Psychopharmacology, 90,* 488–493.

Goodwin, G. M., Green, A. R., & Johnson, P. (1984). 5-HT$_2$ receptor characteristics in frontal cortex and 5-HT$_2$ receptor-mediated head-twitch behaviour following antidepressant treatment in mice. *Br. J. Pharmacol., 83,* 235–242.

Grahame-Smith, D. G., & Green, A. R. (1974). The role of brain 5-hydroxytryptamine in the hyperactivity produced in rats by lithium and monoamine oxidase inhibitors. *Br. J. Pharmacol., 52,* 19–26.

Green, A. R., Heal, O. J., & Goodwin, G. M. (1986). The effects of electroconvulsive therapy and antidepressant drugs on monoamine receptors in rodent brain.

In R. Porter, G. Bock and S. Clark (Eds.), *Antidepressant and receptor function* (pp. 246–259). New York: Wiley.

Green, A. R., Heal, D. J., Johnson, P., Lawrence, B. E., & Nimgaonkar, V. L. (1983). Antidepressant treatments: Effects in rodents on dose response curves of 5-hydroxy-tryptamine and dopamine mediated behaviors and $5HT_2$ receptor number in frontal cortex. *Br. J. Pharmacol., 80,* 377–385.

Green, A. R., Johnson, P., & Nimgaonkar, V. L. (1983). Increased $5-HT_2$ receptor number in brain as a probable explanation for the enhanced 5-hydroxytryptamine-mediated behaviour following repeated electroconvulsive shock administration to rats. *Br. J. Pharmacol., 80,* 173–177.

Green, A. R., & Nutt, D. J. (1985). Antidepressants. In. D. G. Grahame-Smith (Ed.), *Psychopharmacology 2, part I: Preclinical psychopharmacology* (pp. 1–34). Amsterdam, Holland: Elsevier Science Publishers B.V.

Gudelsky, G. A., Koenig, J. I., Jackman, H., & Meltzer, H. T. (1986). Suppression of the hypo- and hyperthermic responses to 5-HT agonists following the repeated administration of monoamine oxidase inhibitors. *Psychopharmacology, 90,* 403–407.

Handley, S. L., & Singh, L. (1986). The modulation of head-twitch behaviour by drugs acting on beta-adrenoceptors: Evidence for the involvement of both $beta_1$- and $beta_2$-adrenoceptors. *Psychopharmacology, 88,* 320–324.

Heal, D. J., Philpot, J., O'Shaughnessy, K. M., & Davies, C. L. (1986). The influence of central noradrenergic function on $5HT_2$-mediated head-twitch responses in mice: Possible implications for the actions of antidepressant drugs. *Psychopharmacology, 89,* 414–420.

Heninger, G. R., Charney, D. S., & Smith, A. (1986). Comparison of the 5HT agonists, tryptophan, MCPP, buspirone and gepirone, on prolactin, growth hormone and cortisol release in rhesus monkeys: Effects of lithium. *Soc. Neurosci. Abstr.,* 16th Annual Meeting, *12* (1) 574.

Heninger, G. R., Charney, D. S., & Smith, A. (1987). Effects of serotonin receptor agonists and antagonists on neuroendocrine function in rhesus monkeys. *Soc. Neurosci. Abstr., 224*(9) 801.

Heninger, G. R., Charney, D. S., & Sternberg, D. E. (1983). Lithium carbonate augmentation of antidepressant treatment: An effective prescription for treatment-refractory depression. *Arch. Gen. Psychiatry, 40,* 1335–1342.

Holmeste, D. M., & Tang, S. W. (1983). Unusual acute effects of antidepressants and neuroleptics on S_2 serotonergic receptors. *Life Sci., 33,* 2527–2533.

Hotta, I., & Yamawaki, S. (1986). Lithium decreases $5HT_1$ receptors but increases 5HT-sensitive adenylate cyclase activity in rat hippocampus. *Biol. Psychiatry, 21,* 1382–1390.

Hrdina, P. D. (1984). ^{3}H-Imipramine high-affinity binding sites in brain down-regulated by chronic nortriptyline and haloperidol but not mianserin treatment. *Psychiat. Res., 11,* 271–278.

Hyttel, J., Overo, K. F., & Arnt, J. (1984). Biochemical effects and drug levels in rats after long-term treatment with the specific 5-HT uptake inhibitor, citalopram. *Psychopharmacology, 83,* 20–27.

Janowsky, A., Okada, F., Manier, D., Applegate, C., & Sulser, F. (1982). Role of serotonergic input in the regulation of the beta-adrenergic receptor-coupled adenylate cyclase system. *Science, 218,* 900–901.

Joyce, P. R. (1985). Mood response to methylphenidate and the dexamethasone suppression test as predictors of treatment response to zimelidine and lithium in major depression. *Biol. Psychiatry, 20,* 598–604.

Joyce, P. R., Hewland, H. R., & Jones, A. V. (1983). Rapid response to lithium in treatment-resistant depression. *Br. J. Psychiatry, 142,* 204–205.

Kellar, K. J., & Bergstrom, D. A. (1983). Electroconvulsive shock: Effects on biochemical correlates of neurotransmitter receptors in rat brain. *Neuropharmacology, 22,* 401–406.

Kellar, K. J., Cascio, C. S., Butler, J. A., & Kurtzke, R. N. (1981). Differential effects of electroconvulsive shock and antidepressant drugs on serotonin-2 receptors in rat brain. *Eur. J. Pharmacol., 69,* 515–518.

Kendall, D. A., Duman, R., Slopis, J., & Enna, S. J. (1982). Influence of adrenocorticotropin hormone and yohimbine on antidepressant-induced declines in rat brain neurotransmitter receptor binding and function. *J. Pharmacol. Exp. Ther., 222,* 566–571.

Kendall, D. A., & Nahorski, S. R. (1985). 5-Hydroxytryptamine-stimulated inositol phospholipid hydrolysis in rat cerebral cortex slices: Pharmacological characterization and effects of antidepressants. *J. Pharmacol. Exp. Ther., 233,* 473–479.

Kennett, G. A., Dourish, C. T., & Curzon, G. (1987). Antidepressant-like action of 5-HT_{1A} agonists and conventional antidepressants in an animal model of depression. *Eur. J. Pharmacol., 134,* 265–274.

Kinnier, W. J., Chuang, D.-M., & Costa, E. (1980). Down regulation of dihydroalprenolol and imipramine binding sites in brain of rats repeatedly treated with imipramine. *Eur. J. Pharmacol., 67,* 289–294.

Klein, E., Patel, J., McDevitt, R., & Zohar, J. (1987). Chronic lithium treatment increases the phosphorylation of a 64-kDa protein in rat brains. *Brain Res., 407,* 312–316.

Kushnir, S. L. (1986). Lithium-antidepressant combinations in the treatment of depressed, physically ill geriatric patients. *Am. J. Psychiatry, 143,* 378–379.

Lakoski, J. M. & Aghajanian, G. (1985). Effects of ketanserin on neuronal responses to serotonin in the prefrontal cortex, lateral geniculate and dorsal raphe nucleus. *Neuropharmacology, 24,* 265–273.

Langer, S. Z., Galzin, A. M., Lee, C. R., & Schoemaker, H. (1986). Antidepressants: Binding sites in brain and platelets. In R. Porter, G. Bock, and S. Clark (Eds.), *Antidepressants and receptor function* (pp. 3–17). New York: Wiley.

Langer, S. Z., Sechter, D., Loo, H., Raisman, R., & Zarifian, E. (1986). Electroconvulsive shock therapy and B_{max} of platelet ^{3}H-imipramine binding in depression. *Arch. Gen. Psychiatry, 43,* 949–952.

Leysen, J. (1984). Problems in *in vitro* receptor binding studies and identification and role of serotonin receptor sites. *Neuropharmacology, 23,* 247–254.

Leysen, J. E., Van Gompel, P., Gommeren, W., Woestenborghs, R., & Janssen, P. A. J. (1986). Down regulation of serotonin-S_2 receptor sites in rat brain by chronic treatment with the serotonin-S_2 antagonists: Ritanserin and setoperone. *Psychopharmacology, 88,* 434–444.

Louie, A. K., & Meltzer, H. (1984). Lithium potentiation of antidepressant treatment. *J. Clin. Psychopharmacol., 4,* 316–321.

Lucki, I., & Frazer, A. (1982). Prevention of the serotonin syndrome in rats by repeated administration of monoamine oxidase inhibitors but not tricyclic antidepressants. *Psychopharmacology, 77,* 205–211.

Lucki, I., Nobler, M. S., & Frazer, A. (1984). Differential actions of serotonin antagonists in two behavioral models of serotonin receptor activation in the rat. *J. Pharmacol. Exp. Ther., 228,* 133–139.

Manier, D. H., Gillespie, D. D., Sanders-Bush, E., & Sulser, F. (1987). The serotonin/noradrenaline-link in brain. *Naunyn-Schmiedeberg's Arch. Pharmacol., 335,* 109–114.

Mann, J. J., Stanley, M., McBride, A., & McEwen, B. S. (1986). Increased serotonin$_2$ and β-adrenergic receptor binding in the frontal cortices of suicide victims. *Arch. Gen. Psychiatry, 43,* 954–959.

Meltzer, H. Y., Lowy, M., Robertson, A., Goodnick, P., & Perline, R. (1984). Effect of 5-Hydroxytryptophan on serum cortisol levels in major affective disorders. *Arch. Gen. Psychiatry, 41,* 391–397.

Menkes, H. A., Baraban, J. M., Freed, A. N., & Snyder, S. H. (1986). Lithium dampens neurotransmitter response in smooth muscle: Relevance to action in affective illness. *Proc. Natl. Acad. Sci. USA, 83,* 5727–5730.

Meyerson, L. R., Wennogle, L. P., Abel, M. S., Coupet, J., Lippa, A. S., Rauh, C. E., & Beer, B. (1982). Human brain receptor alterations in suicide victims. *Pharmacol. Biochem. Behav., 17,* 159–163.

Muhlbauer, H. D., & Muller-Oerlinghausen, B. (1985). Fenfluramine stimulation of serum cortisol in patients with major affective disorders and healthy controls: Further evidence for a central serotonergic action of lithium in man. *J. Neural Transm., 61, 81–94.*

Nelson, J. C., & Byck, R. (1982). Rapid response to lithium in phenelzine non-responders. Am. J. Psychiatry, 141, 85–86.

Nelson, J. C., & Mazure, C. M. (1986). Lithium augmentation in psychotic depression refractory to combined drug treatment. *Am. J. Psychiatry, 143,* 363–366.

Ng, L. K. Y., Chase, T. N., Colburn, R. W., & Kopin, I. J. (1972). Release of ^{3}H-dopamine by L-5-hydroxytryptophan. *Brain Res., 45,* 499–505.

Nimgaonkar, V. L., Goodwin, G. M., Davis, C. L., & Green, A. R. (1985). Downregulation of β-adrenoceptors in rat cortex by repeated administration of desipramine, electroconvulsive shock and clenbuterol requires 5-HT neurons but not 5-HT. *Neuropharmacology, 24,* 279–283.

Olpe, H. R., & Schellenberg, A. (1981). The sensitivity of cortical neurons to serotonin: Effect of chronic treatment with antidepressants, serotonin-uptake inhibitors and monoamine-oxidase-blocking drugs. *J. Neural Transm., 51,* 233–244.

Pawlowski, L., & Melzacka, M. (1986). Inhibition of head twitch response to quipazine in rats by chronic amitriptyline but not fluvoxamine or citalopram. *Psychopharmacology, 88,* 279–284.

Peroutka, S. J., & Snyder, S. H. (1980). Chronic antidepressant treatment decreases spiroperidol-labeled serotonin receptor binding. *Science, 210,* 88–90.

Perry, E. K., Marshall, E. F., Blessed, G., Tomlinson, B. E., & Perry, R. H. (1983).

Decreased imipramine binding in the brain of patients with depressive illness. *Br. J. Psychiatry, 142,* 188–192.

Plenge, P., & Mellerup, E. T. (1982). ³H-Imipramine high-affinity binding sites in rat brain. Effects of imipramine and lithium. *Psychopharmacology, 77,* 94–97.

Potter, W. Z., Calil, H. M., Extein, I., Gold, P. W., Wehr, T. A., & Goodwin, F. K. (1981). Specific norepinephrine and serotonin uptake inhibitors in man: A cross-over study with pharmacokinetic, biochemical, neuroendocrine, and behavioral parameters. *Acta Psychiatr. Scand., 63*(290) 152–165.

Price, L. H., Charney, D. S., Delgado, P. L., Anderson, G. H., & Heninger, G. R. (Submitted for publication.). Effects of desipramine and fluvoxamine treatment on the prolactin response to L-tryptophan: A test of the serotonergic function enhancement hypothesis of antidepressant action.

Price, L. H., Charney, D. S., Delgado, P. L., & Heninger, G. R. (1987). Enhancement of serotonergic function by lithium in affective disorder patients. *Soc. Neurosci. Abstr., 246*(5) 883.

Price, L. H., Charney, D. S., & Heninger, G. R. (1985). Effects of tranylcypromine treatment on neuroendocrine, behavioral, and autonomic responses to tryptophan in depressed patients. *Life Sci., 37,* 809–818.

Price, L. H., Charney, D. S., & Heninger, G. R. (1986). Variability of response to lithium augmentation in refractory depression. *Am.J. Psychiatry, 143,* 1387–1392.

Price, L. H., Charney, D. S., & Heninger, G. R. (1988). Effects of trazodone treatment of serotonergic function in depressed patients. *Psychiatry Res., 24,* 165–175.

Price, L. H., Conwell, Y., & Nelson, J. C. (1983). Lithium augmentation of combined neuroleptic-tricyclic treatment in delusional depression. *Am. J. Psychiatry, 140,* 318–322.

Quik, M., & Azmita, E. (1983). Selective destruction of the serotonergic fibers of the fornix-fimbria and cingulum bundle increases 5-HT$_1$ but not 5-HT$_2$ receptors in rat midbrain. *Eur. J. Pharmacol., 90,* 377–384.

Raisman, R., Briley, M. S., & Langer, S. Z. (1980). Specific tricyclic antidepressant binding sites in rat brain characterized by high-affinity ³H-imipramine binding. *Eur. J. Pharmacol., 61,* 373–380.

Raisman, R., Sechter, D., Briley, M. S., Zarifian, E., & Langer, S. Z. (1981). HIgh affinity (3)H-imipramine binding in platelets from untreated and treated depressed patients compared to healthy volunteers. *Psychopharmacology, 75,* 368–371.

Rappaport, A., Sturtz, F., & Guicheney, P. (1985). Regulation of central α-adrenoceptors by serotoninergic denervation. *Brain Res., 344,* 158–161.

Rowan, M. J., & Anwyl, R. (1985). The effect of prolonged treatment with tricyclic antidepressants on the actions of 5-hydroxytryptamine in the hippocampal slice of the rat. *Neuropharmacology, 24,* 131–137.

Roy, A., & Pickar, D. (1985). Lithium potentiation of imipramine in treatment resistant depression. *Br. J. Psychiatry, 147,* 582–583.

Sangdee, C., & Franz, D. N. (1980). Lithium enhancement of 5-HT transmission induced by 5-HT precursors. *Biol. Psychiatry, 15,* 59–75.

Schotte, A., Maloteaux, J. M., & Laduron, P. M. (1983). Characterization and regional distribution of serotonin S$_2$ receptors in human brain. *Brain Res., 276,* 231–235.

Schrader, G. D., & Levien, H. E. M. (1985). Response to sequential administration of clomipramine and lithium carbonate in treatment-resistant depression. *Br. J. Psychiatry, 147,* 573–575.

Scott, J. A., & Crews, F. T. (1986). Down-regulation of serotonin$_2$, but not of beta-adrenergic receptors during chronic treatment with amitriptyline is independent of stimulation of serotonin$_2$ and beta-adrenergic receptors. *Neuropharmacology, 25,* 1301–1306.

Severson, J. A., & Anderson, B. (1986). Chronic antidepressant treatment and mouse brain H-Imipramine binding. *J. Neurosci. Res., 16,* 429–438.

Sharma, I. J., Venkitasubramanian, T. A., & Agnihotri, B. R. (1986). 3-MHPG as a non-predictor of antidepressant response to imipramine and electroconvulsive therapy. *Acta Psychiatr. Scand., 74,* 252–254.

Shopsin, B., Friedman, E., & Gershon, S. (1976). Parachlorophenylalanine reversal of tranylcypromine effects in depressed patients. *Arch. Gen. Psychiatry, 33,* 811–819.

Shopsin, B., Friedman, E., Goldstein, M., & Gershon, S. (1975). The uses of synthesis inhibitors in determining a role for biogenic amines during imipramine treatment in depressed patients. *Psychopharmacol. Commun., 1,* 239–249.

Siever, L. J., & Davis, K. L. (1985). Overview: Towards dysregulation hypothesis of depression. *Am. J. Psychiatry, 142,* 1017–1031.

Slater, S., de la Vega, C. E., Skyler, J., & Murphy, D. L. (1976). Plasma prolactin stimulation by fenfluramine and amphetamine. *Psychopharmacol. Bull., 12,* 26–27.

Sprouse, J. S., & Aghajanian, G. K. (1987). Electrophysiological responses of hippocampal pyramidal cells to serotonin 5-HT$_{1a}$ and 5-HT$_{1b}$ selective agonists: A comparative study with dorsal raphe neurons. *Soc. Neurosci. Abstr., 459*(9) 1650.

Sprouse, J. S., & Aghajanian, G. K. (1987). Electrophysiological responses of serotonergic dorsal raphe neurons to 5-HT$_{1a}$ and 5-HT$_{1b}$ agonists. *Synapse, 1,* 3–9.

Stanley, M., Virgillio, S., & Gershon, S. (1982). Tritiated imipramine binding sites are decreased in the frontal cortex of suicides. *Science, 216,* 1337–1339.

Stockmeier, C. A., Martino, A. M., & Kellar, K. J. (1985). A strong influence of serotonin axons on beta-adrenergic receptors in rat brain. *Science, 230,* 323–325.

Stolz, J. F., & Marsden, C. A. (1982). Withdrawal from chronic treatment with metergoline, dl-propranolol and amitriptyline enhances serotonin receptor mediated behaviour in the rat. *Eur. J. Pharmacol., 79,* 17–22.

Stolz, J. F., Marsden, C. A., & Middlemiss, D. N. (1983). Effect of chronic antidepressant treatment and subsequent withdrawal on n[^{3}H]-hydroxytryptamine and [^{3}H]-spiperone binding in rat frontal cortex and serotonin receptor mediated behaviour. *Psychopharmacology, 80,* 150–155.

Sugrue, M. F. (1983). Chronic antidepressant therapy and associated changes in central monoaminergic receptor functioning. *Pharmacol. Ther., 21,* 1–33.

Suranyi-Cadotte, B. E., Quirion, R., Nair, N. P. V., Lafaille, F., & Schwartz, G.

(1985). Imipramine treatment differentially affects ³H-imipramine and serotonin uptake in depressed patients. *Life Sci., 36,* 795–799.

Swann, A. C., Heninger, G. R., Roth, R. M., & Maas, J. W. (1981). Differential effects of short and long-term lithium on tryptophan reuptake and serotonergic function in cat brain. *Life Sci., 28,* 347–354.

Treiser, S., Cascio, C. S., O'Donohue, T. L., & Keller, K. (1981). Lithium increases serotonin release and decreases serotonin receptors in the hippocampus. *Science, 213,* 1529–1531.

Treiser, S., & Kellar, K. J. (1980). Lithium: Effects on serotonin receptors in rat brain. *Eur. J. Pharmacol., 64,* 183–185.

Tricklebank, M. D., Forler, C., & Fozard, J. R. (1984). The involvement of subtypes of the 5-HT₁ receptor and of catecholaminergic systems in the behavioural response to 8-hydroxy-2 (DI-n-propylamino) tetralin in the rat. *Eur. J. Pharmacol., 106,* 271–282.

Turmel, A., & deMontigny, C. (1984). Sensitization of rat forebrain neurons to serotonin by adinazolam, an antidepressant triazolobenzodiazepine. *Eur. J. Pharmacol., 99,* 241–244.

Van de Kar, L. D., Karteszi, M., Bethea, C. L., & Ganong, W. F. (1985). Serotonergic stimulation of prolactin and corticosterone secretion is mediated by different pathways from the mediobasal hypothalamus. *Neuroendocrinology, 41,* 380–384.

Veith, R. C., Bielski, R. J., Bloom, V., Fawcett, J. A., Narasimhachari, N., & Friedel, R. O. (1983). Urinary MHPG excretion and treatment with desipramine or amitriptyline: Prediction of response, effect of treatment, and methodological hazards. *J. Clin. Psychopharmacol., 3,* 18–27.

Vetulani, E., Lebrecht, U., & Pilc, A. (1981). Enhancement of responsiveness of the central serotonergic system and serotonin-2 receptor density in rat frontal cortex by electroconvulsive treatment. *Eur. J. Pharmacol., 76,* 81–85.

Wagner, A., Aberg-Wistedt, A., Asberg, M., Bertilsson, L., Montero, D., & Martensson, B. (1987). Platelet ³H-imipramine binding in depression: Short and long term effects of antidepressant drugs, ECT, and lithium. *Arch. Gen. Psychiatry, 44,* 870–877.

Wander, T. J., Nelson, A., Okazaki, H., & Richelson, E. (1986). Antagonism by antidepressants of serotonin S₁ and S₂ receptors of normal brain in vitro. *Eur. J. Pharmacol., 132,* 115–121.

Wielosz, M. (1985). Increased sensitivity to serotonergic agonists after repeated electroconvulsive shock in rats. *Pharmacol. Biochem. Behav., 22,* 683–687.

Willner, P. (1985). Antidepressants and serotonergic neurotransmission: An integrative review. *Psychopharmacology, 85,* 387–404.

Young, S. W., Smith, S. E., Pihl. R. O. & Ervin, F. R. (1985). Tryptophan depletion causes a rapid lowering of mood in normal males. *Psychopharmacology, 877,* 173–177.

Zanko, M. T., & Biegon, A. (1983). Increased β-adrenergic receptor binding in human frontal cortex of suicide victims. *Neurosci. Abstr., 210*(5) 719.

4

Neuroendocrine Studies in Psychiatric Disorders
The Role of Serotonin

J. FRANK NASH
HERBERT Y. MELTZER

Since the discovery of serotonin (5-hydroxytryptamine; 5-HT) in the brain and its subsequent identification as a neurotransmitter, numerous hypotheses have emerged that suggest that serotonergic dysfunction is an important factor in the etiology of a variety of psychiatric disorders. For example, there is abundant clinical evidence consistent with the hypotheses that: (1) a decrease in central serotonergic activity enhances vulnerability to develop major depression or initiation of an episode of depression (Murphy et al., 1978; Meltzer & Lowy, 1987); and (2) an effect on serotonergic systems is relevant to the action of antidepressant drugs, lithium carbonate, and electroconvulsive treatment (Meltzer et al., 1981b).

Similarly, it was once suggested that abnormalities in 5-HT metabolism could produce endogenous hallucinogens that could be responsible for at least some of the symptoms of schizophrenia (Gillin et al., 1976). Although this proposal has generally been rejected, there is other evidence that 5-HT may be implicated in the pathophysiology of schizophrenia or the mechanism of action of antipsychotic drugs, perhaps via an influence on dopaminergic systems (Costall & Naylor, 1978; van Kammen & Gelernter, 1987). Furthermore, altered serotonergic function has been reported in alcoholics (Ballenger et al., 1979), and more recently in obsessive compulsive disorder (Zohar & Insel, 1987), anxiety (Kahn et al., 1988; Charney et al., 1987), Al-

Supported, in part, by USPHS MH 41684, a USPHS Research Scientist Award to HYM, NARSAD Fellowship Extension to JFN, grants from the Cleveland, Bingham, and Sawyer Foundations, and GCRC MO IRR-00030-25. The authors would like to thank Lee Mason for her excellent secretarial assistance.

zheimer's disease (Whitford, 1986; Morgan et al., 1987), and impulsive behaviors such as suicide (van Praag, 1986) and arson (Virkkunen et al., 1987).

At first glance, it may appear surprising that a single neurotransmitter could play a role in such a wide variety of clinically distinct psychiatric disorders. However, abundant evidence from animal and human studies has demonstrated that 5-HT affects many somatic processes, including sleep, sexual activity, appetite, circadian rhythms, neuroendocrine function, anxiety, motor activity, cognitive function, and mood (Meltzer & Lowy, 1987). Since any one or several of the somatic processes that are 5-HT dependent are disturbed in these disorders, disturbances in serotonergic mechanisms, perhaps in relation to an abnormality of other monoamine neurotransmitters such as dopamine (DA), norepinephrine (NE), and acetylcholine, or peptides (i.e., neurotensin, neuropeptide Y, corticotropin-releasing factor), may contribute to, or be the ultimate basis of, some of the symptoms of a variety of psychiatric disorders, rather than being the cause of the basic syndrome.

The direct study of brain function in humans would be most helpful in clarifying the role of 5-HT in these disorders. However, the methods of studying living patients are currently in the early stages of development. Positron emission tomography (PET) may eventually permit the direct quantification of 5-HT receptor binding sites, 5-HT uptake sites, and 5-HT turnover in living subjects (Wong et al., 1987). Single-photo-emission computerized tomography (SPECT) and magnetic resonance imaging (MRI) may also be useful for measuring receptor density and energy metabolism related to serotonergic activity, but actual application to the study of depression and other psychiatric disorders is still a number of years off (Andreasen, 1988). Neuroendocrine studies offer a readily available means of assessing some aspects of serotonergic function in the brain by providing a measure of the response to exogenous serotonergic agents on endogenous hormone secretion.

The purposes of this chapter are to (1) describe the basic principles behind neuroendocrine challenge studies, (2) review the evidence for the role of 5-HT in hormone secretion, (3) present and critique clinical studies of the effects of various serotonergic challenge drugs on hormone secretion in normal volunteers and psychiatric patients, and (4) discuss the potential contribution of neuroendocrine studies with regard to understanding biological abnormalities in psychiatric disorders and the mechanisms by which thymoleptic drugs may correct or influence these mechanisms.

REGULATION OF HORMONE SECRETION

General Mechanisms

Neuroendocrinology is the study of the neural mechanisms involved in hormone secretion. For readers who may be unfamiliar with the neuroendocrine system, here is a brief description. The hypothalamus is the neural center in which afferent information arising from several brain structures—such as the cortical and limbic systems—converges. Groups of nerve cells, referred to as nuclei, within the hypothalamus integrate this afferent input and coordinate a hormonal response. The neurons in some hypothalamic nuclei have axon projections that terminate at the median eminence; the axons of other nuclei synapse directly onto cells located primarily in the posterior pituitary. The axon processes, which are located in the median eminence, terminate onto a network of capillary blood vessels, the hypophyseal portal vessels. Monoamines (e.g., DA) and hormone-releasing factors, such as corticotrophin-releasing factor (CRF), enter into the hypophyseal portal blood supply for transport to the anterior pituitary, where they interact with specific target cells (e.g., lactotrophes and corticotrophes) to inhibit or stimulate hormone secretion, for example, prolactin (PRL) or adrenocorticotropin (ACTH) respectively. The pituitary hormones themselves provide inhibitory feedback to the hypothalamic nuclei, which limits the further secretion of hypothalamic releasing factors, and hence pituitary hormones. Thus, the hypothalamus represents the final pathway for the central control of the anterior and posterior lobes of the pituitary gland. Moreover, the neuroendocrine system represents a dynamic, integrated physiological system that responds to internal or external stimuli to maintain homeostasis.

Rationale for Neuroendocrine Challenge Studies

From the preceding description, it is quite easy to understand why earlier investigators suggested that the hypothalamus provides a relevant model system to study brain function or the effects of drug treatment on neural systems. Hypothetically, the stimulation or inhibition of a hypothalamic releasing factor, and ultimately a hormone, from the pituitary or other target gland, in response to a monoamine precursor or direct-acting agonist, provides a functional measure of a response of that hypothalamic nucleus to the specific stimulus, and perhaps to other aspects of the monoamine system throughout the neuroaxis.

The effects in the hypothalamus must be generalized with caution, however, and, as reviewed by Meltzer et al. (1982) and by van Praag et al. (1987), certain conditions must be met before we can infer that neuroendocrine challenge studies do indeed reflect the functional state of central 5-HT mechanisms. First, the challenge drug should stimulate or inhibit hormone secretion through direct, highly selective mechanisms. Second, a dose-dependent relationship between the challenge drug and hormone response should be demonstrable. Finally, the drug-induced hormone response should be selectively blocked by its pharmacological antagonist.

These criteria have rarely been met in most of the paradigms that have been utilized.

The lack of specificity of many drugs for a given subtype of 5-HT receptor, as well as effects on non-5-HT systems that may influence hormone secretion, makes it hazardous to draw conclusions concerning 5-HT-receptor–mediated processes. Convergent evidence from a variety of drugs, as well as, preferably, independent evidence of a nonneuroendocrine variety, is a valuable adjunct to validate conclusions about the serotonergic system based on neuroendocrine studies. Nevertheless, as reviewed in the preceding sections, the data obtained in clinical neuroendocrine studies provide important information about the serotonergic system.

Effect of Serotonin on Hormone Secretion

The complex arrangement of the hypothalamus makes the study of the precise control of anterior pituitary function difficult. The hypothalamus is traversed by four major afferent fiber systems: (1) the medial forebrain bundle, (2) the periventricular system, (3) the fornix system, and (4) the stria terminalis (reviewed by Swanson, 1987). The medial forebrain bundle is one of the most important and complex fiber systems in the brain, since the axonal projections, which travel in this tract, arise from more than 50 different cell groups (Steinbusch, 1981). There exists anatomical, physiological, and pharmacological evidence that 5-HT neurons located within the hypothalamus, or projecting to it, play a role in the secretion of several anterior pituitary hormones, including PRL, ACTH, and growth hormone (GH). Although 5-HT has been reported to play a role in the secretion of other pituitary hormones, including thyroid-stimulating hormone (TSH), gonadotropic releasing hormones (i.e., LH-RH), and beta-endorophin, this chapter will be limited to the discussion of the effects of 5-HT on PRL, ACTH, and GH secretion, since these are the hormones that have been most intensively studied in psychiatric disorders. For a more detailed review of the role of 5-HT in hormone secretion, the reader is referred to Tuomisto and Männisto (1985).

The regulation of PRL secretion in mammals has been well characterized. The secretion of DA from tuberoinfundibular DA neurons, located in the arcuate nucleus of the medial basal hypothalamus, into the portal blood vessels, tonically inhibits the secretion of PRL (MacLeod, 1976; Gudelsky, 1981), whereas activation of serotonergic mechanisms stimulates the secretion of PRL (Clemens et al., 1978; Meltzer et al., 1981b; Meltzer et al., 1982). Largely as the result of the study of Lamberts and MacLeod (1978), in which 5-HT had no effect on PRL secretion when incubated with the pituitary in vitro, the effects of 5-HT on PRL secretion are believed to be at the level of the hypothalamus rather than directly at the pituitary. The fact that microinjection of 5-HT into the medial basal hypothalamus stimulates PRL secretion in the rat (Willoughby et al., 1988) and that an intact hypothalamic-pituitary axis is required for 5-HT–induced PRL secretion (Thomas et al., 1987) supports a hypothalamic site of action of 5-HT.

The dorsal and medial raphe nuclei located in the midbrain have been reported to be involved in the regulation of PRL secretion in the rat. Advis et al. (1979) found that destruction of 5-HT–containing cell bodies in the midbrain raphe nucleus decreased PRL secretion and lowered forebrain 5-HT and its major metabolite, 5-hydroxyindoleacetic acid (5-HIAA) concentrations. Similarly, Fessler et al. (1984) reported that electrolytic lesions of the medial and dorsal raphe nucleus significantly attenuated 5-hydroxytryptophan (5-HTP)–induced PRL secretion in rats pretreated with the highly selective 5-HT uptake inhibitor fluoxetine. Moreover, serum PRL concentrations correlated with the accumulation of 5-HT in the median eminence. Finally, lesions of the medial basal hypothalamus or posterolateral cuts, which interrupt input from caudal brain regions, including the midbrain, attenuate the stimulation of PRL secretion following the administration of p-chloroamphetamine (PCA), a 5-HT releasing agent (Van de Kar et al., 1985). These data strongly suggest that 5-HT–induced PRL secretion is the result of stimulation of midbrain raphe nuclei that have axon terminals located in the medial basal hypothalamus.

The hypothalamic-pituitary-adrenocortical (HPA) axis is generally considered the prototypical stress-responsive system in the mammalian organism. Given the evidence that stress may be relevant to the onset of many forms of psychopathology, and given the presence of depressive symptoms observed in patients with massive hypercortisolemia characteristic of patients wih Cushing's syndrome (Starkman et al., 1986), it is not surprising that the status of the HPA axis is frequently monitored in psychiatric disorders.

Both CRF and arginine vasopressin (AVP) seem to be involved in the stimulation of ACTH secretion, which, in turn, stimulates the secretion of glucocorticoids (e.g., cortisol) from the adrenal cortex (Rivier & Vale, 1985). There is considerable pharmacological evidence that suggests that 5-HT stimulates the HPA axis (Fuller, 1981). For example, 5-HT has been shown to cause a dose-dependent release of CRF, in vitro, in the intact rat hypothalamus (Holmes et al., 1982). Similarly, fluoxetine, a 5-HT uptake inhibitor, has been reported to increase CRF and AVP concentrations in hypophyseal portal plasma (Gibbs & Vale, 1983).

As was the case with PRL secretion, lesioning the medial basal hypothalamus significantly attenuated PCA- and quipazine-induced corticosterone secretion in the rat (Meyer et al., 1984; Van de Kar et al., 1985). Therefore, it would appear that 5-HT stimulates the HPA axis at the level of the hypothalamus. Recent histological evidence indicates that serotonergic fibers originating from the dorsal and medial raphe nuclei synapse directly with CRF synthesizing neurons located in the hypothalamus (Liposits et al., 1987); however, the anatomical basis for the serotonergic processes that regulate the HPA axis remains controversial. Unlike the case with PRL, lesions of the midbrain raphe nucleus did not block PCA-induced corticosterone secretion (Van de Kar et al., 1982). Posterolateral deafferentation had no effect on PCA-induced corticosterone secretion (Van de Kar et al., 1985). The fact that several 5-HT agonists have been reported to stimulate HPA activity at different sites of action (Meyer et al., 1984; McElroy et al., 1984) further complicates the identification of the origin of 5-HT–mediated HPA activation. Thus, although the majority of studies support a stimulatory role of 5-HT in the regulation of HPA axis, the precise mechanisms and anatomical location remain unknown.

The secretion of GH is regulated by two hypothalamic hormones, GH-RH, which stimulates, and somatostatin, which inhibits GH secretion. For the most part, 5-HT appears to stimulate GH secretion (Tuomisto & Männisto, 1985), and although it has been suggested that 5-HT inhibits somatostatin secretion, the precise role of 5-HT in GH secretion is not clear. Although studies employing 5-HT challenge drugs have frequently included the measurement of GH, the physiological mechanisms that control GH secretion are largely unknown.

Identification of Multiple 5-HT Binding Sites

In 1957, Gaddum and Picarelli demonstrated that various peripheral effects of 5-HT could be selectively antagonized by different pharmacological agents, suggesting the existence of multiple 5-HT receptors. Approximately 20 years later, Peroutka and Snyder (1979), using ligand binding methodology, reported the existence of two distinct 5-HT binding sites in the brain. Since that time, many more types of 5-HT binding sites in the brain have been identified (Peroutka, 1987; see Chapter 2, this volume), although the confirmation of these binding sites as receptors has not progressed as rapidly.

A brief review of 5-HT binding site nomenclature is necessary to follow the development of neuroendocrine challenge studies. Peroutka and Snyder (1979) designated two 5-HT binding sites which they identified as 5-HT_1 and 5-HT_2. The 5-HT_1 site has a high affinity for agonists (e.g., $^3\text{H-5-HT}$) while the 5-HT_2 site has a high affinity for antagonists (e.g., $^3\text{H-spiperone}$ or $^3\text{H-ketanserin}$). The binding sites designated 5-HT_1 were found to be heterogenous and Pedigo et al. (1981) further subdivided them into 5-HT_{1A} and 5-HT_{1B} sites on the basis of the greater affinity of the 5-HT_{1A} site for spiperone. Shortly thereafter, Pazos et al. (1984) designated a third 5-HT_1

binding site, 5-HT_{1C}. Very recently, Kilpatrick et al. (1987) designated a third 5-HT binding site, identified in the brain as 5-HT_3. Although the 5-HT_2 site has a higher affinity for antagonists, the development of [^{3}H]-5-HT$_2$ agonist binding assays (Titeler et al., 1987) has helped to identify potential 5-HT_2 agonists, for example, quipazine and several phenyliso-propylamine derivatives.

EFFECT OF SEROTONERGIC AGENTS ON HORMONE SECRETION

Precursors

Tryptophan

Serotonin is synthesized in neurons from the essential amino acid L-tryptophan (TRP). The role of TRP in the synthesis of 5-HT has been thoroughly reviewed by Fernstrom (1983) and will only be discussed briefly here. Following its dietary or pharmacological administration, TRP enters the general circulation, where 80–90% becomes loosely bound to serum albumin and the remainder circulates in the free form. In order for TRP to enter the central nervous system (CNS), it must be actively transported, which is accomplished by a saturable carrier-mediated process located at the blood–brain barrier. Tryptophan is classified as a large neutral amino acid (LNAA) and, as such, competes for uptake into the CNS with other LNAAs, namely, tyrosine, phenylalanine, leucine, isoleucine, and valine.

Once TRP enters the CNS, it is taken up by serotonergic neurons and converted into 5-HTP by the enzyme tryptophan hydroxylase (TH). The conversion of TRP into 5-HTP represents the rate-limiting step in the synthesis of 5-HT. TH is located exclusively in serotonergic neurons and, thus, represents a highly selective marker of 5-HT neurons. At normal physiological concentrations of brain TRP, TH is unsaturated (Hamon et al., 1979). Changes in TRP availability, therefore, should change TH activity in a similar direction. In fact, administration of TRP has been reported to increase the rate of 5-HTP formation in rat brain (Carlsson & Lindqvist, 1978). From these physiological data, it would appear that L-tryptophan is the ideal probe with which to study the role of 5-HT in hormone secretion. However, several recent studies have questioned the usefulness of TRP as a 5-HT agonist, as will become evident in the following discussion.

The effect of TRP on hormone secretion in normal volunteers has been reviewed (Meltzer et al., 1982; van Praag et al., 1987; Meltzer & Nash, 1988). For the most part, the oral administration of TRP does not consistently stimulate the secretion of PRL, ACTH, or GH. Conversely, its intravenous infusion in doses of 100 mg/kg or greater reliably stimulates the secretion of PRL and, although with much greater variability, GH, without affecting ACTH or cortisol secretion. The intravenous route of TRP administration may produce more consistent effects than oral administration because it reduces the variability associated with erratic gastric absorption and first-pass hepatic metabolism.

Nevertheless, the failure of intravenous TRP to stimulate ACTH and cortisol secretion is in contrast to the greater potency of 5-HTP, the immediate precursor of 5-HT, and direct-acting 5-HT agonists, such as MK-212 (6-chloro-2-[1-piperazinyl]-pyrazine), a $5-HT_2$ agonist, and to a lesser extent, buspirone, a $5-HT_{1A}$ agonist. All of these produce relatively robust effects on cortisol or PRL, or both, but no, or only weak, effects on GH secretion (Meltzer et al., 1984a; Lowy & Meltzer, 1988; Meltzer et al., 1983). This raises the possibility that L-tryptophan may act through a non-5-HT mechanism to stimulate PRL and GH. Additional evidence for this hypothesis will be discussed below.

Charney et al. (1982) reported the effects of intravenous TRP administration on PRL secretion in 10 normal volunteers (six females, four males). Similar results were reported by Koyama and Meltzer (1986). These data confirmed the reliability of intravenous TRP to stimulate PRL secretion as previously reported by MacIndoe and Turkington (1973). The most definitive TRP study to date is the report of Winokur et al. (1986). These authors reported a dose-dependent increase in serum PRL and GH concentrations following the intravenous infusion of TRP. Furthermore, none of the doses of TRP had a significant effect on cortisol or thyrotropin secretion (Koyama & Meltzer, 1986; Winokur et al., 1986). Anderson and Cowen (1986) found that pretreatment with the relatively selective 5-HT uptake inhibitor clomipramine potentiated the effect of TRP on PRL and GH secretion in six normal volunteers, suggesting that the secretion of these hormones is 5-HT mediated.

There is, as yet, only limited evidence that the effect of TRP on PRL and GH secretion can be inhibited by 5-HT antagonists. MacIndoe and Turkington (1973) reported that the nonselective 5-HT antagonist methysergide delayed the rise in PRL following TRP infusion in one female subject. The increase in serum GH secretion following a 5-g oral dose of TRP was antagonized in four female subjects pretreated with cyproheptadine (Fraser et al., 1979). Yet Cowen et al. (1985) reported that pretreatment with cyproheptadine, 4 mg orally, one hour before the intravenous infusion of 7.5 g TRP did not affect the increase in serum PRL and GH compared with a vehicle infusion. However, as noted by the authors, the results were extremely variable, possibly owing to the antidopaminergic, antihistaminergic, or anticholinergic properties of cyproheptadine.

More recently, the PRL response to TRP infusion was reported to be unaffected by pretreatment with either ketanserin (Cowen & Anderson, 1986) or ritanserin (Charig et al., 1986), two highly selective 5-HT$_2$ antagonists (Leysen et al., 1981, 1985). These data suggest that TRP-induced PRL secretion, if it is mediated by 5-HT, may be due to stimulation of 5-HT$_1$ receptors. McCance et al. (1987) found that pretreatment with metergoline (4 mg), which possesses equal binding affinity for 5-HT$_1$ and 5-HT$_2$ binding sites (Leysen et al., 1981), inhibited the increase in PRL secretion following the infusion of 5 g TRP. However, metergoline possesses significant dopaminergic agonist properties (Müller et al., 1983) and PRL secretion was significantly reduced two hours following the administration of metergoline. Thus, the precise receptor mechanisms by which TRP stimulates PRL secretion remain unknown.

The effect of TRP on hormone secretion has been studied in different psychiatric disorders and compared with the responses in normal volunteers. For the most part, the results obtained in studies conducted with depressed patients are in agreement. Heninger et al. (1984) found that the increase in PRL secretion following the intravenous infusion of 7 g TRP was significantly blunted in 25 depressed patients as compared with 19 age- and sex-matched normal volunteers. This finding was confirmed in 20 depressed patients by Koyama and Meltzer (1986), who also reported that the GH response to TRP (100 mg/kg) infusion was even more significantly blunted. Moreover, these studies found that the peak serum TRP concentration, as well as the total area under the curve following TRP infusion, was significantly reduced in the sample of depressed patients as compared with the normal volunteers. When the PRL and GH responses were adjusted for differences in serum TRP concentrations, only the GH response remained blunted in the depressed patients (Koyama, Ohmori, & Meltzer, unpublished observation).

These data suggest that the blunted PRL response to intravenous TRP loads may be the result of altered TRP pharmacokinetics or a reduction in the amount of TRP taken up into the CNS. However, the diminished GH response may be due to some other mechanism. Cowen and Charig (1987) replicated the finding that depressed patients who had lost less than 5 pounds had significantly attenuated PRL and GH responses following infusion of TRP (100 mg/kg). Nevertheless, these authors found no differences between patients and normal volunteers with respect to serum TRP concentrations following intravenous TRP infusion. Regardless, these studies suggest that blunted PRL and/or GH secretion in response to intravenous TRP administration may reflect altered serotonergic mechanisms associated with major depression.

The effect of TRP-induced hormone responses has been evaluated in patients with either obsessive compulsive disorder (OCD) or panic disorder. Charney et al. (1988) found no difference in the hormone responses to intravenous TRP administration in patients with OCD as compared with normal volunteers. Similarly, Charney and Heninger (1986) reported no differences between patients with panic disorder and normal volunteers with respect to TRP-induced hormone secretion. To the best of our knowledge, there are no neuroendocrine studies using TRP in drug-free schizophrenics. However, in one related study, Cowen et al. (1985) reported that six schizophrenic patients chronically treated with antipsychotics had an enhanced PRL and blunted GH response to TRP infusion, as compared with normal volunteers.

The effects of chronic antidepressant treatment on the TRP-induced increase in PRL and GH secretion have provided useful information on the effect of these agents on serotonergic function. For example, in a sample of 13 drug-free depressed patients, infusion of TRP resulted in a blunted PRL response; however, following 28 to 35 days of treatment with either amitriptyline or desipramine, rechallenge with TRP resulted in a significantly enhanced PRL response, as compared with the preceding drug-free period (Charney et al., 1984). Similarly, patients chronically treated with the monoamine oxidase inhibitor (MAOI) tranylcypromine had a significantly greater increase in serum PRL concentrations when tested during treatment as compared with a drug-free period (Price et al., 1985). These studies suggest that at least two forms of antidepressant therapy, tricyclic antidepressants and MAOI, increase serotonergic function in depressed patients, as evidenced by an enhanced PRL response to TRP administration. Cowen et al. (1986) reported that desipramine administration to normal volunteers enhanced the PRL response to TRP, confirming the results obtained in depressed patients and supporting the hypothesis that tricyclic antidepressants act, in part, by enhancing serotonergic function in depressed patients. However, the effect of antidepressant treatment could be secondary to effects on other neurotransmitter systems that indirectly influence the serotonergic system or the antidepressants may potentiate the nonserotonergic effects of TRP.

The blunted PRL and GH responses to TRP infusion would tend to support a hyporesponsive serotonergic system in depression. However, the selectivity of TRP as a 5-HT probe, as well as its ability to increase 5-HT activity, is not completely supported by animal or human studies. For example, although TRP loading in the rat increased the synthesis of 5-HT in discrete nuclei of the hypothalamus, it also increased the intraneuronal metabolism of 5-HT; the release of newly synthesized 5-HT into the synapse did not appear to be increased (Lookingland et al., 1986). Moreover, the direct measurement of 5-HT release in the rat brain following TRP administration was studied using in vivo voltammetry (De Simoni et al., 1987). These authors found that TRP administration enhanced 5-HT synthesis without affecting 5-HT release. Finally, the rate constant (K_m) for the uptake of TRP and other LNAAs is equal to their normal plasma concentration; therefore, even at very high plasma concentrations, the uptake process is limited (Partridge, 1983; DeFeudis, 1987). Van Praag (1983) found that a 5-g oral dose of TRP caused a significant increase in the postprobenecid accumulation of 5-HIAA in the cerebrospinal fluid (CSF) without affecting the concentrations of homovanillic acid (HVA) or 3-methoxy-4-hydroxyphenolglycol (MHPG), the major metabolites of DA and NE respectively. Moreover, Westenberg et al. (1982) found that this dose and route of TRP administration had no effect on serum PRL, cortisol, or GH concentrations. If the same dose of TRP was administered intravenously, however, 5-HIAA concentrations did not increase any further but both HVA and MHPG were significantly reduced (van Praag et al., 1987; Koyama & Meltzer, 1986).

Perhaps not coincidentally and as previously discussed, this dose and route of TRP administration reliably increase PRL secretion. Van Praag et al. (1987) suggest that TRP loading may decrease the influx of tyrosine by competing for uptake into the brain at the LNAA transport site. And finally, Goodwin et al. (1987) reported that dieting (weight loss) significantly enhanced the PRL and GH responses to TRP infusion, suggesting that nonspecific physiological changes alter TRP-induced hormone secretion. This finding is particularly relevant, since severe depression and hospitalization are often accompanied by weight loss.

In conclusion, the intravenous administration of TRP reliably increases PRL and, with much greater variability, GH secretion, without affecting ACTH and cortisol secretion in normal volunteers. In depressed patients, the intravenous administration of TRP increases serum PRL and GH concentrations, but to a lesser extent than it does in normal volunteers. These data have been used to suggest that serotonergic mechanisms may be impaired in depression but not in other psychiatric disorders such as panic disorder, OCD, or schizophrenia. However, the secretion of PRL and GH following intravenous TRP may be the result of TRP interfering with dopaminergic processes and may not provide a valid marker for 5-HT receptor function. Further, validation of this model by inhibition with 5-HT antagonists and clarification of why it does not increase cortisol secretion are essential before it can be accepted.

5-Hydroxytryptophan (5-HTP)

The conversion of L-5-HTP to 5-HT is catalyzed by the enzyme L-aromatic amino acid decarboxylase. The administration of 5-HTP bypasses the rate-limiting step of hydroxylation of tryptophan by TH, resulting in the efficient conversion of 5-HTP to 5-HT. Thus, unlike tryptophan administration, which fails to elicit the "5-HT syndrome" in rodents (Kuhn et al., 1986), 5-HTP–induced behaviors are believed to be mediated by the activation of central 5-HT receptors (Yap & Taylor, 1983). However, L-aromatic amino acid decarboxylase is not confined to serotonergic neurons, but is also found in catecholaminergic neurons. The administration of very high doses of 5-HTP (200–500 mg/kg) in rodents leads to formation of 5-HT in catecholaminergic neurons, which may then act as a false transmitter or by displacement of the catecholamines (Fuxe et al., 1971; Ng et al., 1972). The doses of oral 5-HTP that have been used in neuroendocrine studies in humans (e.g., 1.5–3.0 mg/kg) are much lower and may not alter catecholaminergic neurotransmission via this mechanism.

Over the past 20 years, a number of studies have been performed that examined the effects of 5-HTP on hormone secretion. As previously mentioned, these data have been thoroughly reviewed elsewhere (Meltzer et al., 1982; van Praag et al., 1987; Meltzer & Nash, 1988) and will be mentioned only briefly here. With the exception of one study (Kato et al., 1974), the oral administration of L-5-HTP was found to have little or no effect on PRL secretion in humans (Handwerger et al., 1975; Beck-Peccoz et al., 1976; Westenberg et al., 1982); conversely, the intravenous administration of L-5-HTP has been reported to stimulate PRL secretion (Mashchak et al., 1983; Sueldo et al., 1986). As was the case with TRP, the effect of L-5-HTP administration on GH secretion is quite variable, regardless of the route of administration.

The effects of 5-HTP on ACTH and/or cortisol secretion are somewhat variable. For example, 5-HTP administration has been reported to increase (Imura et al., 1973) or have no effect (Westenberg et al., 1982; Meltzer et al., 1984a) on cortisol secretion in normal volunteers. In the two studies that failed to observe an effect of 5-HTP on cortisol secretion, Westenberg et al. used an enteric-coated tablet, whereas Meltzer et al. used the racemic mixture (DL) of 5-HTP, either of which may have contributed to the negative results. Our laboratory recently found that oral administration of a higher dose of L-5-HTP, 200 mg, reliably stimulates the secretion of ACTH and cortisol in normal volunteers (Meltzer et al., unpublished observation).

There have been very few studies of the effect of putative 5-HT antagonists on the 5-HTP–induced increase in hormone secretion. Kato et al. (1974) found that oral administration of 5-HTP, 200 mg, stimulated the secretion of PRL, which was partially attenuated by pretreatment with the nonselective 5-HT antagonist cyproheptadine. Facchinetti et al. (1987) examined the effect of pretreatment with the 5-HT$_2$ antagonist ritanserin (10 mg twice a day for two days, followed by 10 mg per day for two days) on 5-HTP–induced cortisol secretion in eight normal volunteers. Although ritanserin did not significantly reduce 5-HTP–induced cortisol response in this study, there was a trend toward a diminished mean cortisol response in the ritanserin pretreatment group.

In contrast to human studies, an abundance of rodent data exist in which 5-HTP–induced behavioral effects such as "wet dog" shakes are blocked by selective 5-HT$_2$ antagonists, such as ketanserin and pirenperone (Colpaert & Janssen, 1983; Yap & Taylor, 1983; Lucki et al., 1984). Similarly, L-5-HTP–induced corticosterone secretion in rodents is blocked by ketanserin pretreatment (Nash & Meltzer, personal communication). Nash et al. (1988) found that the atypical antipsychotic clozapine blocked 5-HT$_2$-receptor–mediated hyperthermia and corticosterone secretion in rats.

As a direct extension of these studies, schizophrenic patients maintained, on either clozapine or typical antipsychotics such as haloperidol, chlorpromazine, or fluphenazine were challenged with L-5-HTP, 200 mg orally, or placebo. Clozapine completely blocked 5-HTP–induced cortisol secretion, whereas the typical antipsychotic had no effect (Meltzer et al., in preparation). These data suggest that the effect of 5-HTP on cortisol secretion is mediated, in part, by 5-HT$_2$ receptors. However, as previously discussed, the possibility that catecholaminergic mechanisms are also involved must be considered.

Takahashi et al. (1974) were the first to examine the neuroendocrine effects of 5-HTP administration in depressed patients. In this study, the oral administration of 200 mg of L-5-HTP was found to stimulate the secretion of GH in normal volunteers. In contrast, in 12 depressed patients studied, the GH response to 5-HTP administration was blunted, whereas in four manic patients, the GH response was not significantly different from control values. In another study, Westenberg et al. (1982) compared the effect of 5-HTP on hormone secretion in normal volunteers and depressed patients. Both groups were pretreated with the peripheral decarboxylase inhibitor carbidopa (150 mg) for three days, followed by the oral administration of 200 mg of L-5-HTP; carbidopa blocks the peripheral conversion of 5-HTP to 5-HT, which should increase the availability of 5-HTP for conversion in the CNS. Nevertheless, the authors found that L-5-HTP administration did not stimulate the secretion of either PRL, GH, or cortisol in either group tested.

These negative results could most probably be explained on the basis of the time at which serum samples were obtained. That is, 200 mg L-5-HTP was administered at 9:00 A.M. in an enteric-coated tablet and blood samples were obtained at 20-minute intervals for three hours. Measurements of serum 5-HTP concentrations revealed that drug absorption occurred during the 120–180-minute time period. However, hormone measurements were discontinued at 180 minutes (during peak absorption), thus decreasing the chance of observing hormone secretion. To test this, the authors obtained serum samples at 1300–1800 hours, but again reported no differences between groups. Nevertheless, the negative results reported by Westenberg et al. (1982) do not eliminate the possibility that the hormone responses did occur; they only show that at the times sampled in this study, no hormone responses were observed. Alternatively, pretreatment with carbidopa could interfere with the secretion of pituitary hormones. For example, the administration of carbidopa alters hormone secretion by itself (Garfinkel et al., 1979).

The most extensive studies of the effects of 5-HTP on hormone secretion in psychiatric patients have been carried out by Meltzer et al. (1984a, 1984b, 1984c), who reported that the administration of 200 mg of DL-5-HTP to 15 normal volunteers had little or no effect on the serum concentrations of PRL, GH, or cortisol. Conversely, in the 31 depressed patients and 16 manic patients studied, administration of DL-5-HTP significantly increased serum cortisol concentrations as compared with the normal volunteers. In addition, the cortisol response to DL-5-HTP administration was positively correlated with the Schedule for Affective Disorders and Schizophrenia-Change (SADS-C) Depression Subscale and was significantly greater in seven patients who had attempted suicide than in those who had not (Meltzer et al., 1984b). The authors hypothesized that the enhanced cortisol response to DL-5-HTP in depressed and manic patients resulted from the stimulation of supersensitive 5-HT receptors. This hypothesis is based on the abundant evidence suggesting diminished serotonergic function associated with depression (Meltzer & Lowy, 1987) and animal studies in which the depletion of central 5-HT concentrations results in enhanced behavioral and endocrine responses following an acute challenge with 5-HT agonists (Trulson et al., 1976; Samanin et al., 1980; Kuhn et al., 1981; Quattrone et al., 1981). Finally, Koyama et al. (1987) found that in a sample of nine depressed patients, the cortisol response to DL-5-HTP was negatively correlated with CSF 5-HIAA concentrations but not with CSF levels of other monoamine metabolites. Thus, these data support the hypothesis that decreased concentrations of central 5-HT lead to compensatory changes in 5-HT receptor sensitivity, as reflected by enhanced hormone response to a 5-HT challenge drug. Moreover, these results suggest that peripheral measures of hormone secretion may provide evidence of altered central serotonergic activity.

The results obtained by Meltzer et al. (1984a) have been confirmed and extended. Maes et al. (1987) examined the effect of 5-HTP on cortisol secretion in a sample of 65 depressed patients, who were classified according to the third edition of the *Diagnostic and Statistical Manual of Mental Disorders* (DSM-III) as major or minor depressives. In the patients with minor depression who were administered 200 mg L-5-HTP orally, twice the dose of the active form of 5-HTP used by Meltzer et al. (1984a), no significant increase in serum cortisol was observed. These data correspond to the findings of Meltzer et al. (1984a) in normal subjects. Conversely, the patients diagnosed as major depressives had a significantly greater cortisol response to 5-HTP, as compared with the minor depressives. Interestingly, there was a significant sex effect in this study; specifically, women, but not men, with major depression had a significantly greater cortisol response to 5-HTP, compared with depressed men and women with minor depression.

Few studies have been reported on the effects of 5-HTP on hormone secretion in psychiatric disorders other than depression. Jacobsen et al. (1987) reported the effect of 5-HTP on hormone responses in 10 patients with seasonal affective (mood) disorder (SAD). The administration of 200 mg L-5-HTP significantly elevated serum cortisol concentrations, decreased serum PRL levels, and did not affect GH or melatonin secretion; however, no differences were observed between the normal volunteers and the SAD patients.

In depressed patients chronically treated with tricyclic antidepressants, 5-HTP-induced cortisol response was diminished when compared with the drug-free response pattern (Meltzer et al., 1984c). In the same study, 5-HTP-induced cortisol response was enhanced in manic or depressed patients chronically treated with lithium or MAOIs respectively. Chronic antidepressant administration in rodents has been reported to decrease the number of $5-HT_2$ binding sites (Peroutka & Snyder, 1980; Fuxe et al., 1983). These data suggest that the attenuated cortisol response to 5-HTP administration in depressed patients chronically treated with tricyclic antidepressants may reflect a downregulation of $5-HT_2$ receptors. Similarly, the antimanic effects of lithium may be due to enhanced serotonergic activity (Bunney & Garland-Bunney, 1987), which is reflected in the enhanced cortisol response following 5-HTP administration in patients chronically maintained on lithium. Both clinical and preclinical studies currently being conducted in our laboratory are testing the $5-HT_2$ receptor supersensitivity hypothesis and the effect of antidepressants and lithium on these mechanisms.

Interactions between 5-HTP and other pharmacotherapies are virtually nonexistent. Isolated case reports, such as that of Irwin et al. (1986), have found that chronic antipsychotic treatment enhances 5-HTP–mediated responses. Preliminary studies currently under way in our laboratory are investigating the hormone-response patterns to 5-HTP administration in schizophrenic patients chronically treated with antipsychotics. Studies such as these may provide insight with regard to the increasing evidence that 5-

HT mechanisms play a key role in the psychopathology and the pharmaco-therapy of schizophrenia.

In conclusion, the oral administration of 5-HTP does not affect PRL or GH secretion, but does elevate serum ACTH and cortisol concentrations. This finding may be the result of postsynaptic receptor stimulation. However, 5-HTP may not be a selective 5-HT agonist at high doses and may cause the release of DA as suggested by increased homovanillic acid levels in CSF samples obtained following its oral administration (van Praag et al., 1987). However, further studies are needed to clarify these issues and thus to determine the usefulness of 5-HTP as a 5-HT probe in neuroendocrine studies.

5-HT Releasers

A number of compounds structurally related to amphetamines have been reported to release 5-HT, or inhibit its reuptake, or both (Fuxe et al., 1975). Although some of these agents appear to have toxic effects on 5-HT neurons (Fuller, 1978), one such agent, fenfluramine, has been used for a number of years as an appetite suppressant (Rowland & Carlton, 1986). It is well established that fenfluramine increases 5-HT release and inhibits its uptake; however, fenfluramine has also been reported to increase HVA and 3,4-dihydroxy-phenylacetic acid (DOPAC), two metabolites of DA (Jori & Benardi, 1972; Fuller et al., 1976), which could be due to its ability to block dopamine receptors. The d- and 1-isomers of fenfluramine have been reported to have different effects on 5-HT and DA neurons (Crunelli et al., 1980; Invernizzi et al., 1986). Specifically, the d-isomer of fenfluramine preferentially interacts with 5-HT neuronal mechanisms, whereas the 1-isomer interacts with dopaminergic systems. Moreover, 1-fenfluramine blocks amphetamine- and apomorphine-induced stereotypies (Bendotti et al., 1980) and blocks striatal DA receptors in a manner indistinguishable from that of haloperidol (Bettini et al., 1987). Despite this complex range of action, fenfluramine has been used as a serotonergic challenge drug in neuroendocrine studies.

As reviewed by Meltzer and Nash (1988), fenfluramine administration, whether oral or intravenous, reliably stimulates the secretion of PRL (Quattrone et al., 1983; Casanueva et al., 1984). This effect of fenfluramine on PRL secretion is dose-dependent (Quattrone et al., 1983; Scarduelli et al., 1985). Fenfluramine's effect on cortisol secretion has been infrequently studied. Fenfluramine was reported to produce a dose-dependent increase in serum ACTH and cortisol concentrations in humans in one study (Lewis & Sherman, 1984), but not in another (Mühlbauer & Müller-Oerlinghausen, 1985). Studies conducted in our laboratory suggest that fenfluramine (60 mg, orally) stimulated the secretion of PRL, but not cortisol, in normal volunteers (Meltzer, unpublished observation).

Several studies have demonstrated that the effects of fenfluramine on hormone secretion are blocked by 5-HT antagonists. For example, Quattrone et al. (1983) found that metergoline pretreatment completely blocked fenfluramine-induced PRL secretion. However, as previously mentioned, metergoline, which is also a DA agonist, significantly reduced serum PRL concentrations by itself; therefore, the ability of metergoline to block the fenfluramine-induced PRL secretion could be due to its dopamine agonist properties. On the other hand, Lewis and Sherman (1984) found that pretreatment with the nonselective 5-HT antagonist cyproheptadine significantly blunted fenfluramine-induced ACTH and cortisol secretion. Foresta et al. (1985) reported that the opiate antagonist naloxone significantly reduced fenfluramine-induced PRL secretion, which further complicates the interpretation of fenfluramine neuroendocrine studies by suggesting that fenfluramine may directly or indirectly stimulate the secretion of endogenous opiates. Finally, fenfluramine-stimulated cortisol secretion was completely blocked by pretreatment with the 5-HT$_2$ antagonist ketanserin in a study conducted in dogs (Barbieri et al., 1984).

Very few studies have examined the effects of fenfluramine on hormone secretion in psychiatric disorders. Siever et al. (1984) studied the effects of orally administered fenfluramine, 60 mg, on PRL secretion in 18 depressed patients and 10 normal volunteers. PRL secretion was measured over a five-hour period. Fenfluramine produced a significant increase in serum PRL in both patients and normal controls; however, the PRL response in the depressed patients was significantly lower than that of the normal volunteers. These data are consistent with the hypothesis that a decrease in central 5-HT mechanisms occurs in depression.

However, studies with fenfluramine reflect more than presynaptic stores of 5-HT, since this agent also inhibits 5-HT uptake. The effect of fenfluramine on HPA axis function has been reported in one study. Mühlbauer and Müller-Oerlinghausen (1985) measured serum cortisol in 12 normal volunteers and eight drug-free manic-depressives following the oral administration of 60 mg of fenfluramine. In contrast to the results of Lewis and Sherman (1984), in this study, fenfluramine failed to elevate serum cortisol concentration significantly above basal levels. Mühlbauer and Müeller-Oerlinghausen (1985) did find that the normal decline in serum cortisol concentrations was reversed following fenfluramine administration to manic-depressive patients maintained on lithium. The authors suggest that these data reflect enhanced serotonergic responsiveness related to the mechanism of action of lithium.

Recently, Asnis et al. (1988) reported no difference in PRL or cortisol secretion between 15 depressed patients and 10 normal controls who were administered 60 mg of fenfluramine orally. These authors question the 5-HT selectivity of fenfluramine, and their hypothesis appears to be supported by their finding that chronic desipramine treatment does not enhance fenfluramine-induced hormone response. Similarly, results obtained in our laboratory suggest that fenfluramine-induced PRL secretion does not differ between depressed patients and normal volunteers and that neither group displays a consistent cortisol response to fenfluramine (Meltzer & Nash, unpublished observation).

In conclusion, the use of fenfluramine as a selective 5-HT neuroendocrine probe is difficult to assess, since studies have used the racemic mixture of fenfluramine, which possesses dopaminergic antagonist properties that could effect PRL secretion in particular. Thus, a combination of 5-HT release and blockade of DA receptors could account for the PRL response to fenfluramine, making interpretation of the blunted response in depression difficult. However, the cortisol response to fenfluramine may be more indicative of the serotonergic system. As was the case with TRP and 5-HTP, the lack of specificity detracts from the usefulness of fenfluramine as a probe of central 5-HT mechanisms.

Direct 5-HT Agonists

In addition to the rather nonselective effects of TRP, 5-HTP, and fenfluramine, the use of these probes as 5-HT challenge agents in neuroendocrine studies is limited, owing to the indirect nature of these drugs. Alternatively, direct 5-HT agonists should provide a much clearer assessment of postsynaptic 5-HT function as measured by hormone response patterns. Until recently, the majority of direct 5-HT agonists possessed hallucinogenic activity and so were unsuitable for human use (Meltzer et al., 1981a, 1981b). However, novel 5-HT agonists that do not have hallucinogenic effects have now been developed and employed in neuroendocrine studies.

As discussed earlier, radioligand binding studies suggest that several different 5-HT binding sites are present in the CNS. Thus, 5-HT agonists are classified by their affinity for a given binding site. However, the most important criterion used to define the receptor subtype by which an agonist mediates its effect is the ability of a selective antagonist to block pharmacological responses. Unfortunately, the availability of selective 5-HT antagonists is quite limited. The relatively selective 5-HT$_2$ antagonists, such as ketanserin and ritanserin, are the best-defined agents to date and are not readily available for use in clinical studies. Nevertheless, as discussed in the subsequent sections, the use of direct-acting 5-HT agonists has provided valuable information on the role of 5-HT in hormone secretion.

A summary of the effects of direct 5-HT agonists on neuroendocrine responses is provided in van Praag et al. (1987) and Meltzer and Nash (1988). For the most part, the administration of 5-HT agonists produces consistent increases in PRL and cortisol secretion, with variable effects on serum GH concentrations. For the purpose of this review, the neuroendocrine effects of recently investigated 5-HT agonists will be presented. The agents will be classified according to their binding affinity for one or several of the 5-HT receptor subtypes. For additional information on the ligand binding profile of these agents, see Peroutka (1985, 1987) or Glennon (1987).

Buspirone (Buspar^R), a nonbenzodiazepine anxiolytic, possesses significant affinity for the 5-HT$_{1A}$ binding site (Peroutka, 1985). Its administration to rats produces a dose-dependent increase in PRL and cortisol secretion (Urban et al., 1986; Koenig et al., 1988). In humans, the oral administration of buspirone stimulates the secretion of PRL, cortisol, and, more variably, GH, in a dose-related manner (Meltzer et al., 1983). Buspirone also has some DA antagonist properties that could contribute to its potent effect on PRL secretion, but the affinity for the D-2 dopamine receptor is so weak that this is not likely to account for the PRL increases attributable to buspirone at oral doses as low as 30 mg (approximately 0.3–0.7 mg/kg) (Meltzer et al., 1983).

The neuroendocrine effects of m-chlorophenylpiperazine (mCPP), a metabolite of the antidepressant trazodone (Caccia et al., 1982), has been studied in humans. Although mCPP was originally believed to possess selective affinity for 5-HT$_{1B}$ binding sites, it has recently been reported to have equal affinity for 5-HT$_1$ and 5-HT$_2$ binding sites in human brain (Hamik & Peroutka, 1987). Mueller et al. (1985) reported that mCPP stimulates the secretion of PRL and cortisol, which is presumably dose related. These findings were confirmed and extended by demonstrating that mCPP also stimulated ACTH secretion, but did not affect serum GH concentrations (Mueller et al., 1986).

Quipazine has been reported to stimulate cortisol secretion without altering serum PRL or GH concentrations (Parati et al., 1980). The radioligand binding profile of quipazine is mixed, as it displays equal affinity for both 5-HT$_1$ and 5-HT$_2$ binding sites. However, animal studies have found that quipazine-induced corticosterone secretion is blocked by the 5-HT$_2$ antagonist ketanserin, suggesting that this effect is mediated by 5-HT$_2$ receptor mechanisms (Fuller & Snoddy, 1984).

Finally, Lowy and Meltzer (1988) reported that 6-chloro-2-(1-piperazinyl) pyrazine (MK-212) administered orally produced a dose-dependent increase in cortisol, and a less potent increase in PRL secretion without affecting serum GH concentrations. MK-212 displays little affinity for either 5-HT$_1$ or 5-HT$_2$ binding sites, but has been repeatedly shown to have potent 5-HT agonist properties (Clineschmidt et al., 1985). Moreover, MK-212-induced corticosterone secretion and hyperthermia are blocked by pretreatment with 5-HT$_2$ antagonists, such as ritanserin, ketanserin, and pirenperone, in rodents (Koenig et al., 1987; Gudelsky et al., 1986). These data have led us to conclude that MK-212 stimulates ACTH and cortisol secretion via 5-HT$_2$-mediated mechanisms.

Few studies have examined the interaction between direct 5-HT agonists and antagonists that are selective for either 5-HT$_1$ or 5-HT$_2$ binding sites, because of the limited clinical availability of the selective 5-HT$_2$ antagonists (i.e., ketanserin or ritanserin) and the lack of selective 5-HT$_1$ antagonists. Mueller et al. (1986), however, found that metergoline completely blocked mCPP-induced ACTH, cortisol, and PRL secretion. Interestingly, the interaction between metergoline and mCPP significantly reduced serum PRL values as compared with a placebo and mCPP, and although the results of metergoline and placebo control studies were not reported, these data suggest that metergoline has DA agonist properties in vivo.

However, the DA agonist properties of metergoline do not account for its ability to block mCPP-induced cortisol secretion, suggesting that at least some of the endocrine responses to mCPP are serotonergically mediated. Similarly, as mentioned previously, the effects of MK-212 on cortisol secretion have been examined in patients pretreated with either the atypical antipsychotic clozapine or one of several typical antipsychotics, such as haloperidol, thiothixene, or chlorpromazine. Clozapine, which possesses a high affinity for 5-HT$_2$ receptors (Altar et al., 1986), and which is a potent 5-HT$_2$ antagonist in vivo (Nash et al., 1988), significantly blocked MK-212-induced cortisol secretion in humans (Meltzer et al., 1987). Conversely, the typical antipsychotics had no effect on MK-212-induced cortisol secretion.

The beta-antagonists propranolol and (-)pindolol have considerable affinity for 5-HT$_1$ binding sites in vitro (Nahorski & Willcocks, 1983). Similarly, these agents have been reported to block several physiological responses to 5-HT$_1$ agonists (Sprouse & Aghajanian, 1986; Kennett et al., 1987). The use of either propranolol or (-)pindolol as 5-HT$_{1A}$ antagonists may provide valuable information with regard to the 5-HT receptor subtype responsible for hormone secretion and its potential role in psychiatric disorders.

The effects of direct 5-HT agonists on hormone response patterns in patients with psychiatric disorders are just beginning to be reported in the literature. For example, Zohar et al. (1987) studied the behavioral and hormone responses to mCPP administration in OCD patients and normal controls. Patients who were administered mCPP experienced an exacerbation of OCD symptoms that was not observed when they were given placebo. Both serum PRL and cortisol concentrations increased significantly following mCPP administration; however, OCD patients had a blunted cortisol response to mCPP as compared with normal volunteers, but the PRL response was similar in both groups. Chronic treatment with the potent 5-HT uptake inhibitor clomipramine significantly reduced the behavioral responses to mCPP administration (Zohar et al., 1988).

Interestingly, chronic clomipramine administration significantly elevated serum PRL levels in OCD patients without affecting the response pattern to mCPP. More important, the blunted cortisol response to mCPP was apparently still present in OCD patients chronically treated with clomipramine. The authors of these studies suggest that the exacerbation of OCD symptoms reflects an increased serotonergic responsiveness and that chronic clomipramine treatment decreases responsivity to 5-HT even further. The blunted cortisol response may reflect on inadequate "stress" response; however, further studies are necessary to confirm this hypothesis. Studies conducted in our laboratory suggest that OCD patients have a blunted cortisol response to MK-212 (20 mg, orally) as well as a blunted PRL response to buspirone (30 mg, orally) administration (Bastani, Nash, & Meltzer, in press). These data suggest that hyporesponsive serotonergic mechanisms exist in OCD patients, which is consistent with the finding of Zohar et al. (1988) regarding hormone responses.

In another study, the effect of mCPP on behavioral and hormonal responses was assessed in normal volunteers, agoraphobics, and panic disorder patients (Charney et al., 1987). For the most part, no differences in ratings of anxiety and stimulation of the secretion of PRL, cortisol, and GH were reported between the normal volunteers and the patients studied. However, this study did reveal that mCPP induced feelings of anxiety in both groups, suggesting that serotonergic mechanisms play a role in anxiety.

5-HT Uptake Inhibitors

A number of tricyclic antidepressants are believed to enhance serotonergic transmission by inhibiting the reuptake process, which is the primary means of terminating the effects of 5-HT at postsynaptic receptors (Willner, 1985). Most of these agents are relatively nonselective in that they also inhibit the uptake of NE. However, the development of selective 5-HT uptake inhibitors such as citalopram, zimelidine, fluvoxamine, and fluoxetine makes these logical candidates for studying the role of 5-HT in hormone secretion. Moreover, given their selectivity and the established role of 5-HT in the control of hormone secretion, changes in hormone responses following the administration of these 5-HT uptake inhibitors may provide valuable information with regard to their time course of action, therapeutic efficacy, or both.

In the majority of studies, the acute administration of 5-HT uptake inhibitors has little or no effect on PRL, cortisol, or GH secretion (Meltzer and Nash, 1988). For example, neither zimelidine nor fluvoxamine significantly increased PRL or cortisol secretion in normal volunteers (Syvälahti et al., 1979). Thus, the specificity of these 5-HT uptake inhibitors makes them attractive for use in neuroendocrine studies, although, to date, this potential has not been realized.

To the best of our knowledge, the antagonism of the effects of 5-HT uptake inhibitors is limited to preclinical studies. Similarly, studies on the neuroendocrine effects of these agents in psychiatric disorders are rare. Overall, the utility of selective 5-HT uptake inhibitors as 5-HT neuroendocrine probes is rather limited, mainly because the assumption must be made that the release of 5-HT is similar in normal volunteers and psychiatric patients if differences in neuroendocrine responses are detected.

HORMONES AND 5-HT FUNCTION

The main focus of this chapter has been on the role of 5-HT in the control of hormone secretion with possible applications to the study of psychiatric disorders. However, this discussion would be incomplete without a brief overview of the influence that hormones such as prolactin and cortisol have on 5-HT synthesis and turnover. This is particularly relevant and must be taken into consideration when interpreting neuroendocrine response patterns in psychiatric patients. For example, one of the most consistent neuroendocrine findings observed in patients with depression is HPA disinhibition as reflected by elevated serum cortisol and a blunted circadian rhythm (Carroll et al., 1976; Sachar et al., 1980). Although abnormalities in the serotonergic system are in part believed to mediate many aspects of hypercortisolism, it is noteworthy that adrenalglucocorticoids have been reported to affect brain 5-HT metabolism. Thus, neuroendocrine studies may reflect a consequence of the disease processes rather than the underlying cause.

The effect of PRL on 5-HT synthesis or metabolism has been infrequently studied. In one study, 5-HT synthesis was determined in hypophysectomized rats with and without supplemental administration of PRL (King et al., 1985). These authors found that PRL reduced 5-HT synthesis, which involved an intermediary DA component. Thus, chronic elevations in serum PRL, as are seen following typical antipsychotic treatment or, more recently, with selective 5-HT uptake inhibitors such as clomipramine (Zohar et al., 1987), may confound 5-HT-mediated neuroendocrine responses and result in erroneous conclusions. The relationship between PRL and 5-HT metabolism requires further study.

Although there are some conflicting studies, for the most part, glucocorticoids appear to increase 5-HT synthesis and turnover, as reviewed by McEwen (1987). Glucocorticoid receptors have been identified in 5-HT neurons (Härfstrand et al., 1986). Presumably, glucocorticoids act via these receptor mechanisms to stimulate tryptophan hydroxylase activity (Azmitia & McEwen, 1974). Glucocorticoids have been reported to exert additional effects on serotonergic mechanisms. For example, hypophysectomy and adrenalectomy reduce 5-HT uptake into neuronal synaptosomes. This process is reversed by glucocorticoid administration, suggesting that glucocorticoids play a key role in 5-HT neuronal uptake (Tukiainen, 1981). Similarly, adrenalectomy increases the number of 5-HT$_1$ receptors in the hypothalamus, and this effect can be reversed by administering corticosterone (De Kloet et al., 1986).

Collectively, these data suggest that glucocorticoids activate serotonergic mechanisms. Thus, diminished serotonergic mechanisms may result in elevated serum concentrations of glucocorticoids as a compensatory mechanism. Alternatively, desensitization of central glucocorticoid receptors may reduce 5-HT function, resulting in an increase in 5-HT receptor density. Regardless of the precise interactions, it is clear that future studies on the interaction between HPA function and central serotonergic mechanisms will provide important insights into the origin of psychiatric disorders.

CONCLUSION

The use of the neuroendocrine challenge strategy as a means of studying psychiatric illness has steadily increased over the past decade. For the most part, the probes used to stimulate the serotonergic system are still nonselective, which diminishes the significance of the results. The development of more specific agonists and antagonists will increase the usefulness of neuroendocrine challenge studies. A key question is whether the serotonergic mechanisms that participate in hormone secretion can accurately mirror serotonergic mechanisms that directly take part in symptom or syndrome formation. Such contradictory findings as blunted cortisol and PRL responses to mCPP and MK-212 in obsessive compulsives and a worsening of symptoms with mCPP and no effect on symptoms with MK-212 indicate the care with which hormone responses must be interpreted. It is possible to interpret these results only in the context of other types of evidence that suggest that diminished serotonergic activity is important in the etiology of OCD. The hormone profile shown in serotonergic challenges may prove to have diagnostic specificity as the range of available agents increases. Finally, the hormone responses to serotonergic agents may reveal the effect of psychotropic drugs on specific receptor systems.

REFERENCES

Advis, J. P., Simpkins, J. W., Bennett, J., & Meites, J. (1979). Serotonergic control of prolactin release in male rats. *Life Sci., 24,* 359–366.

Altar, C. A., Wasley, A. M., Neale, R. F., & Stone, G. A. (1986). Typical and atypical antipsychotic occupancy of D_2 and S_2 receptors: An autoradiographic analysis in rat brain. *Brain Res. Bull., 16,* 517–525.

Anderson, I. M., & Cowen, P. J. (1986). Clomipramine enhances prolactin and growth hormone responses to L-tryptophan. *Psychopharm., 89,* 131–133.

Andreasen, N. C. (1988). Brain imaging: Applications in psychiatry. *Science, 239,* 1381–1388.

Asnis, G. M., Eisenberg, J., van Praag, H. M., Lemus, C. Z., Harkavy-Friedman, J. M., & Miller, A. H. (1988). The neuroendocrine response to fenfluramine in depressives and normal controls. *Biol. Psychiatry, 24,* 117–120.

Azmitia, E., & McEwen, B. S. (1974). Adrenalcortical influence on rat brain tryptophan hydroxylase activity. *Brain Res., 78,* 291–302.

Ballenger, J. C., Goodwin, F. K., Major, L. F., & Brown, G. L. (1979). Alcohol and central serotonin metabolism in man. *Arch. Gen. Psych., 36,* 224–227.

Barbieri, C., Sala, M., Bigatti, G., Rauhe, W. G., Guffanti, A., Diena, A., Scorza, D., Beuilacqua, M., & Norbiato, G. (1984). Serotonergic regulation of cortisol secretion in dogs. *Endocrinol., 115,* 748–751.

Bastani, B., Nash, J. F., & Meltzer, H. Y. (in press). Prolactin and cortisol responses to MK-212, a serotonin agonist, in obsessive-compulsive disorder. *Arch. Gen. Psychiatry.*

Beck-Peccoz, P., Ferrari, C., Rondena, M., Paracchi, A., & Faglia, G. (1976). Failure of oral 5-hydroxytryptophan administration to affect prolactin secretion in man. *Hormone Res., 7,* 303–307.

Bendotti, C., Borsini, F., Zanini, M. G., Samanin, R., & Garattini, S. (1980). Effect of fenfluramine and norfenfluramine stereoisomers on stimulant effects of d-amphetamine and apomorphine in the rat. *Pharmac. Res. Comm., 12,* 567–574.

Bettini, E., Ceci, A., Spinelli, R., & Samanin, R. (1987). Neuroleptic-like effects of the 1-isomer of fenfluramine on striatal dopamine release in freely moving rats. *Biochem. Pharmacol., 36,* 2387–2391.

Bunney, W. E., & Garland-Bunney, B. L. (1987). Mechanisms of action of lithium in affective illness: Basic and clinical implications. In H. Y. Meltzer (Ed.), *Psychopharmacology: The third generation of progress* (pp. 553–566). New York: Raven Press.

Caccia, S., Fong, M. H., Garattinis, V., & Zanini, M. G. (1982). Plasma concentrations of trazodone and 1-(3-chlorophenyl)piperazine in man after a single oral dose of trazodone. *J. Pharm. Pharmac., 34,* 605–606.

Carlsson, A., & Lindqvist, M. (1978). Dependence of 5-HT and catecholamine synthesis on concentrations of precursor amino-acids in rat brain. *Naunyn-Schmiedeberg's Arch. Pharmacol., 303,* 157–164.

Carroll, B. J., Curtis, G. C., & Mendels, J. (1976). Neuroendocrine regulation in depression. I. Limbic system-adrenocortical dysfunction. *Arch. Gen. Psych., 33,* 1039–1044.

Casanueva, F. F., Villanueva, L., PeNalva, H., & Cabezas-Cerrato, J. (1984). Depending on the stimulus, central serotonergic activation by fenfluramine blocks or does not alter growth hormone secretion in man. *Neuroendocrinol., 38,* 302–308.

Charig, E. M., Anderson, I. M., Robinson, J. M., Nutt, D. J., & Cowen, P. J. (1986). L-tryptophan and prolactin release: Evidence for interaction between 5-HT$_1$ and 5-HT$_2$ receptors. *Hum. Psychopharm., 1,* 93–97.

Charney, D. S., Goodman, W. K., Price, L., H., Woods, S. W., Rasmussen, S. A., & Heninger, G. R. (1988). Serotonin function in obsessive-compulsive disorder. A comparison of the effects of tryptophan and m-chlorophenylpiperazine in patients and healthy subjects. *Arch. Gen. Psych., 45,* 177–185.

Charney, D. S., & Heninger, G. R. (1986). Serotonin function in panic disorders. The effect of intravenous tryptophan in healthy subjects and patients with panic disorder before and during alprazolam treatment. *Arch. Gen. Psych., 43,* 1059–1065.

Charney, D. S., Heninger, G. R., Reinhard, J. F., Sternberg, D. E., & Hafstead, K. M. (1982). The effect of intravenous L-tryptophan on prolactin and growth hormone and mood in healthy subjects. *Psychopharm., 77,* 217–222.

Charney, D. S., Heninger, G. R., & Sternberg, D. E. (1984). Serotonin function and mechanism of action of antidepressant treatment. *Arch. Gen. Psych., 41,* 359–365.

Charney, D. S., Woods, S. W., Goodman, W. K., & Heninger, G. R. (1987). Serotonin function in anxiety. II. Effects of the serotonin agonist mCPP in panic disorder patients and healthy subjects. *Psychopharm., 92,* 14–24.

Clemens, J. A., Roush, M. E., & Fuller, R. W. (1978). Evidence that serotonin neurons stimulate secretion of prolactin releasing factor. *Life Sci., 22,* 2209–2214.

Clineschmidt, B. V., Reiss, D. R., Pettibone, D. J., & Robinson, J. L. (1985). Characterization of 5-hydroxytryptamine receptors in rat stomach fundus. *J. Pharmacol. Exp. Ther., 235,* 696–708.

Colpaert, F. C., & Janssen, P. A. J. (1983). The head-twitch response to intraperitoneal injection of 5-hydroxytryptophan in the rat: Antagonist effects of purported 5-hydroxytryptamine antagonists and of pirenperone, an LSD antagonist. *Neuropharm., 22,* 993–1000.

Costall, B., & Naylor, R. J. (1978). Neuroleptic interaction with the serotonergic-dopaminergic mechanisms in the nucleus accumbens. *J. Pharm. Pharmac., 30,* 257–259.

Cowen, P. J., & Anderson, I. M. (1986). 5-HT neuroendocrinology. In J. F. N. Deakin (Ed.), *The biology of depression* (pp. 71–89). London: Royal College of Psychiatrists.

Cowen, P. J., & Charig, E. M. (1987). Neuroendocrine responses to intravenous tryptophan in major depression. *Arch. Gen. Psych., 44,* 958–966.

Cowen, P. J., Gadhvi, H., Gosden, B., & Kolakowska, T. (1985). Responses of prolactin and growth hormone to L-tryptophan infusion: Effects in normal subjects and schizophrenic patients receiving neuroleptics. *Psychopharm., 86,* 164–169.

Cowen, P. J., Geaney, D. P., Schächter, M., Green, A. R., & Elliott, J. M. (1986). Desipramine treatment in normal subjects: Effects on neuroendocrine responses to tryptophan and on platelet serotonin (5-HT) related receptors. *Arch. Gen. Psych., 43,* 61–67.

Crunelli, V., Bernasconi, S., & Samanin, R. (1980). Effects of d- and l-fenfluramine on striatal homovanillic acid concentrations in rats after pharmacological manipulation of brain serotonin. *Pharmacol. Res. Commun., 12,* 215–223.

DeFeudis, F. V. (1987). The brain is protected from nutrient excess. *Life Sci., 40,* 1–9.

De Kloet, E. R., Sybesma, H., & Reul, H. M. (1986). Selective control by corticosterone of serotonin₁ receptor capacity in raphe-hippocampal system. *Neuroendo., 42,* 513–521.

De Simoni, M. G., Sokola, A., Fodritto, F., Dal Toso, G., & Algeri, S. (1987). Functional meaning of tryptophan-induced increase of 5-HT metabolism as clarified by in vivo voltammetry. *Brain Res., 411,* 89–94.

Facchinetti, F., Martignoni, E., Nappi, G., Marini, S., Petraglia, F., Sandrini, G., & Genazzani, A. R. (1987). Ritanserin, a serotonin-S₂ receptor antagonist, does not prevent 5-hydroxytryptophan-induced β-EP, β-LPH and cortisol secretion. *Hormone Res., 27,* 42–46.

Fernstrom, J. D. (1983). Role of precursor availability in control of monoamine biosynthesis in brain. *Physiol. Rev., 63,* 484–546.

Fessler, R. G., Deyo, S. N., Meltzer, H. Y., & Miller, R. J. (1984). Evidence that the medial and dorsal raphe nuclei mediate serotonergically-induced increases in prolactin release from the pituitary. *Brain Res., 299,* 231–237.

Foresta, C., Scanelli, G., Indino, M., Federspil, G., & Scandellari, C. (1985). Naloxone reduces the fenfluramine-induced prolactin release in man. *Clin. Endocrinol., 22,* 539–543.

Fraser, W. M., Tucker, H. S. T., Grubb, S. R., Wigand, J. P., & Blackard, W. G. (1979). Effect of L-tryptophan on growth hormone and prolactin release in normal volunteers and patients with secretory pituitary tumors. *Horm. Metab. Res., 11,* 149–155.

Fuller, R. W. (1978). Structure-activity relationships among the halogenated amphetamines. In J. H. Jacoby & L. D. Lytle (Eds.), *Serotonin neurotoxins* (pp. 147–159). New York: New York Academy of Sciences.

Fuller, R. W. (1981). Serotonergic stimulation of pituitary-adrenocortical function in rats. *Neuroendocrinol., 32,* 118–127.

Fuller, R. W., Perry, K. W., & Clemens, J. A. (1976). Elevation of 3, 4-dihydroxyphenylacetic acid concentrations in rat brain and stimulation of prolactin secretion by fenfluramine: Evidence for antagonism at dopamine receptor sites. *J. Pharm. Pharmac., 28,* 643–644.

Fuller, R. W., & Snoddy, H. D. (1984). Central serotonin antagonist activity of ketanserin. *Res. Comm. Chem. Path. Pharmacol., 46,* 151–154.

Fuxe, K., Butcher, L. L., & Engel, J. (1971). DL-5-hydroxytryptophan-induced changes in central monoamine neurons after peripheral decarboxylase inhibition. *J. Pharm. Pharmac., 23,* 420–424.

Fuxe, K., Farnebo, L.-O., Harnberger, B., & Ogren, S.-O. (1975). On the *in vivo* and *in vitro* actions of fenfluramine and its derivatives on central monoamine neurons, especially 5-hydroxytryptamine neurons, and their relation to the anorectic activity of fenfluramine. *J. Postgrad. Med., 51,* 35–45.

Fuxe, K., Ogren, S.-O., Agnati, L. F., Benfenati, F., Fredholm, B., Andersson, K., Zini, I., & Eneroth, P. (1983). Chronic antidepressant treatment and central 5-HT synapses. *Neuropharm., 22,* 389–400.

Gaddum, J. H., & Picarelli, Z. P. (1957). Two kinds of tryptamine receptors. *Br. J. Phrmacol., 12,* 323–328.

Garfinkel, P. E., Brown, G. M., Warsh, J. J., & Stancer, H. C. (1979). Neuroendocrine responses to carbidopa in primary affective disorders. *Psychoneuroendo, 4,* 13–20.

Gibbs, D. M., & Vale, W. (1983). Effect of serotonin reuptake inhibitor fluoxetine on corticotropin-releasing factor and vasopressin secretion into hypophysial portal blood. *Brain Res., 280,* 176–179.

Gillin, J. C., Kaplan, J., Stillman, R., & Wyatt, R. J. (1976). The psychedelic model of schizophrenia: The case of N,N-dimethyltryptamine. *Am. J. Psych., 153,* 203–208.

Glennon, R. A. (1987). Central serotonin receptors as targets for drug research. *J. Med. Chem., 30,* 1–12.

Goodwin, G. M., Fairburn, C. G., & Cowen, P. J. (1987). The effects of dieting and weight loss on neuroendocrine responses to tryptophan, clonidine and apomorphine in volunteers. Important implications for neuroendocrine investigations in depression. *Arch. Gen. Psych., 44,* 952–957.

Gudelsky, G. A. (1981). Tuberoinfundibular dopamine neurons and the regulation of prolactin secretion. *Psychoneuroendo., 6,* 3–16.

Gudelsky, G. A., Koening, J. I., & Melter, H. Y. (1986). Thermoregulatory responses to serotonin [5-HT] receptor stimulation in the rat: Evidence for opposing role of $5-HT_2$ and $5-HT_{1A}$ receptors. Neuropharmacology, *25,* 1307–1313.

Hamik, A., & Peroutka, S. J. (1987). 1-(m-chlorophenyl)piperazine (mCPP) interactions with neurotransmitter receptors in human brain. *Soc. Neurosci. Abst., 13,* 1237.

Hamon, M., Bourgoin, S., & Youdim, M. B. H. (1979). Tryptophan hydroxylation in the central nervous system and other tissues. In. M. B. H. Youdim (Ed.), *Aromatic amino acid hydroxylases and mental disease* (pp. 223–297). New York: Wiley.

Handwerger, S., Plonk, J. W., Lebovits, H. E., Bivens, C. H., & Feldman, J. M. (1975). Failure of 5-hydroxytryptophan to stimulate prolactin and growth hormone secretion in man. *Hormone Metab. Res., 7,* 214–216.

Härfstrand, A., Fuxe, K., Cintra, A., Agnati, L. F., Zini, I., Wikström, A.-C., Okret, S., Yu, Z.-Y., Goldstein, M., Steinbusch, H., Verhofstad, A., & Gustafsson, J.-A. (1986). Glucocorticoid receptor immunoreactivity in monoaminergic neurons in rat brain. *Proc. Natl. Acad. Sci., 83,* 9779–9783.

Heninger, G. R., Charney, D. J., & Sternberg, D. E. (1984). Serotonergic function in depression. Prolactin response to intravenous tryptophan in depressed patients and healthy subjects. *Arch. Gen. Psych., 41,* 398–402.

Holmes, M. C., Di Renzo, G. D., Beckford, B., Gillham, B., & Jones, M. T. (1982).

Role of serotonin in the control of secretion of corticotropin-releasing factor. *J. Endocrinol., 93,* 151–160.

Imura, H., Nakai, Y., & Yoshimi, T. (1973). Effect of 5-HTP on growth hormone and ACTH release in man. *J. Clin. Endocrinol. Metab., 36,* 204–206.

Invernizzi, R., Berettera, C., Garattini, S., & Samanin, R. (1986). D- and l-isomers of fenfluramine differ markedly in their interaction with brain serotonin and catecholamines in the rat. *Eur. J. Pharmacol., 120,* 9–15.

Irwin, M., Fuentenebro, F., Marder, S. R., & Yuwiler, A. (1986). L-5-Hydroxytryptophan-induced delirium. *Biol. Psych., 21,* 673–676.

Jacobsen, F. M., Sack, D. A., Wehr, T. A., Rogers, S., & Rosenthal, N. E. (1987). Neuroendocrine response to 5-hydroxytryptophan in seasonal affective disorder. *Arch. Gen. Psych., 44,* 1086–1091.

Jori, A., & Benardi, D. (1972). Further studies on the increase of striatal homovanillic acid induced by amphetamine and fenfluramine. (1972) *Eur. J. Pharmacol., 19,* 276–280.

Kahn, R. S., van Praag, H. M., Wetzler, S., Asnis, G. M., & Barr, G. (1988). Serotonin and anxiety revisited. *Biol. Psych., 23,* 189–208.

Kato, Y., Nakai, Y., Imura, H., Chihara, K., & Ohgo, S. (1974). Effects of 5-hydroxytryptophan on plasma prolactin levels in man. *J. Clin. Endocrinol., 38,* 695–697.

Kennett, G. A., Dourish, C. T., & Curzon, G. (1987). 5-HT$_{1B}$ agonists induce anorexia at a postsynaptic site. *Eur. J. Pharmacol., 141,* 429–435.

Kilpatrick, G. L., Jones, B. J., & Tyers, M. B. (1987). Identification and distribution of 5-HT$_3$ receptors in rat brain using radioligand binding. *Nature, 330,* 746–748.

King, T. J., Steger, R. W., & Morgan, W. W. (1985). Effect of hypophysectomy and subsequent prolactin administration on hypothalamic 5-hydroxytryptamine synthesis in ovariectomized rats. *Endocrinol., 116,* 485–491.

Koenig, J. I., Gudelsky, G. A., & Meltzer, H. Y. (1987). Stimulation of corticosterone and β-endorphin secretion in the rat by selective 5-HT receptor subtype activation. *Eur. J. Pharmacol., 137,* 1–8.

Koenig, J. I., Meltzer, H. Y., & Gudelsky, G. A. (1988). 5-Hydroxytryptamine$_{1A}$ receptor-mediated effects of buspirone, gepirone and ipsapirone. *Pharm. Biochem. Behav., 29,* 711–715.

Koyama, T., Lowy, M. T., & Meltzer, H.Y. (1987). 5-Hydroxytryptophan-induced cortisol response and CSF 5-HIAA. *Am.J. Psych., 144,* 334–347.

Koyama, T., & Meltzer, H. Y. (1986). A biochemical and neuroendocrine study of the serotonergic system in depression. In H. Hippius et al. (Eds.), *New results in depression research* (pp. 169–188). Berlin-Heidelberg: Springer-Verlag.

Kuhn, C. M., Vogel, R. A., Mailman, R. B., Mueller, R. A., Schanberg, S. M., & Breese, G. R. (1981). Effect of 5,7-dihydroxytryptamine on serotonergic control of prolactin secretion and behavior in rats. *Psychopharm., 73,* 188–193.

Kuhn, D. M., Wolf, W., & Youdim, M. B. H. (1986). Serotonin neurochemistry revisited: A new look at some old axioms. *Neurochem. Int., 8,* 141–154.

Lamberts, S. W. J., & MacLeod, R. M. (1978). The interaction of the serotonergic and dopaminergic systems on prolactin secretion in the rat. *Endocrinol., 103,* 287–295.

Lewis, D. A., & Sherman, B. M. (1984). Serotonergic stimulation of adrenocortico-tropin secretion in man. *J. Clin. Endocrinol. Metab., 58,* 458–462.

Leysen, J. E., Awouter, F., Kennis, L., Laduron, P. M., Vandenberk, J., & Janssen, P. A. J. (1981). Receptor binding profile of R 41 468, a novel antagonist at 5-HT₂ receptors. *Life Sci., 28,* 1015–1022.

Leysen, J. E., Gommeren, W., Van Gompel, P., Wynants, J., Janssen, P. F. M., & Laduron, P. M. (1985). Receptor-binding properties *in vitro* and *in vivo* of ritanserin, a very potent and long-acting serotonin-S₂ antagonist. *Mol. Pharmacol., 27,* 600–611.

Liposits, Z. S., Phelix, C., & Paull, W. K. (1987). Synaptic interaction of serotonergic axons and corticotropin releasing factor (CRF) synthesizing neurons in the hypothalamic paraventricular nucleus of the rat. *Histochemistry, 86,* 541–549.

Lookingland, K. J., Shannon, N. J., Chapin, D. J., & Moore, K. E. (1986). Exogenous tryptophan increases synthesis, storage, and intraneuronal metabolism of 5-hydroxytryptamine in the rat hypothalamus. *J. Neurochem., 47,* 205–212.

Lowy, M. T., & Meltzer, H. Y. (1988). Stimulation of serum cortisol and prolactin secretion in man by MK-212, a centrally active serotonin agonist. *Biol. Psych., 23,* 818–828.

Lucki, I., Nobler, M. S., & Frazer, A. (1984). Differential actions of serotonin antagonists on two behavioral models of serotonin receptor activation in the rat. *J. Pharmacol. Exp. Ther., 228,* 133–139.

MacIndoe, J. H., & Turkington, R. W. (1973). Stimulation of human prolactin secretion by intravenous infusion of L-tryptophan. *J. Clin. Invest., 53,* 1972–1978.

MacLeod, R. M. (1976). Regulation of prolactin secretion. In L. Martini and W. F. Ganong (Eds.), *Frontiers in neuroendocrinology,* Vol. 4 (pp. 169–184). New York: Raven Press.

Maes, M., De Ruyter, M., Claes, R., Bosma, G., & Suy, F. (1987). The cortisol responses to 5-hydroxytryptophan, orally, inn depressive inpatients. *J. Affec. Disorders, 13,* 23–30.

Mashchak, C. A., Kletsky, O. A., Spencer, C., & Artal, R. (1983). Transient effect of L-5-hydroxytryptophan on pituitary function in men and women. *J. Clin. Endocrinol. Metab., 56,* 170–176.

McCance, S. L., Cowen, P. J., & Grahame-Smith, D. G. (1987). Metergoline attenuates the prolactin responses to L-tryptophan. *Br. J. Clin. Pharmacol., 23,* 607–608.

McElroy, J. F., Miller, J. M., & Meyer, J. S. (1984). Fenfluramine, p-chloroamphetamine and p-fluoroamphetamine stimulation of pituitary-adrenocortical activity in rat: Evidence for differences in site and mechanism of action. *J. Pharmacol. Exp. Ther., 228,* 593–599.

McEwen, B. S. (1987). Glucocorticoid-biogenic amine interactions in relation to mood and behavior. *Biochem. Pharmacol., 36,* 1755–1763.

Meltzer, H. Y. (1988). Clozapine: Clinical advantages and biological mechanisms. In C. Schulz & C. Tamminga (Eds.), *Schizophrenia: A scientific focus.* International Conference on Schizophrenia. (pp. 302–309). New York: Oxford.

Meltzer, H. Y., Fleming, R., & Robertson, A. (1983). The effect of buspirone on prolactin and growth hormone in man. *Arch. Gen. Psych., 40,* 1099–1102.

Meltzer, H. Y., Gudelsky, G., Koenig, J., & Lowy, M. (1988). Neuroendocrine effects of buspirone: Mediation by dopaminergic and serotonergic mechanisms. In G. Tunnicliff, A. Eison, & D. Taylor (Eds.), *Buspirone: Mechanisms and clinical aspects.* New York: Academic Press.

Meltzer, H. Y., Kwon, B., Ramirez, L., & Nash, J. F. (1987). Clozapine as a 5-HT$_2$ antagonist in man. *Soc. Neurosci. Abst., 13,* 800.

Meltzer, H. Y., & Lowy, M. T. (1987). The serotonin hypothesis of depression. In H. Y. Meltzer (Ed.), *Psychopharmacology: The third generation of progress* (pp. 513–526). New York: Raven Press.

Meltzer, H. Y., Lowy, M. T., Goodnick, P., Robertson, A., & Perline, R. (1984c). Effect of 5-hydroxytryptophan on serum cortisol levels in major affective disorders. III. Effect of antidepressants and lithium carbonate. *Arch. Gen. Psych., 41,* 391–397.

Meltzer, H.Y., & Nash, J. F. (1988). Serotonin and mood: Neuroendocrine aspects. In D. Granten & D. Pfaff (Eds.), *Current topics in neuroendocrinology* (pp. 183–210). Heidelberg, Germany: Springer-Verlag.

Meltzer, H.Y., Perline, R., Tricou, B. J., Lowy, M., & Robertson, A. (1984b). Effect of 5-hydroxytryptophan on serum cortisol levels in major affective disorders. II. Relation to suicide, psychosis and depressive symptoms. *Arch. Gen. Psych., 41,* 379–387.

Meltzer, H. Y., Simonovic, M., Fang, V. S., & Goode, D.J. (1981a). Neuroendocrine effects of psychotomimetic drugs. *J. McLean Hosp., 6,* 115–137.

Meltzer, H. Y., Simonovic, M., Sturgeon, R. D., & Fang, V. (1981b). Effects of antidepressants, lithium and electroconvulsive treatment on rat serum prolactin levels. *Acta Psychiat. Scan., 63,* 100–121 (Suppl 290).

Meltzer, H. Y., Umberkoman-Wiita, B., Robertson, A., Tricou, B. J., Lowy, M., & Perline, R. (1984a). Effect of 5-hydroxytryptophan on serum cortisol levels in major affective disorders. I. Enhanced response in depression and mania. *Arch. Gen. Psych., 41,* 366–374.

Meltzer, H. Y., Wiita, B., Tricou, B. J., Simonovic, M., Fang, V., & Manov, G. (1982). Effect of serotonin precursors and serotonin agonists on plasma hormone levels. In B. T. Ho (Ed.), *Serotonin in biological psychiatry* (pp. 117–138). New York: Raven Press.

Meyer, J. S., McElroy, J. F., Yehuda, R., & Miller, J. (1984). Serotonergic stimulation of pituitary-adrenocortical activity in rats: Evidence for multiple sites of action. *Life Sci., 34,* 1891–1898.

Morgan, D. G., May, P. C., & Finch, C. E. (1987). Dopamine and serotonin systems in human and rodent brain: Effects of age and neurodegenerative disease. *J. Am. Geriatric Soc., 35,* 334–345.

Mueller, E. A., Murphy, D. L., & Sunderland, T. (1985). Neuroendocrine effects of m-chlorophenylpiperazine, a serotonin agonist, in human. *J. Clin. Endocrinol. Metab., 61,* 1179–1184.

Mueller, E. A., Murphy, D. L., & Sunderland, T. (1986). Further studies of the putative serotonin agonist, m-chlorophenylpiperazine: Evidence for a serotonin receptor-mediated mechanism of action in humans. *Psychopharm., 89,* 388–391.

Mühlbauer, H. D., & Müller-Oerlinghausen, B. (1985). Fenfluramine stimulation of serum cortisol in patients with major affective disorders and healthy controls: Further evidence for a central serotonergic action of lithium in man. *J. Neural. Transm., 61,* 81–94.

Müller, E. E., Locatelli, V., Cellas, S., Penalva, A., Novelli, A., & Cocchi, D. (1983). Prolactin-lowering and releasing drugs: Mechanisms of action and therapeutic applications. *Drugs, 25,* 399–432.

Murphy, D. L., Campbell, I. C., & Costa, J. L. (1978). The brain serotonergic system in the affective disorders. *Prog. Neuropsychopharmacol., 2,* 1–31.

Nahorski, S. R., & Willcocks, A. L. (1983). Interactions of β-adrenoreceptor antagonists with 5-hydroxytryptamine receptor subtypes in rat cerebral cortex. *Br. J. Pharmacol., 78,* 107P.

Nash, J. F., Meltzer, H. Y., & Gudelsky, G. A. (1988). Antagonism of serotonin receptor mediated neuroendocrine and temperature responses by atypical neuroleptics in the rat. *Eur. J. Pharmacol., 151,* 463–469.

Ng, L. K. Y., Chase, T. N., Colburn, R. W., & Kopin, I. (1972). Release of [³H]dopamine by L-5-hydroxytryptophan. *Brain Res., 45,* 499–505.

Parati, E. A., Zanardi, P., Cocchi, D., Caracini, T., & Müller, E. E. (1980). Neuroendocrine effects of quipazine in man in health state or with neurological disorders. *J. Neural. Transm., 47,* 273–297.

Pardridge, W. M. (1983). Brain metabolism: A perspective from the blood-brainbarrier. *Physiol. Rev., 63,* 1481–1535.

Pazos, A., Hoyer, D., & Palacios, J. M. (1984). The binding of serotonergic ligands to the porcine choroid plexus: Characterization of a new type of serotonin recognition site. *Eur. J. Pharmacol., 106,* 539–546.

Pedigo, N. W., Yamamura, H. I., & Nelson, D. L. (1981). Discrimination of multiple [³H]5-hydroxytryptamine binding sites by the neuroleptic spiperone in rat brain. *J. Neurochem., 36,* 220–226.

Peroutka, S. J. (1985). Selective labeling of 5-HT$_{1A}$ and 5 = HT$_{1B}$ binding sites in bovine brain. *Brain Res., 344,* 167–171.

Peroutka, S. J. (1987). Serotonin receptors. In H. Y. Meltzer (Ed.), *Psychopharmacology: The third generation of progress.* (pp. 303–311). New York: Raven Press.

Peroutka, S. J., & Snyder, S. H. (1979). Multiple serotonin receptors: Differential finding of [³H]5-hydroxytryptamine, [³H]lysergic acid diethylamide and [³H]spiroperidol. *Mol. Pharmacol., 16,* 687–699.

Peroutka, S. J., & Snyder, S. H. (1980). Regulation of serotonin$_2$ (5-HT$_2$) receptors labeled with [³H]spiroperidol by chronic treatment with the antidepressant amitriptyline. *J. Pharmacol. Exp. Ther., 215,* 582–587.

Price, L. H., Charney, D. J., & Heninger, G. R. (1985). Effects of tranylcypromine treatment on neuroendocrine, behavioral, and autonomic responses to tryptophan in depressed patients. *Life Sci., 37,* 809–818.

Quattrone, A., Tedeschi, G., Aguglia, V., Scopacasa, F., Di Renzo, G. E., & Annunziato, L. (1983). Prolactin secretion in man: A useful tool to evaluate the activity of drugs on central 5-hydroxytryptaminergic neurons. Studies with fenfluramine. *Br. J. Clin. Pharmac., 16,* 471–475.

Rivier, C., & Vale, W. (1985). Effects of corticotropin-releasing factor, neurohypophyseal peptides, and catecholamines on pituitary function. *Fed. Proc., 44,* 189–196.

Rowland, N. E., & Carlton, J. (1986). Neurobiology of an anorectic drug: Fenfluramine. *Prog. Neurobiol., 27,* 13–62.

Samanin, R., Mennini, T., Ferraris, A., Bendotti, C., & Borsini, F. (1980). Hyper- and hyposensitivity of central serotonin receptors: [^{3}H]serotonin binding and functional studies in the rat. *Brain Res., 189,* 449–457.

Sachar, E. J., Asnis, G., Halbreich, U., Nathan, R. S., & Halpern, F. (1980). Recent studies in the neuroendocrinology of major depressive disorders. *Psychiatric Clinics of North America, 3,* 313–329.

Scarduelli, C., Matlei, A. M., Brambilla, G., Zavaglia, C., Adelasco, P., Cavioni, V., & Ferrari, C. (1985). Effect of fenfluramine oral administration on serum prolactin levels in healthy and hyperprolactinemic women. *Gynecol. Obstet. Invest., 19,* 92–96.

Siever, L. J., Murphy, D. L., Slater, S., de la Vega, E., & Lipper, S. (1984). Plasma prolactin changes following fenfluramine in depressed patients compared to controls: An evaluation of central serotonergic responsivity in depression. *Life Sci., 34,* 1029–1039.

Sprouse, J. S., & Aghajanian, G. K. (1986). (-)Propranolol blocks the inhibition of serotonergic dorsal raphe cell firing by 5-HT$_{1A}$ selective agonists. *Eur. J. Pharmacol., 128,* 295–298.

Starkman, M. N., Schteingart, D. E., & Schork, M. A. (1986). Cushing's syndrome after treatment: Changes in cortisol and ACTH levels, and amelioration of the depressive syndrome. *Psychiatry Res., 19,* 177–188.

Steinbusch, H. W. M. (1981). Distribution of serotonin immunoreactivity in the central nervous system of the rat: Cell bodies and terminals. *Neurosci., 6,* 557–618.

Sueldo, C. E., Duda, M., & Kletsky, O. A. (1986). Influence of sequential doses of 5-hydroxytryptophan on prolactin release. *Am. J. Obstet. Gynecol., 154,* 424–427.

Swanson, L. W. (1987). *Handbook of chemical neuroanatomy* (pp. 1–104). Vol. 5: Integrated systems of the CNS. Part I. Hypothalamus, hippocampus, amygdala, retina. A. Björkland, T. Hökfelt, & L. W. Swanson (Eds.). New York: Elsevier.

Syvälahti, E., Nagy, A., & van Praag, H. M. (1979). Effects of zimelidine, a selective 5-HT uptake inhibitor, on serum prolactin levels in man. *Psychopharm., 64,* 251–253.

Takahashi, S., Kondo, H., Yoshimura, M., & Ochi, Y. (1974). Growth hormone responses to administration of L-5-hydroxytryptophan (L-5-HTP) in manic-depressive psychoses. Psychoneuroendocrinology Workshop Conf. Int. Soc. Psychoneuroendocrinol. (pp. 32–38), Basel: Karger.

Thomas, G. B., Cummins, J. T., & Clarke, I. J. (1987). Secretion of prolactin in response to serotonin requires an intact hypothalamo-pituitary axis in the ewe. *Neurosci. Lett., 83,* 323–326.

Titler, M., Lyon, R. A., Davis, K. H., & Glennon, R. A. (1987). Selectivity of serotonergic drugs for multiple brain serotonin receptors. Role of [^{3}H]-4-bromo-2,5-dimethoxyphenylisopropylamine ([^{3}H] DOB), a 5-HT$_2$ agonist radioligand. *Biochem. Pharmacol., 36,* 3265–3271.

Trulson, M. E., Eubanks, E. E., & Jacobs, B. L. (1976). Behavioral evidence for supersensitivity following destruction of central serotonergic nerve terminals by 5,7-dihydroxytryptamine. *J. Pharmacol. Exp. Ther., 198,* 23–32.

Tukiainen, E. (1981). Effect of hypophysectomy and adrenalectomy on 5-hydroxytryptamine uptake by rat hypothalamic synaptosomes and blood platelets. *Acta Pharmacol. et Toxicol., 48,* 139–144.

Tuomisto, J., & Männisto, P. (1985). Neurotransmitter regulation of anterior pituitary hormones. *Pharmacol. Res., 37,* 251–332.

Urban, J. H., Van de Kar, L. D., Lorens, S. A., & Bethea, C. L. (1986). Effect of the anxiolytic drug buspirone on prolactin and corticosterone secretion in stressed and unstressed rats. *Pharmacol. Biochem. Behav., 25,* 457–462.

Van de Kar, L. D., Karteszi, M., Bethea, C. L., & Ganong, W. F. (1985). Serotonergic stimulation of prolactin and corticosterone secretion is mediated by different pathways from the mediobasal hypothalamus. *Neuroendocrinol., 41,* 380–385.

Van de Kar, L. D., Wilkinson, C. W., Skrobik, Y., Brownfield, M. S., & Ganong, W. F. (1982). Evidence that serotonergic neurons in the dorsal raphe nucleus exert a stimulatory effect on the secretion of renin but not of corticosterone. *Brain Res., 235,* 233–247.

van Kammen, D. P., & Gelernter, J. (1987). Biochemical instability in schizophrenia. II: The serotonin and gamma-aminobutyric acid systems. In H. Y. Meltzer (Ed.), *Psychopharmacology: The third generation of progress* (pp. 753–758). New York: Raven Press.

van Praag, H. M. (1983). In search of the mode of action of antidepressants. 5-HTP/tyrosine mixtures in depressions. *Neuropharm., 22,* 433–440.

van Praag, H. M., Lemus, C., & Kahn, R. (1987). Hormonal probes of central serotonergic activity: Do they really exist? *Biol. Psych., 22,* 86–98.

van Praag, H. M. (1986). Biological suicide research: Outcome and limitation. *Biol. Psych., 21,* 1305–1323.

Virkkunen, M., Nuutila, A., Goodwin, F. K., & Linnoila, M. (1987). Cerebrospinal fluid monoamine metabolite levels in male arsonists. *Arch. Gen. Psych., 44,* 241–247.

Westenberg, H. G. M., van Praag, H. M., deJong, T. V. M., & Thijssen, J. H. H. (1982). Postsynaptic activity in depressive serotonergic patients: Evaluation of the neuroendocrine strategy. *Psych. Res., 7,* 361–371.

Whitford, G. M. (1986). Alzheimer's disease and serotonin: A review. *Pharmacopsych., 15,* 133–142.

Willner, P. (1985). Antidepressants and serotonergic neurotransmission: An integrative review. *Psychopharm., 85,* 387–404.

Willoughby, J. O., Menadue, M. F., & Liebelt, H. J. (1988). Activation of 5-HT-1 serotonin receptors in the medial basal hypothalamus stimulates prolactin secretion in the unanesthetized rat. *Neuroendocrinol., 47,* 83–87.

Winokur, A., Lindberg, N. D., Lucki, I., Phillips, J., & Amsterdam, J. D. (1986).

Hormonal and behavioral effects associated with intravenous L-tryptophan administration. *Psychopharm., 88,* 213–219.

Wong, D. F., Lever, J.R., Hartig, P. R., Dannals, R. F., Villemagne, V., Hoffman, B. J., Wilson, A. A., Ravert, H. T., Links, J. M., Scheffel, U., & Wagner, H. T., Jr. (1987). Localization of serotonin 5-HT$_2$ receptors in living human brain positron emission tomography using N1-([^{11}C]-methyl)-2-Br-LSD. *Synapse, 1,* 393–398.

Yap, C. Y., & Taylor, D. A. (1983). Involvement of 5-HT$_2$ receptors in the wet-dog shake behavior induced by 5-hydroxytryptophan in the rat. *Neuropharm., 22,* 801–804.

Zohar, J., & Insel, T. R. (1987). Obsessive-compulsive disorder: Psychobiological approaches to diagnosis, treatment, and pathophysiology. *Biol. Psych., 22,* 667–687.

Zohar, J., Insel, T. R., Zohar-Kadouch, R. C., Hill, J. L., & Murphy, D. L. (1988). Serotonergic responsivity in obsessive-compulsive disorder. Effects of chronic clomipramine treatment. *Arch. Gen. Psych., 45,* 167–172.

Zohar, J., Mueller, E. A., Insel, T. R., Zohar-Kadouch, R. C., & Murphy, D. L. (1987). Serotonergic responsitivity in obsessive-compulsive disorder. Comparisons of patients and healthy controls. *Arch. Gen. Psych., 44,* 946–951.

5

The Monoamine
Hypothesis
of Depression
The Case for Serotonin

SERENA-LYNN BROWN

AVRAHAM BLEICH

HERMAN M. VAN PRAAG

With the discovery several decades ago that both the tricyclic antidepressants (TCAs) and the monoamine oxidase (MAO) inhibitors provide clinical efficacy in the treatment of depression, and the subsequent demonstration that imipramine and amitriptyline inhibit in vivo monoamine (MA) uptake in MAergic nerve cells in the central nervous system (CNS) (Glowinski & Axelrod, 1964), the monoamine hypothesis of depression was proposed (Bunney & Davis, 1965; Schildkraut, 1965). This hypothesis suggests that at least some depressions result from an absolute or relative deficiency of MAs, and particularly norepinephrine (NE), at functionally important brain receptor sites. Van Praag and Leijnse (1963a, 1963b), Coppen (1967), and subsequently Maas (1975) extended this hypothesis to include the important role of a proposed deficiency of serotonin, or 5-hydroxytryptamine (5-HT), in this disorder. This suggested the possibility that some depressed patients had more of a "noradrenergic" depression, whereas others had more of a "serotonergic" depression (Maas, 1975).

Over the last 25 years, research into the biology of depression proliferated. As the role of the MAs in depression was investigated further, several problems with the monamine hypothesis emerged: (1) There is a significantly delayed onset of clinical response after antidepressant treatment. Whereas MAO inhibition and the NE or 5-HT reuptake blockade effects of the antidepressants occur within hours of initial administration, clinical improvement usually requires between one and four weeks of treatment (Iversen & Mackay, 1979; Stahl, 1984). (2) Several drugs that appear to have no effect on MA reuptake, such as mianserin (Goodlet et al., 1977) and iprindole (Gluckman & Baum, 1969; Lahti & Maickel, 1971), nevertheless are effective antidepressants (Zis & Goodwin, 1979; Sugrue, 1983a, 1983b). (3) Compounds that have been shown to be effective MA reuptake inhibitors, such as amphetamines and cocaine, do not possess effective antidepressant properties (Overall et al., 1962; Post et al., 1974; Heninger & Charney, 1982; Sugrue, 1983a).

Such clinical data suggest that the therapeutic efficacy of antidepressant treatment (TCAs, MAO inhibitors, atypical antidepressants, and electroconvulsive therapy, or ECS) may not be elucidated by preclinical examination of the short-term effects of these compounds upon NE or 5-HT availability. Therefore, more recently, investigators have focused upon specific receptor changes induced by chronic administration of various antidepressants, with emphasis upon the NEergic and the 5-HTergic systems. Other researchers have examined both presynaptic and postsynaptic parameters in drug-free as well as medicated depressed patients, in the attempt to determine the role played by these neurotransmitter receptor systems in depressive disorder.

PRESYNAPTIC 5-HT FUNCTION

5-HT Metabolism

Postmortem Brain Studies

The direct analysis of levels of 5-HT and its primary metabolite 5-hydroxyindoleacetic acid (5-HIAA) provides a crude means of assessing 5-HT metabolism in postmortem brain specimens of depressed patients or of suicide victims. Data from such studies, however, are difficult to interpret because of the differences in type of control group, cause of death, length of drug-free interval before death, age, food intake, time elapsing between death and autopsy, regions of brain sampled, and dissection and laboratory techniques utilized.

The majority of investigators have shown a reduction in levels of 5-HT and 5-HIAA in midbrain raphe nuclei (the major loci of 5-HT-containing neuronal cell bodies) in postmortem brain specimens of depressed patients who died of natural causes and suicide victims (Shaw et al., 1967; Bourne et al., 1968; Lloyd et al., 1974; Birkmayer & Riederer, 1975; Beskow et al., 1976; Cochran et al., 1976). In contrast to these relatively consistent findings in the raphe nuclei, no consistent findings have been reported in forebrain areas (Lloyd et al., 1974; Beskow et al., 1976; Cochran et al., 1976; Korpi et al., 1986).

It should be noted, however, that most of the investigated subjects died as a consequence of suicide, and a body of data is accumulating that suggests the possibility that the psychopathological correlate of 5-HT dysfunction might be suicidality itself, rather than depression per se, irrespective of diagnosis (van Praag et al., 1987a).

Cerebrospinal Fluid Studies

Another means of investigating CNS 5-HT metabolism in humans involves measurement of 5-HIAA in the cerebrospinal fluid (CSF). Baseline CSF 5-HIAA has been measured, as well as 5-HIAA accumulation after the administration of probenecid, which inhibits the transport of 5-HIAA from the CNS, including the CSF, to the bloodstream. Probenecid-induced 5-HIAA accumulation in the CSF is considered to provide a crude indication of 5-HT metabolism in the CNS as a whole. With appropriate doses of probenecid, almost complete inhibition of the active transport of 5-HIAA is achieved (Emanuelsson et al., 1987). Thus, postprobenecid CSF 5-HIAA is thought to reflect some degree of presynaptic 5-HT function, although, of course, CSF formation and absorption processes also play a role in determining the concentration of this metabolite.

Most investigators have found decreased postprobenecid 5-HIAA accumulation in the CSF of depressed patients as compared with normals, suggesting decreased 5-HT metabolism (van Praag et al., 1970; Sjostrom, 1973; van Praag et al., 1973a, 1973b; Bowers, 1974a). It has also been suggested that decreased CSF 5-HIAA may be correlated with severity of depression (Coppen et al., 1972b; Goodwin et al., 1973; Bowers, 1974a; Asberg et al., 1976a; Banki, 1977; Agren, 1980a, 1980b).

Over the past decade, a number of researchers have demonstrated a high correlation between decreased CSF 5-HIAA and history of suicide attempts, especially those that involve a violent component (Asberg et al., 1976a, 1976b; Oreland et al., 1981; Traskman et al., 1981; van Praag, 1982a, 1982b; Agren, 1983; Roy-Byrne et al., 1983). Since a correlation between CSF 5-HIAA and suicidality has also been demonstrated among schizophrenics and nondepressed patients with a variety of personality disorders, these findings may indicate that the psychopathological correlate of decreased CSF 5-HIAA might involve suicidality, regardless of the psychiatric diagnosis (van Praag, 1986a).

Effects of Antidepressant Treatment

Investigators have consistently found decreased CSF 5-HIAA in depressed patients after chronic administration of antidepressant medications, including the TCAs, atypical antidepressants, and MAO inhibitors (Papeschi & McClure, 1971; Kupfer & Bowers, 1972; Bowers, 1974b; Post & Goodwin, 1974; Bertilsson et al., 1976; Siwers et al., 1976; Asberg et al., 1977; Traskman et al., 1979; Mendlewicz et al., 1982). ECS has not been shown to produce consistent changes in CSF 5-HIAA (Ashcroft et al., 1966; Bowers et al., 1969; Nordin et al., 1971; Abrams et al., 1976).

Plasma Tryptophan

Tryptophan is the primary dietary precursor of 5-HT. It is taken up actively by the CNS, and other neutral amino acids, including tyrosine, phenylalanine, leucine, isoleucine, and valine, compete for the same transport mechanism. Thus, levels of CNS tryptophan are a function of the ratio of plasma tryptophan to the plasma levels of these competing amino acids (Wurtman, 1982). Tryptophan availability is one of the major factors determining the rate of 5-HT synthesis in the CNS.

A few preliminary investigations have reported that, in a subgroup of depressed patients (particularly those with endogenous features), the plasma ratio of tryptophan to competing amino acids is decreased (Moller et al., 1976, 1980; Moller & Kirk, 1981). A reduced plasma tryptophan ratio would give rise to a reduction of tryptophan influx into and availability within the CNS, and would lead to lowered 5-HT synthesis. No studies correlating plasma tryptophan and CSF 5-HIAA have been published.

Regulation of 5-HT Release

The release of 5-HT into the synaptic cleft is assumed to be under the control of presynaptic 5-HTergic inhibitory autoreceptors (Haigler & Aghajanian, 1974). Decreased sensitivity of these receptors increases 5-HT release, whereas increased sensitivity decreases 5-HT release. As of yet, only animal data are available on this subject. A number of investigators have reported increased 5-HT concentration in rodent brain after electroconvulsive shock (ECS) (Breitner et al., 1961; 1964; Essman, 1968, 1973). Recently, Goodwin et al. (1985) showed that in mice a wide range of antidepressant drugs and ECS decrease the response mediated by presynaptic 5-HT (possibly 5-HT_{1A}) autoreceptors. Essman (1986) has also demonstrated that ECS produces increased density of presynaptic 5-HT_1, but not 5-HT_2 receptor sites.

5-HT Uptake, ³H-Imipramine Binding, and 5-HT₂ Binding

Over the past decade, the human blood platelet, which is a neuroectodermal derivative, has emerged as a peripheral model for the study of the transport, storage, metabolism, and release of 5-HT by 5-HTergic nerve endings (Sneddon, 1973; Stahl, 1977). Because of biochemical and morphological similarities between platelets and CNS 5-HT synapses, and because of data suggesting that virtually all 5-HT in blood is associated with the platelets (Yuwiler et al., 1981), it is felt that direct evaluation of 5-HT uptake can be obtained by measuring incorporation of radiolabeled 5-HT into human platelets or synaptosomal preparations.

Platelet 5-HT Uptake

The human blood platelet possesses a high-affinity active transport system that is thought to be coupled to the sodium/potassium ATPase system and to be related to and dependent on intracellular sodium concentration (Sneddon, 1969; Stahl & Meltzer, 1978). The kinetic parameters of this system are V_{max}, indicating the number of carrier molecules, and K_m, a measure of the affinity of the carrier molecules for 5-HT. This transport system closely resembles the reuptake mechanism for 5-HT in 5-HTergic nerve terminals (Sneddon, 1973; Tuomisto et al., 1979).

During the past 10 years, investigators have consistently found that platelet 5-HT uptake is reduced in unmedicated depressed patients (Tuomisto, 1974; Hallstrom et al., 1976; Mulgirigama, 1976; Tuomisto & Tukiainen, 1976; Coppen et al., 1981; Tuomisto et al., 1979; Born et al., 1980; Mirkin & Coppen, 1980; Meltzer et al., 1981; Wood et al., 1983a; Suranyi-Cadotte et al., 1985). All of these groups have shown decreased platelet 5-HT uptake, expressed by a decrease in active transport, or V_{max}, with no change in affinity, or K_m, although Kaplan and Mann (1982) have shown an increase in affinity in unmedicated depressed patients.

It should be noted that there are accumulating data suggesting that circadian rhythmicity may be a prominent factor influencing 5-HT uptake dynamics in depressed patients (Oxenkrug et al., 1978; Wirz-Justice & Puhringer, 1978; Rausch et al., 1982; Humphries et al., 1985; Modai et al., 1986). Other investigators have reported seasonal variations in platelet 5-HT uptake in normal and depressed patients (Swade & Coppen, 1981; Arora et al., 1984; Egrise et al., 1986).

Effects of Antidepressant Treatment

Data on the effects of antidepressant treatment on 5-HT uptake have generally shown that TCAs, zimelidine, and lithium cause a (further) decrease in platelet 5-HT uptake after several weeks of treatment (Coppen & Wood, 1980; Ross et al., 1980; Coppen et al., 1981; Meltzer et al., 1981, 1983a; Willner 1985). On the other hand, some investigators have reported no significant change in or normalization of 5-HT uptake after antidepressant treatments such as TCAs, atypical antidepressants, ECS, and lithium (Tuomisto et al., 1979; Born et al., 1980; Giret et al., 1980; Meltzer et al.,

1981; Wood et al., 1983b; Suranyi-Cadotte et al., 1985; Healy & Leonard, 1987).

It should be noted that although the human blood platelet is generally accepted as a peripheral model for the study of 5-HTergic nerve endings, the exact relationship between platelet 5-HT uptake and synaptic kinetic parameters, and thus the functional significance of findings concerning platelet 5-HT uptake, is not clear at this time.

³H-Imipramine Binding Sites

Recently, high-affinity and saturable binding sites for ³H-imipramine have been found on human platelets and on 5-HT nerve terminals. These sites appear to be specific for TCAs and their active metabolites, and seem to have a functional relationship with the 5-HT uptake or transport site, probably modulating inhibition of 5-HT uptake.

Most investigators have found a consistent and significant decrease in platelet ³H-imipramine binding in unmedicated depressed patients, as compared with controls. This decrease in binding has been expressed as a decrease in B_{max}, or number of binding sites, without change in K_d, or affinity of the binding sites for the ligand (Asarch et al., 1980; Briley et al., 1980; Coppen & Wood, 1980; Paul et al., 1981; Raisman et al., 1981, 1982; Kaplan & Mann, 1982; Baron et al., 1983; Langer & Raisman, 1983; Stanley & Mann, 1983; Suranyi-Cadotte et al., 1983, 1985; Wood et al., 1983a; Roy et al., 1987). One team of investigators recently reported both a decrease in B_{max} and a slight decrease in apparent affinity of binding for platelets of such individuals (Innis et al., 1987). Several other investigators, however, have failed to find differences in platelet ³H-imipramine binding between depressives and controls (Whitaker et al., 1984; Tang & Morris, 1985; Carstens et al., 1986; Egrise et al., 1986).

Effect of Antidepressant Treatment

The few studies of the effects of chronic antidepressant treatment on platelet ³H-imipramine binding in humans have produced variable results. In normal subjects, platelet ³H-imipramine binding sites were shown to be decreased after clomipramine (Poirier et al., 1987) and increased after desipramine (Cowen et al., 1986). Studies with depressed patients show the same variability. While one study found no effect of chronic TCA treatment on ³H-imipramine binding in depressed patients (Langer & Raisman, 1983), another study has shown the opposite (Suranyi-Cadotte et al., 1985), and a more recent study has demonstrated increased B_{max} with 5-HT uptake blockers, not returning to baseline even when patients had been drug-free and clinically recovered one to two years later (Wagner et al., 1987).

Several groups of investigators have examined ³H-imipramine binding in postmortem brain specimens of depressed individuals (who died either from natural causes or as a consequence of suicide) and normal controls, and have shown a reduction in the number of ^{3}H-imipramine binding sites in the depressed group that was unrelated to age, delay of assay, type of terminal illness, or cause of death (Langer et al., 1981). Perry et al. (1983), Stanley et al. (1982), and Stanley and Mann (1983) have also reported a decrease in presynaptic ^{3}H–imipramine binding sites in the hippocampus and occipital cortex of suicide victims. These findings, however, were not replicated by Meyerson et al. (1982). Problems with postmortem brain studies have been referred to above.

It should be noted that, at present, the exact role of the platelet ^{3}H-imipramine binding site and its functional relationship to both its central counterpart (the 5-HT nerve ending) and specific modulation of platelet 5-HT uptake have not been clearly elucidated. Whereas the ^{3}H–imipramine binding site is believed to be associated with the 5-HT reuptake site in membranes of both platelet and brain, until more work is done in this area, we can only speculate about the significance of such findings.

Platelet 5-HT$_2$ Receptor Binding

Several recent studies have examined platelet 5-HT$_2$ receptor binding. Using ^{3}H–ketanserin, Biegon et al. (1987) demonstrated increased B$_{max}$ with no change in K$_d$ in patients with major depression, with a decrease of B$_{max}$ to control levels after four weeks of treatment with antidepressants. Arora and Meltzer (1989) also found increased B$_{max}$ without change in K$_d$ in the platelets of depressed patients as compared with normal controls using ^{3}H-lysergic acid diethylamide, but noted that this increase in B$_{max}$ was based on data from only the female depressed patients. This is an avenue of study that warrants further development.

POSTSYNAPTIC 5-HT RECEPTOR FUNCTION

5-HT Receptor Binding

5-HT receptors differ according to their central or peripheral location, their occurrence on neurons or on other cells (e.g., platelets), and their location either presynaptically or postsynaptically. 5-HT receptors in brain have been divided into three subtypes—5-HT$_1$, 5-HT$_2$, and 5-HT$_3$—by binding studies utilizing different radioligands (Peroutka et al., 1981; Peroutka, 1989). Chapter 2 of this book provides a full description of the differences between these receptor subtypes. Our present understanding of the functional significance of the different 5-HT receptor subtypes is far from complete.

Several postmortem brain studies of suicide victims have reported increased density of postsynaptic 5-HT$_2$ receptors (McKeith et al., 1987), along with reduced density of presynaptic imipramine binding sites in frontal cortex (Stanley et al., 1982; Stanley & Mann, 1983; Mann et al., 1986).

Effects of Antidepressant Treatment

Only animal data are available at this time concerning the effects of antidepressant treatment on brain 5-HT$_1$ and 5-HT$_2$ receptors. Chronic TCA treatment (Peroutka & Snyder, 1980; Fuxe et al., 1982; Stolz et al., 1983; Stockmeier & Kellar, 1986), treatment with MAO inhibitors (Peroutka & Snyder, 1980; Kellar et al., 1981; Koshikawa et al., 1985), and treatment with atypical antidepressants (Peroutka & Snyder, 1980; Fuxe et al., 1982; Stolz et al., 1983) consistently cause a decrease in postsynaptic 5-HT$_2$ receptor binding. In contrast, ECS treatment has been shown to cause an increase in 5-HT$_2$ receptor binding (Kellar et al., 1981; Vetulani et al., 1981; Stockmeier & Kellar, 1986).

In general, no change has been seen in 5-HT$_1$ receptor binding with the administration of a wide range of TCA and atypical antidepressant medications or ECS (Peroutka & Snyder, 1980; Blackshear & Sanders-Bush, 1982; Fuxe et al., 1982; Lucki & Frazer, 1982; Stolz et al., 1983) although MAO inhibitors (Peroutka & Snyder, 1980; Lucki & Frazer, 1982) and two atypical antidepressants, mianserin (Segawa et al., 1982) and zimelidine (Fuxe et al., 1979, 1981), have been found to cause decreased binding to these receptors.

Challenge Studies

The neuroendocrine challenge or probe provides a "window" on central MA function, enabling investigators to evaluate receptor function indirectly in vivo. This paradigm involves the administration of a selective 5-HT agonist or antagonist, with subsequent ongoing measurements of pituitary hormones thought to be under 5-HTergic control, such as ACTH, cortisol, prolactin, and growth hormone. It is believed that the magnitude of the hormonal response provides an indirect measurement of 5-HT receptor sensitivity or function.

The studies conducted on depressed patients are limited in number and have provided variable results. The biochemical challengers generally used have been the 5-HT precursors L-tryptophan and 5-hydroxytryptophan (5-HTP), both thought to cause an increase in 5-HT synthesis and function, and thus both expected to produce an elevated release of the aforementioned hormones. However, neither L-tryptophan nor 5-HTP is 5-HT selective. Both influence catecholamine (CA) metabolism significantly and differentially. L-tryptophan appears either to have no effect or, in high doses, to cause a decrease in CA synthesis and function, probably owing to decreased influx of tyrosine into the CNS because of competition with tryptophan for the same carrier mechanism (Wurtman, 1982; van Praag et al., 1987b).

5-HTP, however, increases both 5-HT and NE synthesis. 5-HTP is decarboxylated to 5-HT by the nonspecific enzyme aromatic amino-acid decarboxylase. This enzyme is not specific to the 5-HT neurons. It is believed that 5-HTP is converted to 5-HT in catecholaminergic neurons, ultimately acting as a false transmitter. CA metabolism is thought to increase as a consequence. The net effect of increased CA synthesis and false transmitter production is probably increased CA function.

Prolactin

Depressed patients have been reported to show a blunted release of prolactin in response to administration of high intravenous doses of L-tryptophan, interpreted as attributable to subsensitive postsynaptic 5-HT receptors (Charney et al., 1984; Heninger et al., 1984), although some investigators have found no significant change in the prolactin response to considerably lower doses of L-tryptophan or to 5-HTP (Kato et al., 1974; Handwerger et al., 1975; Woolf & Lee, 1977; Wiebe et al., 1977; Fraser et al., 1979; Hyyppa et al., 1979; Glass et al., 1980; Charney et al., 1982; Westenberg et al., 1982). Similarly, intravenous administration of high dosages of 5-HTP after pretreatment with a peripheral decarboxylase inhibitor appears to cause an increased release of prolactin in normals (Lancranjan et al., 1977; van Praag, 1983). In depressed patients, oral 5-HTP administration seems to have no effect on serum prolactin concentrations (Westenberg et al., 1982; Meltzer et al., 1983).

Fenfluramine (considered to be a 5-HT–agonistic compound during short-term usage through increased release and decreased uptake) has also been shown to produce a blunted prolactin response in 18 depressed patients, compared with 10 normal controls (Siever et al., 1984), although this finding was not replicated in a recent study (Asnis et al., 1988).

Chronic treatment with amitriptyline or desipramine (Charney et al., 1984) and with tranylcypromine (Price et al., 1985a) has been shown to produce an enhanced prolactin response to L-tryptophan in depressed patients. Charney et al. (1984) have postulated that such long-term antidepressant treatment may cause enhancement of postsynaptic 5-HT receptor sensitivity through compensatory changes in receptor function and chronic postsynaptic receptor blockade (e.g., with amitriptyline), or via effects on the NE system (e.g., with desipramine), or at the level of the effector system itself (e.g., 5-HT–sensitive adenylate cyclase). It has also been reported that lithium enhances the prolactin response to fenfluramine administration in depressed individuals (Slater et al., 1976), and its short-term, but not long-term, administration enhances the prolactin response to L-tryptophan in such patients (Price et al., 1983). Shapira et al. (1989) also have shown that imipramine enhances the prolactin response to fenfluramine in depressed patients.

Cortisol.

In depressed patients, oral 5-HTP has been reported to produce significantly enhanced serum cortisol levels, which has been interpreted as a possible consequence of 5-HT postsynaptic receptor hypersensitivity (Meltzer et al., 1983c; Meltzer 1984). On the other hand, it has also been reported that there is no change in plasma cortisol in depressed patients after administration of L-tryptophan and 5-HTP (Westenberg et al., 1982). A possible explanation for such a discrepancy in data involves differences in the 5-HTP dosage utilized, so that higher doses of 5-HTP used in the second study may have produced increased synthesis of NE, thus inhibiting cortisol (van Praag et al., 1987b).

Meltzer (1984) has further attempted to assess the effects of various antidepressant compounds on the cortisol response to 5-HTP in depressed patients. Whereas the members of his group found an enhanced cortisol response to 5-HTP after a three- to five-week course of treatment with lithium or MAO inhibitors, they also showed that the cortisol response was reduced after the same period of treatment with TCAs (Meltzer et al., 1984a). These data are contradictory and appear to be uninterpretable at this time.

Growth Hormone

One early preliminary report that 5-HTP produces a blunted growth hormone (GH) response in depressed patients (Takahashi et al., 1976) could not be confirmed by another recent study that demonstrated no changes in plasma GH after either L-tryptophan or 5-HTP in depressed patients (Westenberg et al., 1982).

Thus, because of the limited number of neuroendocrine challenge studies in depressed patients, and the variability of the results obtained, few definitive answers have been found. Van Praag et al. (1987b) recently reviewed the present state of 5-HT challenge studies, delineating two major pitfalls: nonselectivity of the 5-HT biochemical challengers generally utilized and noncomparability of studies because of variations in dosage and route of administration of the challenging agents.

Electrophysiological Studies

To investigate 5-HTergic transmission directly, electrophysiological single-unit recording studies have been utilized to evaluate postsynaptic responses to iontophoretically applied neurotransmitter (5-HT). These studies have been conducted on animal preparations only and involve the measurement of the effects of antidepressant treatments.

Chronic antidepressant treatments such as TCAs (deMontigny & Aghajanian, 1978; Gallager & Bunney, 1979; Menkes & Aghajanian, 1981), atypical antidepressants such as iprindole and mianserin (Menkes & Aghajanian, 1981; Blier & deMontigny, 1984), and ECS (deMontigny, 1984) have all been shown to enhance postsynaptic response to iontophoretically applied 5-HT. Such an enhanced postsynaptic response has also been reported after iontophoretic administration of 5-methoxy-dimethyltryptamine (5-MeO-DMT), a direct postsynaptic receptor agonist that is not a substrate of the 5-HT reuptake system. Thus, this phenomenon may reflect supersensitivity of the postsynaptic 5-HT receptor, and not an effect of increased availability of the neurotransmitter in the synaptic cleft. It should be noted, however, that these observations of enhanced responsiveness were all related to subcortical areas, and not to cortex (Olpe & Schellenberg, 1981), which might suggest antidepressant variability of action on 5-HT receptors in different regions of the brain. These findings are in contrast to receptor binding data showing that chronic antidepressant treatment causes a reduction in postsynaptic 5-HT$_2$ receptor binding.

Behavioral Studies

The evaluation of behavioral models, particularly the "serotonin syndrome" in rats (defined by Straub tail, piloerection, hindlimb abduction or rigidity, lateral head weaving, tremor, hyperactivity, salivation, and repetitive forepaw treading) (Grahame-Smith, 1971; Jacobs, 1976; Sloviter et al., 1978), believed to express 5-HT function in the CNS, has provided another means of indirectly evaluating the degree of responsivity of this neurotransmitter system (Charney et al., 1981; Willner, 1985). Such studies have been done in animals, measuring the effects of antidepressant treatment on these variables.

Chronic administration of antidepressant treatments such as TCAs (Friedman & Dallob, 1979; Mogilnicka & Klimek, 1979; Jones, 1980; Fuxe et al., 1982; Lucki & Frazer, 1982; Stolz et al., 1983), atypical antidepressants (Mogilnicka & Klimek, 1979; Jones, 1980; Fuxe et al., 1983), ECS (Green et al., 1977; Vetulani et al., 1981) but not MAO inhibitors (Lucki & Frazer, 1982) was found to enhance the effect of 5-HT precursors such as L-tryptophan and 5-HTP and direct 5-HT agonists such as 5-MeO-DMT on the aforementioned behaviors.

Treatment Studies

5-HT Precursors

Tryptophan

The results of using L-tryptophan as an antidepressant treatment have been equivocal, as some investigators have shown antidepressant efficacy whereas others have not (Coppen et al., 1972a; Murphy et al., 1974; Dunner & Fieve, 1975; Jenssen et al., 1975; Mendels et al., 1975; Farkas et al., 1976; Herrington et al., 1976; Rao & Broadhurst, 1976; Wirz-Justice, 1977; Chouinard et al., 1979; Cooper, 1979; Growdon, 1979; Lindberg et al., 1979; Cole et al., 1980; Thomson et al., 1982; van Praag, 1986a, 1987c). It has been proposed that inadequacy of study design, heterogeneity of patients, lack of control of plasma concentrations of other competing neutral amino acids, interactions with concurrently administered antidepressant medications, and dosage either above or below the "therapeutic window" found for L-tryptophan might account for the lack of clear answers concerning the use of this primary 5-HT precursor in the treatment of depression (Gelenberg et al., 1982). However, it has been demonstrated that L-tryptophan can potentiate the antidepressant effects of MAO inhibitors (Coppen et al., 1963), clomipramine (Walinder et al., 1976), and ECS (D'Elia et al., 1977; Raotma, 1978), although it should also be noted that, clinically, it is contraindicated to give L-tryptophan along with an MAO inhibitor because of possible hypertensive side effects or LSD-like decompensation. In addition, because of the recently identified "eosinophilia-myalgia syndrome" seen in some patients taking L-tryptophan (Claurn et al., 1990; Hertzmen et al., 1990), this dietary supplement has been recalled by the FDA, and such studies are no longer in progress, awaiting an explanation for the etiology of this association.

5-HTP

Results on the efficacy of 5-HTP in the treatment of depression are more clear cut. It has been reported that 5-HTP has effective antidepressant activity, both acutely and, possibly, prophylactically (Sano, 1972; Angst et al., 1977; van Hiele, 1980), although a few researchers who utilized short-term treatment have questioned such efficacy (Brodie et al., 1973; Takahashi et al., 1976). Van Praag (1984) conducted a double-blind comparison of 5-HTP and L-tryptophan in the treatment of depression, and found that 5-HTP treatment was significantly more effective than either L-tryptophan or placebo.

The antidepressant efficacy of 5-HTP has been found to be potentiated by tyrosine, the CA precursor of both NE and DA (van Praag, 1983), suggesting that its net effect is to increase both 5-HT and CA synthesis and function, and that this combined effect is responsible for its antidepressant efficacy. The fact that high dosages of tryptophan decrease CA synthesis might be another possible explanation for the relative ineffectiveness of tryptophan as an antidepressant as compared with 5-HTP.

Several other studies have shown superior clinical efficacy of 5-HTP in combination with antidepressants, particularly with clomipramine, and possibly with the MAO inhibitors (van Praag et al., 1974; Lopez-Ibor et al., 1976) in comparison with either agent alone. It should be noted that, in the above treatment studies, 5-HTP was generally administered concurrently with a peripheral decarboxylase inhibitor, in order to reduce the required dosage and thus side effects. Finally, it should be noted that several investigators have observed that the administration of 5-HTP to normal subjects can produce euphoria (Trimble et al., 1975; Puhringer et al., 1976a, 1976b), further lending evidence to the proposed mood-elevating effects of 5-HTP.

A possible explanation for this disparity between these two 5-HT precursors' antidepressant efficacy involves the differential effect of these two compounds on the CAergic system. Whereas high doses of L-tryptophan may cause a decrease in central CA synthesis by reducing the ratio of tyrosine to the competing amino acids, the administration of 5-HTP has been shown to cause an increase in the metabolism of 5-HT, DA, and NE, thus raising CAergic as well as 5-HTergic tone (van Praag et al., 1987b). It has been postulated that these dual effects may provide the best conditions for antidepressant activity.

5-HT Depleting Agents
pCPA

Parachlorophenylalanine (pCPA) is a tryptophan hydroxylase inhibitor that causes a significant decrease in central 5-HT and 5-HIAA in animals and humans (Cremata & Koe, 1966; Koe & Weissman, 1966; Goodwin & Post, 1973, 1975). In one study to date, pCPA was reported to cause an increase in depressive symptomatology in depressed patients, and to antagonize the therapeutic effects of the MAO inhibitor tranylcypromine (Shopsin et al., 1976).

Fenfluramine

Fenfluramine, an anorectic agent, is known to cause a rapid release of 5-HT at the synapse, to inhibit 5-HT uptake, and to have weak direct agonist activity at the 5-HT receptor (Murphy et al., 1986). Longer-term administration of fenfluramine has been found to reduce central 5-HT and 5-HIAA levels (Shoulson & Chase, 1975; Clineschmidt et al., 1978). Ward et al. (1985) have reported that fenfluramine may possess some antidepressant efficacy based on a short-term study of a small group of depressed patients, although this may well be attributable to its acute 5-HT agonistic effects, and longer-term treatment and follow-up in such a study are required to elucidate this more fully.

"Selective" 5-HT Agents and Lithium Augmentation

The 5-HT reuptake inhibitors have been described as indirect 5-HT agonists. These agents enhance 5-HTergic transmission by increasing the concentration of 5-HT available postsynaptically, inhibiting inactivation of the neurotransmitter through uptake back into the nerve terminal, and producing most of the same effects as direct agonists while being dependent on neuronal 5-HT release for their actions (Fuller, 1986).

Zimelidine, the best-documented selective 5-HT reuptake inhibitor, was released and then withdrawn from the market because of its severe side effects. Zimelidine and its primary metabolite norzimelidine have been shown to be potent 5-HT uptake blockers; norzimelidine also possesses weak NE uptake blockade effects (Bertilsson et al., 1980; Asberg et al., 1986). This drug has been shown to downregulate both 5-HT$_1$ and 5-HT$_2$ receptors with differential affinities of binding (Fuxe et al., 1983). The antidepressant effects of zimelidine have been demonstrated to be superior to placebo (Norman et al., 1983) and comparable to imipramine (Meredith & Feighner, 1983), amitriptyline (Claghorn et al., 1983), desipramine (Aberg-Wistedt, 1982), and maprotilene (Nystrom & Hallstrom, 1985).

Fluvoxamine is a potent and selective presynaptic 5-HT reuptake inhibitor, structurally dissimilar from the tricyclics, with little NE uptake inhibition at normal doses (Claassen et al., 1977), and high 5-HT$_2$ receptor affinity (Ogren et al., 1979; Maj, 1981; Fuller, 1987). This compound has been shown to possess clinical efficacy comparable to that of imipramine (Norton et al., 1984; Dominguez et al., 1985) and clomipramine (Klok et al., 1981; DeWilde et al., 1983; Dick & Ferrero, 1983), and to be superior to placebo (Cottevanger, 1984; Benfield & Ward, 1986; Mendels, 1987), particularly when clinical trials of longer than four weeks are utilized (Quitkin et al., 1984; Asberg et al., 1986).

Fluoxetine, released in the United States in the late 1980's and now widely prescribed, possesses pharmacological properties similar to those shown by fluvoxamine, and has also been shown to have an antidepressant effect comparable to that of imipramine or amitriptyline and superior to placebo (Bremner, 1984; Chouinard, 1985; Cohn & Wilcox, 1985; Stark & Hardison, 1985).

Clomipramine, recently released for use in the United States, is a potent 5-HT reuptake blocker. However, its primary metabolite, clordesipramine, possesses potent NE uptake inhibitory properties (Fuller, 1987), but its effects on 5-HT receptor subtypes have not been demonstrated (Lucki & Frazer, 1982; Willner, 1985).

Trazodone, an antidepressant with proved efficacy (Kane & Lieberman, 1984) that is widely prescribed in both the United States and abroad, is both a 5-HT uptake blocker and a 5-HT receptor agonist (Maj et al., 1979), and it has adrenergic effects as well (Richelson & Nelson, 1984). At the same time, the primary metabolite of trazodone, m-chlorophenylpiperazine (mCPP), is known to be a highly selective 5-HT$_1$ agonist (Mueller et al.,

1985). Thus, it can be seen that one medication can act at several different locations within the synapse, and the net effect on neuronal transmission represents a summation of these various actions.

At the present time, several other "selective" 5-HT compounds are under clinical investigation (Asberg et al., 1986; Mendels, 1987). These include 5-HT uptake blockers such as femoxetine, paroxetine, cianopramine, citalopram, and sertraline.

The recent availability for human use of selective and/or potent 5-HT$_2$ receptor antagonists, including ketanserin, ritanserin, setoperone, pirenpirone, and altanserin (Janssen, 1985; Fuller, 1986), may allow the further exploration of the 5-HT receptor function and its clinical correlates in depression.

It should be noted that cyproheptadine, another 5-HT$_2$ antagonist, has shown some efficacy in improving both eating behavior and depressive symptomatology in a study of anorectics and bulimics (Halmi et al., 1986), although much further work remains to be done in the area of depression.

Recently, lithium, which possesses moderate antidepressant efficacy on its own (Ramsey & Mendels, 1981), has been shown also to augment significantly clinical response to TCAs, MAO inhibitors, or a combination of the two (Price et al., 1983, 1985a, 1985b; Nelson & Mazure, 1986; Thompson & Thomas, 1986). It is currently believed that lithium may enhance 5-HT transmission across the synapse (deMontigny et al., 1981), either by presynaptic effects, such as increasing the uptake of tryptophan or 5-HTP into 5-HTergic nerve endings, thus presumably increasing 5-HT synthesis (Meltzer et al., 1984a), or inhibiting 5-HT uptake, thus increasing 5-HT synaptic concentration (Meltzer et al., 1983a), or by augmenting sensitivity of postsynaptic receptors (Friedman & Dallob, 1979; Meltzer et al., 1984a, 1984b). Some work has also suggested that lithium may exert a number of its effects on the 5-HT system through its effects on calcium as a second messenger, transducing stimuli from the 5-HTergic and NEergic systems (Meltzer, 1986).

Thus, it appears that "selective" 5-HT uptake inhibitors, which presumably enhance 5-HT activity, possess antidepressant efficacy. The effects of lithium, thought to augment the clinical efficacy of antidepressants by increasing 5-HT transmission, lend support to the hypothesis that increasing 5-HTergic activity may mediate some aspects of antidepressant effects, and may be a common (5-HTergic) mechanism of action of antidepressant activity.

5-HT HYPOTHESES OF DEPRESSION

According to the data presented here, it seems likely that 5-HT dysfunction is related to depression. However, given the diverse and heterogenous nature of these findings, it appears most suitable to integrate the data in a dichotomous way, favoring either hypofunction or hyperfunction of the 5-HTergic system in depression, rather than attempt to force these findings into an overall unidirectional hypothesis.

The classical "monoamine hypothesis" of depression suggests that this disorder is caused by decreased availability and diminished function of the MAergic system, and thus antidepressant treatments exert therapeutic action by increasing synaptic MA availability and neurotransmission.

Evidence for "5-HT hypofunction" in depression includes data suggesting the following:

1. Decreased CNS 5-HT synthesis and metabolism in depression (as reflected in lowered concentrations of 5-HT and 5-HIAA in postmortem brain and CSF studies and reduced ratio of plasma tryptophan to competing neutral amino acids).

2. Increased 5-HT receptor sensitivity, neurotransmission, and function in depressives after antidepressant treatment (as expressed by an enhanced prolactin response to neuroendocrine challenge after such treatment, and by data from electrophysiological recording studies and behavioral models suggesting enhanced postsynaptic 5-HT function after chronic antidepressant treatment.

3. Antidepressant efficacy shown by 5-HT precursors that increase 5-HT synthesis/function and by selective 5-HT reuptake inhibitors.

4. Augmentation of antidepressant treatment by lithium, which is believed to enhance 5-HT neurotransmission.

5. Depressogenic effects shown by 5-HT depleting agents.

Evidence also exists for the "5-HT hyperfunction" hypothesis of depression, which suggests that 5-HT neurotransmission is enhanced in depression, presumably as a consequence of hypersensitive postsynaptic 5-HT receptors. If such hypersensitivity is primary, it might account for a (compensatory) decrease in brain 5-HT metabolism found in unmedicated depressed patients, although, of course, the opposite mechanism is also possible. Evidence supporting this hypothesis includes data suggesting the following:

1. Platelet 5-HT uptake is decreased in depressed patients, which increases the availability of 5-HT at the synapse and thus serves to enhance 5-HT neurotransmission.

2. Antidepressants produce further decreases in presynaptic 5-HT availability (as reflected in further decreases in CSF 5-HIAA, and normalized platelet uptake found in several studies).

3. There is an increased density of postsynaptic 5-HT$_2$ receptors in the frontal cortex of depressed patients and suicide victims.

4. There is decreased binding to postsynaptic 5-HT$_2$ receptors after chronic antidepressant treatment as seen in animals (although it is not clear that such changes are directly related to antidepressant activity, as it has been shown that ECS produces increased postsynaptic 5-HT$_2$ binding).

5. Increased sensitivity of postsynaptic 5-HT receptors is seen in depressed patients, as suggested by neuroendocrine challenge data showing an enhanced cortisol response to 5-HTP at baseline, with reduction in the cortisol response to 5-HTP after tricyclic antidepressant treatment.

Thus, to sum up, the 5-HT hypotheses of depression propose that either the 5-HT system is underfunctional in depression, and thus antidepressant treatments act to enhance 5-HT neurotransmission (via presynaptic and postsynaptic effects), or that the 5-HT system is overfunctional in depression, primarily because of hypersensitive postsynaptic receptors, and thus antidepressant treatments act to decrease 5-HT neurotransmission. It should be noted that understanding the data concerning these two theories is made more difficult by the fact that some processes are primary and some are secondary, or compensatory, and it is not really possible at this time to differentiate between the two. Thus, as discussed above, an abnormality in presynaptic 5-HT mechanisms could cause a compensatory increase in postsynaptic receptor sensitivity, while an abnormality or defect at the 5-HT receptor site itself might result in consequent changes in 5-HT production and turnover. Since net neuronal transmission is determined by both presynaptic and postsynaptic processes, it is probably overly simplistic to attempt to decide on a 5-HT hypofunction or hyperfunction hypothesis of depression on the basis of measurements of only one of these sets of variables.

Another important possibility in considering the MA hypotheses of depression is that we may not be dealing with a primary dysfunction of the MA system itself, but instead may be observing the end results of a dysregulation of the human biological clock, which regulates endogenous biorhythms. It is well documented that the occurrence of depressive episodes may be strongly influenced by seasonal variability. Within each episode there are also well-documented biological, as well as psychopathological, changes that appear to vary according to circadian rhythmicity. Recent studies in depressed individuals now suggest that synaptic processes, such as 5-HT uptake and ^{3}H-imipramine binding, may also reflect circadian and seasonal variability (Healy & Leonard, 1987). Thus it is also possible that a common locus of antidepressant action may be to restore the premorbid function of the biological clock, which is then secondarily expressed as a change in MA function. It is possible as well that 5-HT hypofunction and 5-HT hyperfunction may relate to different stages within a depressive episode.

DIMENSIONAL SIGNIFICANCE OF 5-HT DYSFUNCTIONS

We have previously suggested that the specificity of 5-HT dysfunctions might be better related to certain psychopathological phenomena than to depression per se.

Initially, disturbances in serotonergic function were implicated in depressive disorder, primarily with endogenous or melancholic features. Subsequent data have suggested that serotonergic dysfunction might be related to suicidality in depression, to suicidality in general (van Praag, 1986b), and, finally, to dysregulation of aggression (Valzelli, 1984), possibly as a consequence of impulse control disorder. In addition, serotonergic dysfunction has been linked to the symptoms of anxiety and depressive mood (van Praag et al., 1987c). Studies showing 5-HT disturbances in nondepressed persons, such as violent criminals, also suggest that the neurotransmitter system dysfunction may have broader significance than involvement in a single psychiatric disorder.

These findings suggest that the specificity of the biological variable (serotonergic disturbance) may be more closely related, on the functional or dimensional level, to psychopathological dimensions or to psychological dysfunction than to nosological categories (diseases).

Biological research in psychiatry has a strong nosological orientation. It would appear, however, that use of the functional or dimensional approach, complementary to the nosological approach, could increase our understanding of biological variables in psychiatric disorders.

POSSIBLE CA/5-HT INTERACTIONS IN DEPRESSION

While recent research has shown that treatment-resistant depressed patients may respond to "selective" 5-HT agents (Asberg et al., 1986), most available data suggest that a mixed treatment aimed at augmenting both 5-HT and NE availability may be more effective in the treatment of depression (van Praag et al., 1987a). This is particularly interesting in light of Maas's original hypothesis that there may be two subtypes of depressions, one 5-HTergic and one NEergic in nature (Maas, 1975). Although the emphasis of this chapter is on the 5-HTergic system, clearly the study of one neurotransmitter system in isolation cannot entirely explain the pathogenesis of such a complex disease.

NE and 5-HT.

The classical monoamine hypothesis of depression initially proposed that decreased availability of NE and hypofunction of the NEergic system are causally related to depressive illness. With advances in molecular research strategies, this hypothesis has been modified to focus on the function of specific NE receptors. Sulser (1987) has proposed that primary hypersensitivity of beta-adrenergic receptors may be causally related to depression, and that antidepressant treatments exert clinical efficacy through downregulation of these receptors. This hypothesis has been supported by Charney et al. (1981), who have suggested that antidepressant treatments decrease beta-adrenergic receptor sensitivity and function. The question then arises regarding the nature of the role that 5-HT might play in these processes.

There is an increasing body of data showing anatomical as well as functional interactions between 5-HT neurons originating in the midbrain raphe and cerebral cortex and NE neurons in the locus coeruleus (Dahlstrom & Fuxe, 1964; Levitt & Moore, 1978; Morrison et al., 1982). There is also well-documented evidence of certain mutual modulation effects between these two systems (Brunello et al., 1982; Janowsky et al., 1982; Dumbrille-Ross & Tang, 1983; Nimgaonkar et al., 1985; Scott & Crews, 1985, 1986).

Recently, it has been suggested that an intact 5-HT system is needed for the downregulation of beta-adrenergic receptors by antidepressant treatment (Sulser, 1986, 1987). It has also been shown that selective 5-HT agents can indirectly stimulate the NE system, subsequently causing beta-adrenergic receptor downregulation in discrete brain regions (Wamsley et al., 1987). Kellar and Stockmeier (1986) have presented data suggesting that while some antidepressant treatments may require the presence of intact 5-HTergic neurons to mediate downregulation of beta-adrenergic receptors, other antidepressant treatments, such as ECS, can decrease beta-adrenergic receptor binding after lesioning of 5-HTergic neurons, suggesting that the influence of 5-HTergic axons on beta-adrenergic receptors may extend beyond a simple influence upon downregulation by antidepressant medications. It thus appears that an alternative and critical role of 5-HT in antidepressant treatments may be the mediation of antidepressant effects on the NE system.

DA and 5-HT.

Up until now, data on the role of dopamine (DA) have not delineated any clear role for this neurotransmitter in depression. For example, antidepressant medications appear to exert minimal effect on DA neurotransmission

(Charney et al., 1981). However, it has been suggested that decreased DA function [as expressed by decreased CSF homovanillic acid (HVA), the primary metabolite of DA] may mediate certain depressive symptoms, such as hypoactivity and lack of initiative, with L-dopa causing an increase in CSF HVA and improving psychomotor retardation (van Praag et al., 1975).

Since a complex anatomical and functional interaction is known to exist between the DAergic and the 5-HTergic neuronal systems in the forebrain, and since it is assumed that 5-HT imposes an inhibitory modulatory tone on these DAergic circuits (Jenner et al., 1983), enhancing 5-HT neurotransmission by antidepressants is assumed to (further) decrease DAergic function. If such a mode of interaction does exist, this does not favor the direct involvement of DAergic hypofunction in depression, although DA/5-HT interactions, again, are highly likely in this disorder, and may be of greater importance in certain specific dimensions of symptomatology, such as decreased motility.

CONCLUSION

From the foregoing data, it certainly appears that 5-HT dysfunction is involved in depression. When the body of biological data in this area is comprehensively reviewed, it becomes clear that many of the results are contradictory, and can be interpreted as lending support to either the "5-HT hypofunction" hypothesis or to the "5-HT hyperfunction" hypothesis of depression. Future research in biological psychiatry is needed to resolve this dilemma, and should address the question through the use of neuroendocrine challenge tests, employing selective 5-HT agonists, such as mCPP, which is a direct activator of the 5-HT (primarily the 5-HT$_1$) receptor (Mueller et al., 1985; Murphy et al., 1986), and antagonists such as ritanserin, a selective 5-HT$_2$ receptor blocker (Leysen et al., 1985), that have now become available. Such tests will help to elucidate the functional state of the 5-HTergic system in depressed patients, and to explore the biological effects of different antidepressant treatments in these patients.

Another interpretation of 5-HT dysfunction in depression involves the possibility that such dysfunction might mediate certain psychopathological phenomena (e.g., aggression dysregulation, anxiety, and disturbances of mood and impulse control) across nosological dimensions, rather than being related to depression per se. Correlating the outcome of neuroendocrine challenge tests and other 5-HT-related variables with these various psychopathological dimensions will help further to explain their relationship to 5-HTergic dysfunctions.

Finally, although the emphasis of this chapter has been on the 5-HTergic system, it is evident that no single isolated neurotransmitter system can account for the pathogenesis of depression. Rather, this issue should be explored in the context of the complex functional interactions among the various neurotransmitter systems, particularly between 5-HT and NE. Experimental results concerning the molecular interrelationships between 5-HT and NE synaptic models suggest several possibilities for such interactions. Future research should simultaneously explore the state of the 5-HT and the NE systems, as well as the response of the NE system to what have until now been assumed to be purely 5-HTergic manipulations. For example, future challenge studies might employ 5-HT agonists combined with NE antagonists, or 5-HT antagonists combined with NE agonists, in order to help to understand more clearly the various roles of these two systems in the neuroendocrinological/hormonal abnormalities reported in depressed patients.

With the elucidation of some of the complex modulatory interactions between the 5-HT and the NE systems, it will become more possible to develop an understanding of which specific physiological abnormalities may be etiologically related to depressive illness, and which specific effects of antidepressant treatments may actually mediate clinical efficacy. Such advances in understanding will then make it possible to greatly improve our clinical treatment of this extremely disabling disorder.

REFERENCES

Aberg-Wistedt, A. (1982). Comparison between zimelidine and desipramine in endogenous depression: A cross-over study. *Acta Psychiatr. Scand., 66,* 129–138.

Abrams, R., Essman, W. B., Taylor, M. A., & Fink, M. (1976). Concentration of 5-hydroxyindoleacetic acid, homovanillic acid, and tryptophan in the cerebrospinal fluid of depressed patients before and after ECT. *Biol. Psychiatry, 11,* 85–90.

Agren, H. (1980a). Symptom patterns in unipolar and bipolar depression correlating with monamine metabolites in the cerebrospinal fluid: I. General patterns. *Psychiatry Res., 3,* 211–223.

Agren, H. (1980b). Symptom patterns in unipolar and bipolar depression correlating with monoamine metabolites in the cerebrospinal fluid: II. Suicide. *Psychiatry Res., 3,* 225–236.

Agren, H. (1983). Life at risk: Markers of suicidality in depression. *Psychiatr. Dev., 1,* 87–104.

Angst, J., Woggon, B., & Schoepf, J. (1977). The treatment of depressions with L-5-hydroxytryptophan versus imipramine. *Arch. Psychiatr., Nervenkr., 24,* 175–186.

Arora, R. C., Kriegel, L., & Meltzer, H. Y. (1984). Seasonal variation of serotonin uptake in normal controls and depressed patients. *Biol. Psychiatry, 19,* 795–804.

Arora, R. C., & Meltzer, H. Y. (1989). Increased serotonin 2 (5HT2) receptor binding as measured by 3H-lysergic acid diethylamide (3H-LSD) in the blood platelets of depressed patients. *Life Sci., 44,* 725–734.

Asarch, K. B., Shih, J. C., & Kulcsar, A. (1980). Decreased 3H-imipramine binding in depressed males and females. *Commun. Psychopharmacol., 4,* 425–432.

Asberg, M., Eriksson, B., Martensson, B., Traskman-Bendz, L., & Wagner, A. (1986). Therapeutic effects of serotonin uptake inhibitors in depression. *J. Clin. Psychiatry, 47*(4, suppl), 23–35.

Asberg, M., Ringberger, V. A., Sjoqvist, F., Thoren, P., Traskman, L., & Tuck, J. R. (1977). Monoamine metabolites in cerebrospinal fluid and serotonin uptake inhibition during treatment with chlorimipramine. *Clin. Pharmacol. Ther., 21,* 201–207.

Asberg, M., Thoren, P., Traskman, L., Bertilsson, L., & Ringberger, V. (1976b). Serotonin depression: A biochemical subgroup within the affective disorders. *Science, 191,* 478–480.

Asberg, M., Traskman, L., & Thoren, P. (1976a). 5HIAA in the cerebrospinal fluid: A biochemical suicide predictor? *Arch. Gen. Psychiatry, 33,* 1193–1197.

Ashcroft, G. W., Crawford, T. B. B., Eccleston, D., Sharman, D. F., MacDougall, E. J., Stanton, J. B., & Binns, J. K. (1966). 5-Hydroxyindole compounds in the cerebrospinal fluid of patients with psychiatric or neurological diseases. *Lancet, 2,* 1049–1052.

Asnis, G. M., Eisenberg, J., van Praag, H. M., & Lemus, C. Z. (1988). The neuroendocrine response to fenfluramine in depressive and normal controls. *Biol. Psychiatry, 24,* 117–120.

Banki, C. M. (1977). Correlation of anxiety and related symptoms with cerebrospinal fluid 5-hydroxyindoleacetic acid in depressed women. *J. Neural Transm., 41,* 135–143.

Baron, M., Barkai, A., Gruen, R., Kowalik, S., & Quitkin, F. (1983). 3H-imipramine platelet binding sites in unipolar depression. *Biol. Psychiatry, 18,* 1403–1409.

Benfield, P., & Ward, A. (1986). Fluvoxamine: A review of its pharmacodynamic and pharmacokinetic properties, and therapeutic efficacy in depressive illness. *Drugs, 32,* 313–334.

Bertilsson, L., Asberg, M., & Thoren, P. (1976). Differential effect of chlorimipramine and nortriptyline on cerebrospinal fluid metabolites of serotonin and noradrenaline in depression. *Eur. J. Clin. Pharmacol., 21,* 194–200.

Bertilsson, L., Tuck, J. R., & Siwers, B. (1980). Biochemical effects of zimelidine in man. *Eur. J. Clin. Pharmacol., 18,* 483–487.

Beskow, J., Gottfries, C. G., Roos, B. E., & Winblad, D. B. (1976). Determination of monoamine and monoamine metabolites in the human brain: Postmortem studies in a group of suicides and in a control group. *Acta Psychiatr. Scand., 53,* 7–20.

Biegon, A., Weizman, A., Karp, L., Ram, A., Tiano, S., & Wolff, M. (1987). Serotonin 5-HT2 receptor binding on blood platelets—A peripheral marker for depression? *Life Sci., 41,* 2485–2492.

Birkmayer, W., & Riederer, P. (1975). Biochemical post-mortem findings in depressed patients. *J. Neural Transm., 37,* 95–109.

Blackshear, M. A., & Sanders-Bush, E. (1982). Serotonin receptor sensitivity after acute and chronic treatment with mianserin. *J. Pharmacol. Exp. Ther., 221,* 303–308.

Blier, P., & DeMontigny, C. (1984). Enhancement of serotonergic neurotransmission by non-tricyclic antidepressant drugs: Single cell studies in the rat. Abstr, *14th Collegium Internationale Neuro-Psychopharmacologicum* (p. 829), Florence, Italy.

Born, G. V. R., Grignani, G., & Martin, K. (1980). Long-term effect of lithium on the uptake of 5-hydroxytryptamine by human platelets. *Br. J. Clin. Pharmacol., 9,* 321–325.

Bourne, H. R., Bunney, W. E., Jr., & Colburn, R. W. (1968). Noradrenaline, 5-hydroxytryptamine and 5-hydroxyindoleacetic acid in hindbrains of suicidal patients. *Lancet, 2,* 805–808.

Bowers, M. B. (1974a). Lumbar CSF 5-hydroxyindoleacetic acid and homovanillic acid in affective syndromes. *J. Nerv. Ment. Dis., 158,* 325–330.

Bowers, M. B. (1974b). Amitriptyline in man: Decreased formation of central 5-hydroxyindoleacetic acid. *Clin. Pharmacol. Ther., 15,* 167–170.

Bowers, M. B., Heninger, G. R., & Gerbode, F. A. (1969). Cerebrospinal fluid 5-hydroxyindoleacetic acid and homovanillic acid in psychiatric patients. *Int. J. Neuropharmacol., 8,* 255–262.

Breitner, C., Picchioni, A., Chin, L., & Burton, L. E. (1961). The effect of electrostimulation on brain 5-hydroxytryptamine concentration. *Dis. Nerv. Syst., 22,* 93–96.

Breitner, C., Picchioni, A., & Chin, L. (1964). Neurohormone levels in brain after CNS stimulation including electrotherapy. *J. Neuropsychiatry, 5,* 153–158.

Bremner, J. D. (1984). Fluoxetine in depressed patients: A comparison with imipramine. *J. Clin. Psychiatry, 45,* 414–419.

Briley, M. S., Langer, S. Z., Raisman, R., Sechter, D., & Zarifian, E. (1980). Tritiated imipramine binding sites are decreased in platelets of untreated depressed patients. *Science, 209,* 303–305.

Brodie, H. K. H., Sack, R., & Siever, L. (1973). Clinical studies of L-5-hydroxytryptophan in depression. In J. Barchas, & E. Usdin (Eds.), *Serotonin and behavior.* (pp. 549–559). New York: Academic Press.

Brunello, N., Barbaccia, M. L., Chuang, D. M., & Costa, E. (1982). Down-regulation of beta-adrenergic receptors following repeated injections of desmethylimipramine: Permissive role of serotonergic axons. *Neuropharmacol., 21,* 1145–1149.

Bunney, W. E., & Davis, J. M. (1965). Norepinephrine in depressive reactions: A review. *Arch. Gen. Psychiatry, 13,* 483–494.

Carlsson, A., Gottfries, C. G., Holmberg, G., Modigh, K., Svensson, T., & Ogren, S. O. (1981). Recent advances in the treatment of depression. *Acta Psychiatr. Scand., 63*(Suppl 290), 1–477.

Carstens, M., Engelbrecht, A., Russell, V., Aalbers, C., Gagiano, C. A., Chalton, D. D., & Talgaard, J. J. F. (1986). Imipramine binding sites on platelets of patients with major depressive disorder. *Psychiatry Res., 18,* 333–342.

Charney, D. S., Heninger, G. R., Reinhard, J. F., Sternberg, D., & Hafstead, K. M. (1982). The effect of intravenous L-tryptophan on prolactin, growth hormone, and mood in healthy subjects. *Psychopharmacology, 78,* 38–43.

Charney, D. S., Heninger, G. R., & Sternberg, D. E. (1984). Serotonin function and mechanism of action of antidepressant treatment. *Arch. Gen. Psychiatry, 41,* 359–365.

Charney, D. S., Menkes, D. B., & Heninger, G. R. (1981). Receptor sensitivity and the mechanism of action of antidepressant treatment: Implications for the etiology and therapy of depression. *Arch. Gen. Psychiatry, 38,* 1160–1180.

Chouinard, G. (1985). A double-blind controlled clinical trial of fluoxetine and amitriptyline in the treatment of outpatients with major depressive disorder. *J. Clin. Psychiatry, 46,* 32–37.

Chouinard, G., Young, S. N., Annable, L., & Sourkes, T. L. (1979). Tryptophan nicotinamide, imipramine and their combination in depression. *Acta Psychiatr., Scand., 59,* 395–414.

Claassen, V., Davies, J. E., Hertting, G., & Placheta, P. (1977). Fluvoxamine, a specific 5-hydroxytryptamine uptake inhibitor. *Br. J. Pharmacol., 60,* 505–516.

Claghorn, J., Gershon, S., Goldstein, B. J., Behrnetz, S., Bush, D. F., & Huitfeldt, B. (1983). A double-blind evaluation of a zimelidine in comparison to placebo and amitriptyline in patients with major depressive disorder. *Prog. Neuropsychopharmacol. Biol. Psychiatry, 7,* 367–382.

Clauw, D. J., Nashel, D. J., Umhau, A., Kate, P. (1990). Tryptophan-associated eosinophilic connective-tissue disease. *JAMA, 263,* 1502–1506.

Clineschmidt, B. V., Zacchei, A. G, Totaro, J. A., Pfleuger, A. B., McGuffin, J. C., & Wishousky, T. I. (1978). Fenfluramine and brain serotonin. *Ann. N.Y. Acad. Sci., 305,* 222–241.

Cochran, E., Robins, E., & Grote, S. (1976). Regional serotonin levels in brain: A comparison of depressive suicides and alcoholic suicides with controls. *Biol. Psychiatry, 11,* 283–294.

Cohn, J. B., & Wilcox, C. (1985). A comparison of fluoxetine, imipramine, and placebo in patients with major depressive disorder. *J. Clin. Psychiatry, 46,* 26–31.

Cole, J. O., Hartmann, E., & Brigham, P. (1980). L-tryptophan: Clinical studies. *McLean Hosp. J., 5,* 37–71.

Cooper, A. J. (1979). Tryptophan antidepressant: Physiological sedative, fact or fancy? *Psychopharmacology (Berlin), 61,* 97–102.

Coppen, A. (1967). The biochemistry of affective disorders. *Br. J. Psychiatry, 113,* 1237–1264.

Coppen, A., Brooksbank, B. W. L., & Peet, M. (1972a). Tryptophan concentration in the cerebrospinal fluid of depressive patients. *Lancet, 1,* 1393.

Coppen, A., Prange, A. J., Hill, C., & Whybrow, P. F. (1972b). Abnormalities of indoleamines in affective disorders. *Arch. Gen. Psychiatry, 26,* 474–478.

Coppen, A., Shaw, D. M., & Farrell, J. P. (1963). Potentiation of the antidepressive effect of a monoamine-oxidase inhibitor by tryptophan. *Lancet, 1,* 79–81.

Coppen, A., Swade, C., & Wood, K. (1981). The action of antidepressant drugs on 5-hydroxytryptamine uptake by platelets—relationship to therapeutic effect. *Acta Psychiatr. Scand., 63*(Suppl 290), 236–243.

Coppen, A., & Wood, K. M. (1980). Peripheral serotonergic and adrenergic responses in depression. *Acta Psychiatr. Scand., 280*(Suppl 61), 21–28.

Cottevanger, E. A. (1984). Fluvoxamine, highly selective 5-HT reuptake inhibitor. In B. W. Duphar (Ed.), Monograph. Worthington, OH: Kali-Duphar Laboratory.

Cowen, P. J., Geaney, D. P., Schachter, M., Green, A. R., & Elliott, M. (1986). Desipramine treatment in normal subjects. Effects on neuroendocrine responses to tryptophan and on platelet serotonin 5HT-related receptors. *Arch. Gen. Psychiatry, 43,* 61–67.

Cremata, V. Y., & Koe, K. B. (1966). Clinical-pharmacological evaluation of p-chlorophenylalanine: A new serotonin depleting agent. *Clin. Pharmacol. Ther., 7,* 768–776.

Dahlstrom, A., & Fuxe, K. (1964). Evidence for the existence of monoamine-containing neurons in the central nervous system: I. Demonstration of monoamines in the cell bodies of brain stem neurons. *Acta Physiol. Scand., 62*(Suppl 232), 1–55.

D'Elia, G., Lehmann, J., & Raotma, H. (1977). Evaluation of the combination of tryptophan and ECT in the treatment of depression. I. Clinical analysis. *Acta Psychiatr. Scand., 56,* 303–318.

DeMontigny, C. (1984). Electroconvulsive shock treatments enhance responsiveness of forebrain neurons to serotonin. *J. Pharmacol. Exp. Ther., 228,* 230–234.

DeMontigny, C., & Aghajanian, G. K. (1978). Tricyclic antidepressants: Long-term treatment increases responsivity of rat forebrain neurons to serotonin. *Science, 202,* 1303–1306.

DeMontigny, C., Grunberg, F., Mayer, A., & Duschenes, J.-P. (1981). Lithium induces rapid relief of depression in tricyclic antidepressant drug non-responders. *Br. J. Psychiatry, 138,* 252–256.

DeWilde, J. E., Metrens, C., & Wakelin, J. S. (1983). Clinical trials of fluvoxamine vs. chlorimipramine with single and three times daily dosing. *Br. J. Clin. Pharmacol., 15,* 427s–431s.

Dick, P., & Ferrero, E. (1983). A double-blind comparative study of the clinical efficacy of fluvoxamine and chlorimipramine. *Br. J. Clin. Pharmacol., 15,* 419s–425s.

Dominguez, R. A., Goldstein, B. J., Jacobson, A. F., & Steinbrook, R. M. (1985). A double-blind placebo-controlled study of fluvoxamine in depression. *J. Clin. Psychiatry, 46,* 84–87.

Dumbrille-Ross, A., & Tang, S. W. (1983). Noradrenergic and serotonergic input necessary for imipramine induced changes in beta but not S2 receptor densities. *Psychiatry Res., 9,* 207–215.

Dunner, D. L., & Fieve, R. R. (1975). Affective disorders: Studies with amine precursors. *Am. J. Psychiatry, 132,* 180–184.

Egrise, D., Rubinstein, M., Schoutens, A., Cantraine, F., & Mendlewicz, J. (1986). Seasonal variation of platelet serotonin uptake and 3H-imipramine binding in normal and depressed subjects. *Biol. Psychiatry, 21,* 283–292.

Emanuelsson, B.-M., Widerlov, E., Walleus, H., & Paalzow, L. K. (1987). Determinations of 5-hydroxyindoleacetic acid and homovanillic acid in human CSF with monitoring of probenecid levels in CSF and plasma. *Psychopharmacology, 92,* 144–149.

Essman, W. B. (1968). Electroshock induced retrograde amnesia and brain serotonin metabolism: Effect of several antidepressant compounds. *Psychophar-macologia, 13,* 258–266.

Essman, W. B. (1973). *Neurochemistry of cerebral electroshock.* New York: Spectrum.

Essman, W. B. (1986). Effect of electroconvulsive shock on serotonin activity. In S. Malitz & H. A. Sackeim (Eds.), *Electroconvulsive therapy: Clinical and basic research issues,* Vol. 462 (pp. 99–104). New York: Academy of Sciences.

Farkas, T., Dunner, D. L., & Fieve, R. R. (1976). L-tryptophan in depression. *Biol. Psychiatry, 11,* 295–302.

Fraser, W. M., Tucker, H. S., Grubb, S. R., Wigand, J. P., & Blackard, W. G. (1979). Effect of l-tryptophan on growth hormone and prolactin release in normal volunteers and patients with secretory pituitary tumors. *Horm. Metab. Res., 11,* 149–155.

Friedman, E., & Dallob, A. (1979). Enhanced serotonin receptor activity after chronic treatment with imipramine or amitriptyline. *Psychopharmac. Commun., 3,* 89–92.

Fuller, R. W. (1986). Pharmacologic modification of serotonergic function: Drugs for the study and treatment of psychiatric and other disorders. *J. Clin. Psychiatry, 47,* 4–8.

Fuller, R. W. (1987). Pharmacologic properties of serotonergic agents and antidepressant drugs. *J. Clin. Psychiatry, 48*(Suppl), 5–11.

Fuxe, K., Ogren, S.-O., Agnati, L. F., Andersson, K., & Eneroth, P. (1982). Effects of subchronic antidepressant drug treatment on central serotonergic mechanism in the male rat. In E. Costa & G. Racagni (Eds.), *Typical and atypical antidepressants: Molecular mechanisms.* (pp. 91–107). New York: Raven Press.

Fuxe, K., Ogren, S.-O., Agnati, L. F., Benfenati, F., Fredholm, B., Andersson, K., Zini, L., & Eneroth, P. (1983). Chronic antidepressant treatment and central 5-synapses. *Neuropharmacology, 22,* 389–400.

Fuxe, K., Ogren, S.-O., Agnati, L. F., Eneroth, P., Holm, A. C., & Andersson, K. (1981). Long-term treatment with zimelidine leads to a reduction in 5-hydroxytryptamine neurotransmission within the central nervous system of the mouse and rat. *Neurosci. Lett., 21,* 57–62.

Gallager, D. W., & Bunney, W. E., Jr. (1979). Failure of chronic lithium treatment block tricyclic antidepressant-induced 5-HT supersensitivity. *Naunyn-Schmiedebergs Arch. Pharmacol., 307,* 129–133.

Gelenberg, A. J., Gibson, C. J., & Wojcik, J. D. (1982). Neurotransmitter precursors for the treatment of depression. *Psychopharmacol. Bull., 18,* 7–18.

Giret, M., Launay, J. M., Dreux, C., Zarifian, E., Benyacoub, K., & Loo, H. (1980). Modifications of biochemical parameters in blood platelets of schizophrenic and depressive patients. *Neuropsychobiology, 6,* 290–296.

Glass, A. R., Smallridge, R. C., Schaaf, M., & Dimond, R. C. (1980). Absent prolactin response to L-tryptophan in normal and acromegalic subjects. *Psychoneuroendocrinology, 5,* 261–265.

Glowinski, J., & Axelrod, J. (1964). Inhibition of uptake of tritiated noradrenaline in the intact rat brain by imipramine and structurally related compounds. *Nature (Lond.), 204,* 1318–1319.

Gluckman, M. I., & Baum, T. (1969). The pharmacology of iprindole, a new antidepressant. *Psychopharmacologia (Berlin), 15,* 169–185.

Goodlet, F., Mreylees, S. E., & Sugrue, M. F. (1977). Effects of mianserin, a new antidepressant, on the in vitro and in vivo uptake of monoamines. *Br. J. Pharmacol., 61,* 307–313.

Goodwin, G. M., De Souza, R. J., & Green, A. R. (1985). Presynaptic serotonin receptor-mediated response in mice attenuated by antidepressant drugs and electroconvulsive shock. *Nature, 317,* 531–533.

Goodwin, F. K., & Post, R.M. (1973). The use of probenecid in high doses for the estimation of central serotonin turnover in affective illness and addicts on methadone. In J. Barchas & E. Usdin (Eds.), *Serotonin and behavior* (pp. 476–480). New York: Academic Press.

Goodwin, F. K., & Post, R. M. (1975). Studies of amine metabolites in affective illness and in schizophrenia: A comparative analysis. In D. X. Freedman (Ed.), *Biology of the major psychoses,* Vol. 54 (pp. 299–332). New York: Raven Press.

Goodwin, F. K., Post, R. M., Dunner, D. L., & Gordon, E. K. (1973). Cerebrospinal fluid amine metabolites in affective illness: The probenecid technique. *Arch. Gen. Psychiatry, 26,* 57–63.

Grahame-Smith, D. G. (1971). Studies in vivo on the relationship between brain tryptophan, brain 5-HT synthesis and hyperactivity in rats treated with a monoamine oxidase inhibitor and L-tryptophan. *J. Neurochem., 18,* 1053–1066.

Growdon, J. H. (1979). Neurotransmitter precursors in the diet: Their use in the treatment of brain diseases. In R. J. Wurtman & J. J. Wurtman (Eds.), *Nutrition and the brain: Disorders of eating and nutrients in treatment of brain diseases,* Vol. 3 (pp. 117–181). New York: Raven Press.

Haigler, H. J., & Aghajanian, G. K. (1974). Lysergic acid diethylamide and serotonin: A comparison of effects on serotonin neurons receiving a serotonergic input. *J. Pharmacol. Exp. Ther., 188,* 688–689.

Hallstrom, C. O. S., Pare, C. M. B., Rees, W. L., Trenchard, A., & Turner, P. (1976). Platelet uptake of 5-hydroxytryptamine and dopamine in depression. *Postgrad. Med. J. (Suppl), 52*(Suppl 3), 40–44.

Halmi, K. A., Eckert, E., LaDu, T. J., & Cohen, J. (1986). Anorexia nervosa: Treatment efficacy of cyproheptadine and amitriptyline. *Arch. Gen. Psychiatry, 43,* 177–181.

Handwerger, S., Plonk, J. W., Lebovitz, H. E., Bivens, C. H., & Feldman, J. M. (1975). Failure of 5-hydroxytryptophan to stimulate prolactin and growth hormone secretion in man. *Hormon. Metab. Res., 7,* 214–216.

Healy, D., & Leonard, B. E. (1987). Monoamine transport in depression: Kinetics and dynamics. *J. Affect. Disord., 12,* 91–103.

Heninger, G. R., & Charney, D. S. (1982). The monoamine receptor sensitivity hypothesis of antidepressant drug action. *Psychopharmacol. Bull., 18,* 130–135.

Heninger, G. R., Charney, D. S., & Sternberg, D. E. (1984). Serotonergic function in depression. *Arch. Gen. Psychiatry, 41,* 398–402.

Herrington, R. N., Bruce, A., Johnstone, E. C., & Lader, M. H. (1976). Comparative trial of L-tryptophan and amitriptyline in depressive illness. *Psychol. Med., 6,* 673–678.

Hertzman, P. A., Blevins, W. L., Mayer, J., Greenfield, B., Ting, M., Gleich, G. J. (1990). Association of the eosinophilia-myalgia syndrome with the ingestion of tryptophan. *N. Engl. J. Med., 233*, 869–873.

Humphries, L., Shirley, P., Allen, M., Codd, E. E., & Walker, R. F. (1985). Daily patterns of serotonin uptake in platelets from psychiatric patients and control volunteers. *Biol. Psychiatry, 20*, 1073–1081.

Hyyppa, M. T., Jolma, T., Lura, J., Langvik, V. A., & Kytomaki, O. (1979). L-tryptophan treatment and the episodic secretion of pituitary hormones and cortisol. *Psychoneuroendocrinology, 4*, 29–35.

Innis, R. B., Charney, D. S., & Heninger, G. R. (1987). Differential 3H-imipramine platelet binding in patients with panic disorder and depression. *Psychiatry Res., 21*, 33–41.

Iversen, L. L., & Mackay, A. V. P. (1979). Pharmacodynamics of antidepressants and antimanic drugs. In E. S. Paykel & A. Coppen (Eds.), *Psychopharmacology of affective disorders* (pp. 60–90). New York: Oxford University Press.

Jacobs, B. L. (1976). An animal behavior model for studying central serotonergic synapses. *Life Sci., 19*, 777–786.

Janowsky, A., Okada, F., Manier, D., Applegate, C. D., Sulser, F., & Sterankov, L. R. (1982). Role of serotonergic input in the regulation of the beta-adrenergic receptor-coupled adenylate cyclase system. *Science, 218*, 900–901.

Janssen, P. A. J. (1985). Pharmacology of potent and selective S2-serotonergic antagonists. *J. Cardiovasc. Pharmacol., 7*(Suppl 7), S2–S11.

Jenner, P., Sheehy, M., & Marsden, C. D. (1983). Noradrenaline and 5-hydroxytryptamine modulation of brain dopamine function: Implications for the treatment of Parkinson's disease. *Br. J. Clin. Pharmacol., 15*(Suppl), 2779–2898.

Jenssen, K., Fruensgaard, K., Ahlfors, U. G., Pihkanen, T. A., Tuomikoski, S., Ose, E., Dencker, S. J., Lindberg, D., & Nagy, A. (1975). Tryptophanimipramine in depression. *Lancet, 2*, 920.

Jones, R. S. G. (1980). Enhancement of 5-hydroxytryptamine-induced behavioral effects following chronic administration of antidepressant drugs. *Psychopharmacology, 69*, 307–311.

Kane, J. M., & Lieberman, J. (1984). The efficacy of amoxapine, maprotiline, and trazodone in comparison to imipramine and amitriptyline: A review of the literature. *Psychopharmacol. Bull., 20*, 240–249.

Kaplan, R. D., & Mann, J. J. (1982). Altered platelet serotonin uptake kinetics in schizophrenia and depression. *Life Sci., 31*, 583–588.

Kato, Y., Nakai, Y., Imura, H., Chihara, K., & Ohgo, S. (1974). Effect of 5-hydroxytryptophan (5-HTP) on plasma prolactin levels in man. *J. Clin. Endocrinol. Metab., 38*, 695–697.

Kellar, K. J., Cascio, C. S., Butler, J. A., & Kurtzke, R. N. (1981). Differential effects of electroconvulsive shock and antidepressant drugs on serotonin-2 receptors in rat brain. *Eur. J. Pharmacol., 69*, 515–518.

Kellar, K. J., & Stockmeier, C. A. (1986). Effects of electroconvulsive shock and serotonin axon lesions on beta-adrenergic and serotonin-2 receptors in rat brain. In S. Malitz & H. A. Sackeim (Eds.), *Electroconvulsive therapy: Clinical and basic research issues*, Vol. 462 (pp. 76–90). New York: New York Academy of Sciences.

Klok, C. J., Brouwer, G. J., van Praag, H. M., & Doogan, D. (1981). Fluvoxamine and clomipramine in depressed patients. A double-blind clinical study. *Acta Psychiatr. Scand., 64,* 1–11.

Koe, B. K., & Weissman, A. (1966). p-Chlorophenylalanine: A specific depletor of brain serotonin. *J. Pharmacol. Exp. Ther., 154,* 499–516.

Korpi, E. R., Kleinman, J. E., Goodman, S. I., Phillips, I., DeLisi, L. E., Linnoila, M., & Wyatt, R. J. (1986). Serotonin and 5-hydroxyindoleacetic acid in brains of suicide victims: Comparison in chronic schizophrenic patients with suicide as cause of death. *Arch. Gen. Psychiatry, 43,* 594–600.

Koshikawa, F., Koshikawa, N., & Stephenson, J. D. (1985). Effects of antidepressant drug combinations on cortical 5HT2 receptors and wet-dog shakes in rats. *Eur. J. Pharmacol., 118,* 273–281.

Kupfer, D. J., & Bowers, M. B. (1972). REM sleep and central monoamine oxidase inhibition. *Psychopharmacologia, 27,* 182–190.

Lahti, T. A., & Maickel, R. P. (1971). The tricyclic antidepressants—Inhibition of norepinephrine uptake as related to potentiation of norepinephrine uptake as related to potentiation of norepinephrine and clinical efficacy. *Biochem. Pharmacol., 20,* 482–486.

Lancranjan, I., Wirz-Justice, A., Puhringer, W., & Del Pozo, E. (1977). Effect of L-5-hydroxytryptophan infusion on growth hormone and prolactin secretion in man. *J. Clin. Endocrinol. Metab., 45,* 588–593.

Langer, S. Z., Javoy-Agid, F., Raisman, R., Briley, M., & Agid, Y. (1981). Distribution of specific high affinity binding sites for (3H)imipramine in human brain. *J. Neurochem., 37,* 267–271.

Langer, S. Z., & Raisman, R. (1983). Binding of 3H-imipramine and 3H-desipramine as biochemical tools for studies in depression. *Neuropharmacology, 22,* 407–413.

Levitt, P., & Moore, R. Y. (1978). Noradrenaline neuron innervation of the neocortex in the rat. *Brain Res., 139,* 219–232.

Leysen, J. E., Gommeren, W., van Gompel, P., Wynants, J., Janssen, P. F. M., & Laduron, P. M. (1985). Receptor binding properties in vitro and in vivo of ritanserin: A very potent and long-acting serotonin-S2 antagonist. *Mol. Pharmacol., 27,* 600–611.

Leysen, J. E., Niemegeers, C. J. E., Tollenaere, J. P., & Laduron, P. M. (1978). Serotonergic component of neuroleptic receptors. *Nature, 272,* 168–171.

Lindberg, D., Ahlfors, U. G., Dencker, S. J., Fruensgaard, K., Hansten, S., Jensen, K., Ose, E., & Pihkanen, A. (1979). Symptom reduction in depression after treatment with L-tryptophan or imipramine. *Acta Psychiatr. Scand., 60,* 287–294.

Lloyd, K. G., Farley, I. J., Deck, J. H. N., & Horneykiewicz, O. (1974). Serotonin and 5-hydroxyindoleacetic acid in discrete areas of the brainstem of suicide victims and control patients. *Adv. Biochem. Psychopharmacol., 11,* 387–398.

Lopez-Ibor, J. J., Gutierrez, J. J. A., & Iglesias, M. L. M. (1976). 5-Hydroxytryptophan (5-HTP) and an MAOI (nialamide) in the treatment of depression: A double-blind controlled study. *Intern. Pharmacopsychiat., 11,* 8–15.

Lucki, I., & Frazer, A. (1982). Prevention of the serotonin syndrome in rats by repeated administration of monoamine oxidase inhibitors but not tricyclic antidepressants. *Psychopharmacology, 77,* 205–211.

Maas, J. W. (1975). Biogenic amines and depression: Biochemical and pharmacological separation of two types of depression. *Arch. Gen. Psychiatry, 32,* 1357–1361.

Maj, J. (1981). Serotonergic mechanisms of antidepressant drugs. *Pharmacopsychiatry, 14,* 35–39.

Maj, J., Palider, W., & Rawlow, A. (1979). Trazodone, a central serotonin antagonist and agonist. *J. Neural Transm., 44,* 237–248.

Mann, J. J., Stanley, M., McBride, P. A., & McEwen, B. S. (1986). Increased serotonin-2 and beta-adrenergic receptor binding in the frontal cortices of suicide victims. *Arch. Gen. Psychiatry, 43,* 954–959.

McKeith, I. G., Marshall, E. F., Ferrier, I. N., Armstrong, M. M., Kennedy, W. N., Perry, R. H., Perry, E. K., & Eccleston, D. (1987). 5-HT receptor binding in postmortem brain from patients with affective disorder. *J. Affect. Disord., 13,* 67–74.

Meltzer, H.Y. (1984). Serotonergic function in the affective disorders: The effect of antidepressants and lithium on the 5-hydroxytryptophan-induced increase in serum cortisol. *Ann. N. Y. Acad. Sci., 430,* 115–137.

Meltzer, H. Y. (1986). Lithium mechanisms in bipolar illness and altered intracellular calcium functions. *Biol. Psychiatry, 21,* 492–510.

Meltzer, H. Y., Arora, R. C., Baber, R., & Tricou, B. J. (1981). Serotonin uptake in blood platelets of psychiatric patients. *Arch. Gen. Psychiatry, 38,* 1322–1326.

Meltzer, H. Y., Arora, R. C., & Goodnick, P. (1983a). Effect of lithium carbonate on serotonin uptake in blood platelets of patients with affective disorders. *J. Affect. Disord., 5,* 215–221.

Meltzer, H. Y., Lowy, M., Robertson, A., Goodnick, P., & Perline, R. (1984a). Effect of 5-hydroxytryptophan on serum cortisol levels in major affective disorders: III. Effect of antidepressants and lithium carbonate. *Arch. Gen. Psychiatry, 41,* 391–397.

Meltzer, H.Y., Umberkoman-Witta, B., Robertson, A., Tricou, B. J., & Lowy, M. (1983c). Enhanced serum cortisol response to 5-hydroxytryptophan in depression and mania. *Life Sci., 33,* 2541–2549.

Meltzer, H. Y., Umberkoman-Witta, B., Robertson, A., Tricou, B. J., Lowy, M., & Perline, R. (1984b). Effect of 5-hydroxytryptophan on serum cortisol levels in major affective disorders: I. Enhanced response in depression and mania. *Arch. Gen. Psychiatry, 41,* 366–374.

Mendels, J. (1987). Clinical experience with serotonin reuptake inhibiting antidepressants. *J. Clin. Psychiatry, 48*(Suppl), 26–30.

Mendels, J., Stinnett, J. L., Burns, D., & Frazer, A. (1975). Amine precursors and depression. *Arch. Gen. Psychiatry, 32,* 22–30.

Mendlewicz, U., Pinder, R. M., Stulemeijerm, S. M., & Van Dorth, R. (1982). Monoamine metabolites in cerebrospinal fluid of depressed patients during treatment with mianserin or amitriptyline. *J. Affect. Disord., 4,* 219–226.

Menkes, D. B., & Aghajanian, G. K. (1981). Alpha-1-adrenoreceptor-mediated responses in the lateral geniculate nucleus are enhanced by chronic antidepressant treatment. *Eur. J. Pharmacol., 74,* 27–35.

Meredith, C. H., & Feighner, J. P. (1983). A double-blind, controlled evaluation of zimelidine, imipramine and placebo in patients with primary affective disorders. *Acta Psychiatr. Scand., 68*(Suppl 308), 70–79.

Meyerson, L. R., Wennogle, L. P., Abel, M. S., Coupet, J., Lippa, A. S., Rauh, C. E., & Beer, B. (1982). Human brain receptor alternations in suicide victims. *Pharmacol. Biochem. Behav., 17,* 159–163.

Mirkin, A. M., & Coppen, A. (1980). Electrodermal activity in depression: Clinical and biochemical correlates. *Br. J. Psychiatry, 137,* 93–97.

Modai, I., Malmgren, R., Asberg, M., & Bering, H. (1986). Circadian rhythm of serotonin transport in human platelets. *Psychopharmacology, 88,* 493–495.

Mogilnicka, E., & Klimek, V. (1979). Mianserin, danitracen and amitriptyline withdrawal increases the behavioral responses of rats to L-5-HTP. *J. Pharm. Pharmacol., 31,* 704–705.

Moller, S. E., & Kirk, L. (1981). Decreased tryptophan availability in endogenous depression caused by disturbed plasma leucine clearance. *Prog. Neur. Psychopharmacol., 5,* 277–279.

Moller, S. E., Kirk, L., & Fremming, K. H. (1976). Plasma amino acids as an index for subgroups in manic depressive psychosis: Correlation to effect of tryptophan. *Psychopharmacologia, 49,* 205–213.

Moller, S. E., Kirk, L., & Honore, P. (1980). Relationship between plasma ratio of tryptophan to competing amino acids and the response to L-tryptophan treatment in endogenously depressed patients. *J. Affect. Disord., 2,* 47–50.

Morrison, J. H., Foote, S. L., Molliver, M. E., Bloom, F. E., & Lidov, H. G. W. (1982). Noradrenergic and serotonergic fibers innervate complementary layers in monkey primary visual cortex: An immunohistochemical study. *Proc. Natl. Acad. Sci. USA, 79,* 2401–2405.

Mueller, E. A., Murphy, D. L., Sunderland, T., & Jones, J. (1985). A new postsynaptic serotonin receptor agonist suitable for studies in humans. *Psychopharmacol. Bull., 21,* 701–703.

Mulgirigama, L. D. (1976). Significance of uptake studies with biogenic amines. In J. E. Murphy (Ed.), *Research and clinical investigation in depression* (pp. 10–15). Northampton, England: Cambridge Medical Publications.

Murphy, D. L., Baker, M., Goodwin, F. K., Miller, H., Kotin, J., & Bunney, W. E. (1974). L-tryptophan in affective disorders: Indoleamine changes and differential clinical effects. *Psychopharmacologia, 34,* 11–20.

Murphy, D. L., Mueller, E. A., Garrick, N. A., & Aulakh, C. S. (1986). Use of serotonergic agents in the clinical assessment of central serotonin function. *J. Clin. Psychiatry, 47*(Suppl), 9–15.

Nelson, J. C., & Mazure, C. M. (1986). Lithium augmentation in psychotic depression refractory to combined drug treatment. *Am. J. Psychiatry, 143,* 363–366.

Nimgaonkar, V. L., Goodwin, F. K., Davies, C. L., & Green, A. R. (1985). Down-regulation of beta-adrenoceptors in rat cortex by repeated administration of desipramine, electroconvulsive shock and clenbuterol requires 5HT neurones but not 5HT. *Neuropharmacology, 24,* 279–283.

Nordin, G., Ottosson, J. O., & Roos, B. E. (1971). Influence of convulsive therapy on 5-hydroxyindoleacetic acid and homovanillic acid in cerebrospinal fluid in endogenous depression. *Psychopharmacologia, 20,* 315-320.

Norman, T. R., Burrows, G. D., Marriot, P. F., McIntyre, I. M., Davies, B. M., & Moore, R. G. (1983). Zimelidine: A placebo-controlled trial in depression. *Psychiatry Res., 8,* 95-103.

Norton, K. R., Sireling, L. I., Bhat, A. V., Rao, B., & Paykel, E. S. (1984). A double-blind comparison of fluvoxamine, imipramine and placebo in depressed patients. *J. Affect. Disord., 7,* 297-308.

Nystrom, C., & Hallstrom, T. (1985). Double-blind comparison between a serotonin and a noradrenaline reuptake blocker in the treatment of depressed outpatients: Clinical aspects. *Acta Psychiatr. Scand., 72,* 6-15.

Ogren, S. O., Fuxe, K., Agnati, L. F., Gustavsson, J. A., Jonsson, G., & Holm, A. C. (1979). Reevaluation of the indoleamine hypothesis of depression: Evidence for a reduction of functional activity of central 5-HT systems by antidepressant drugs. *J. Neural. Transm., 46,* 85-103.

Olpe, H. R., & Schellenberg, A. (1981). The sensitivity of cortical neurons to serotonin: Effect of chronic treatment with antidepressants, serotonin-uptake inhibitors and monoamine-oxidase-blocking drugs. *J. Neural. Transm., 51,* 233-244.

Oreland, L., Wiberg, A., Asberg, M., Traskman, L., Sjostrand, L., Thoren, P., Bertilsson, L., & Tybring, G. (1981). Platelet MAO activity and monoamine metabolites in cerebrospinal fluid in depressed and suicidal patients and in healthy controls. *Psychiatry Res., 4,* 21-29.

Overall, J. E., Hollister, L. E., Pokorny, A. D., Casey, J. F., & Katz, G. (1962). Drug therapy in depressions: Controlled evaluation of imipramine, isocarboxazid, dextroamphetamine, amobarbital, and placebo. *Clin. Pharmacol. Ther., 3,* 16-22.

Oxenkrug, I. M., Prakhje, J., & Mikhalenko, J. N. (1978). Disturbed circadian rhythms of 5-hydroxytryptamine uptake by blood platelets in depressive psychoses. *Act. Nerv. Super. (Praha), 20,* 66-67.

Papeschi, R., & McClure, D. J. (1971). Homovanillic and 5-hydroxyindoleacetic acid in cerebrospinal fluid of depressed patients. *Arch. Gen. Psychiatry, 25,* 354-358.

Paul, S. M., Rehavi, M., Rice, K. C., Ittah, Y., & Skolnick, P. (1981). Does high affinity (3H)imipramine binding label serotonin reuptake sites in brain and platelet? *Life Sci., 28,* 2753-2760.

Peroutka, S. J. (1989). Central 5HT receptors: Functional correlates and clinical relevance. In S. L. Brown & H. M. van Praag (Eds.), *Serotonin in the psychiatric disorders.* New York: Brunner/Mazel.

Peroutka, S. J., Lebovitz, R. M., & Snyder, S. H. (1981). Two distinct central serotonin receptors with different physiological functions. *Science, 212,* 827-829.

Peroutka, S. J., & Snyder, S. H. (1980). Long term antidepressant treatment decreases spiroperidol-labelled serotonin receptor binding. *Science, 210,* 88-90.

Perry, E. K., Marshall, E. F., Blessed, G., Tomlinson, B. E., & Perry, R. H. (1983). Decreased imipramine binding in the brains of patients with depressive illness. *Br. J. Psychiatry, 142,* 188-192.

Poirier, M. F., Galzin, A. M., Loo, H., Pimoule, C., Segonz, A. C. A., Benkelfat,

C., Sechter, D., Zerifian, E., Schoemaker, H., & Langer, S. Z. (1987). Changes in 3H-5HT uptake and 3H-imipramine binding in platelets after chlorimipramine in healthy volunteers. Comparison with maprotiline and amineptine. *Biol. Psychiatry, 22,* 287–302.

Post, R. M., & Goodwin, F. K. (1974). Effects of amitriptyline and imipramine on amine metabolites in the cerebrospinal fluid of depressed patients. *Arch. Gen. Psychiatry, 30,* 234–239.

Post, R. M., Kopin, J., & Goodwin, F. K. (1974). The effects of cocaine in depressed patients. *Am. J. Psychiatry, 131,* 511–517.

Price, L. H., Charney, D. S., & Heninger, G. R. (1985a). Efficacy of lithium-tranylcypromine treatment in refractory depression. *Am. J. Psychiatry, 142,* 619–623.

Price, L. H., Charney, D. S., & Heninger, G. R. (1985b). Effects of tranylcypromine treatment on neuroendocrine, behavioral, and autonomic responses to tryptophan in depressed patients. *Life Sci., 37,* 809–818.

Price, L. H., Conwell, Y., & Nelson, J. C. (1983). Lithium augmentation of combined neuroleptic-tricyclic treatment in delusional depression. *Am. J. Psychiatry, 140,* 318–322.

Puhringer, W., Wirz-Justice, A., Graw, P., LaCoste, V., & Gastpar, M. (1976a). Intravenous L-5-hydroxytryptophan in normal subjects: An interdisciplinary precursor loading study. Part I: Implication of reproducible mood elevation. *Pharmakopsychiatrie, 9,* 260–268.

Puhringer, W., Wirz-Justice, A., & Lancranjan, I. (1976b). Mood elevation and pituitary stimulation after IV L-5-HTP in normal subjects: Evidence for a common serotonergic mechanism. *Neurosci. Lett., 2,* 349–354.

Quitkin, F. M., Rabkin, J. G., Ross, D., & McGrath, P. J. (1984). Duration of antidepressant drug treatment: What is an adequate trial? *Arch. Gen. Psychiatry, 41,* 238–245.

Raisman, R., Briley, M. S., Bouchami, F., Sechter, D., Zarifian, E., & Langer, S. Z. (1982). 3H-imipramine binding and serotonin uptake in platelets from untreated depressed patients and control volunteers. *Psychopharmacology, 77,* 332–335.

Raisman, R., Sechter, D., Briley, M. S., Zarifian, E., & Langer, S. Z. (1981). High affinity 3H-imipramine binding in platelets from untreated and treated depressed patients compared to healthy volunteers. *Psychopharmacology, 75,* 368–371.

Ramsey, T. A., & Mendels, J. (1981). Lithium ion as an antidepressant. In S. J. Enna, J. B. Malick & E. Richelson (Eds.), *Antidepressants: Neurochemical, behavioral and clinical perspectives* (pp. 175–182). New York: Raven Press.

Rao, B., & Broadhurst, A. D. (1976). Tryptophan and depression. *Br. Med. J., 1,* 460.

Raotma, H. (1978). The combination of tryptophan and electroconvulsive therapy in the treatment of depression. Academic dissertation, University of Gothenburg.

Rausch, J. L., Shah, N. S., Burch, E. A., & Donald, A. G. (1982). Platelet serotonin uptake in depressed patients: Circadian effect. *Biol. Psychiatry, 17,* 121–123.

Richelson, E., & Nelson, A. (1984). Antagonism by antidepressants of neurotransmitter receptors of normal human brain in vitro. *J. Pharmacol. Exp. Ther., 230,* 94–102.

Ross, S. B., Aperia, B., Beck-Friis, J., Jansa, S., Wetterberg, L. & Aberg, A. (1980). Inhibition of 5-hydroxytryptamine uptake in human platelets by antidepressant agents in vivo. *Psychopharmacology, 67,* 1–7.

Roy, A., Everett, D., Pickar, D., & Paul, S. M. (1987). Platelet tritiated imipramine binding and serotonin uptake in depressed patients and controls: Relationship to plasma cortisol levels before and after dexamethasone administration. *Arch. Gen. Psychiatry, 44,* 320–327.

Roy-Byrne, P., Post, R. M., Rubinow, D. R., Linnoila, M., Savard, R., & Davis, D. (1983). CSF 5HIAA and personal and family history of suicide in affectively ill patients: A negative study. *Psychiatry Res., 10,* 263–274.

Sano, I. (1972). L-5-hydroxytryptophan (L-5-HTP) therapy. *Folia Psychiatr. Neurol. Jpn., 26,* 7–17.

Schildkraut, J. J. (1965). The catecholamine hypothesis of affective disorders: A review of supporting evidence. *Am. J. Psychiatry, 122,* 509–522.

Scott, J. A., & Crews, F. T. (1985). Increase in serotonin-2 receptor density in rat cerebral cortex slices by stimulation of beta-adrenergic receptors. *Biochem. Pharmacol., 34,* 1585–1588.

Scott, J. A., & Crews, F. T. (1986). Down-regulation of serotonin-2, but not of beta-adrenergic receptors during chronic treatment with amitriptyline is independent of stimulation of serotonin-2 and beta-adrenergic receptors. *Neuropharmacology, 25,* 1301–1306.

Segawa, T., Mizuta, T., & Uehara, M. (1982). Role of the central serotonergic system as related to the pathogenesis of depression: Effect of antidepressants on rat central serotonergic activity. In S. Z. Langer, R. Takahashi, T. Segawa, & M. Briley (Eds.), *New vistas in depression* (pp. 3–10). New York: Pergamon Press.

Shapira, B., Reiss, A., Kaiser, N., Kindler, S., & Lerer, B. (1989). Effect of imipramine treatment on the prolactin response to fenfluramine and placebo challenge in depressed patients. *J. Affect. Disord., 16,* 1–4.

Shaw, D. M., Camps, F. E., & Eccleston, E. G. (1967). 5-hydroxytryptamine in the hindbrain of depressive suicides. *Br. J. Psychiatry, 113,* 1407–1411.

Shopsin, B., Friedman, E., & Gershon, S. (1976). Parachlorophenylalanine reversal of tranylcypromine effects in depressed patients. *Arch. Gen. Psychiatry, 33,* 811–819.

Shoulson, I., & Chase, T. N. (1975). Fenfluramine in man: Hypophagia associated with diminished serotonin turnover. *Clin. Pharmacol. Ther., 17,* 616–621.

Siever, L. J., Murphy, D. L., Slater, S., de la Vega, E., & Lipper, S. (1984). Plasma prolactin changes following fenfluramine in depressed patients compared to controls: An evaluation of central serotonergic responsivity in depression. *Life Sci., 34,* 1029–1039.

Siwers, B., Ringberger, V. A., Tuck, R., & Sjoqvist, F. (1976). Initial clinical trial based on clinical methodology of zimelidine (a serotonin uptake inhibitor) in depressed patients. *Clin. Pharmacol. Ther., 21,* 194–200.

Sjostrom, R. (1973). 5-hydroxyindole acetic acid and homovanillic acid in cerebrospinal fluid in manic-depressive psychosis and the effect of probenecid treatment. *Eur. J. Clin. Pharmacol., 6,* 75–80.

Slater, S., de la Vega, C. E., Skyler, J., & Murphy, D. L. (1976). Plasma prolactin stimulation by fenfluramine and amphetamine. *Psychopharmacol. Bull., 12,* 26–27.

Sloviter, R. S., Drust, E. G., & Connor, J. D. (1978). Specificity of a rat behavioral model for serotonin receptor activation. *J. Pharmacol. Exp. Ther., 206,* 339–347.

Sneddon, J. M. (1969). Sodium-dependent accumulation of 5-hydroxytryptamine by rat blood platelets. *Br. J. Pharmacol., 37,* 680–688.

Sneddon, J. M. (1973). Blood platelets as a model for monoamine-containing neurons. *Prog. Neurobiol., 1,* 151–198.

Stahl, S. M. (1977). The human platelet. *Arch. Gen. Psychiatry, 34,* 509–516.

Stahl, S. M. (1984). Regulation of neurotransmitter receptors by desipramine and other antidepressant drugs: The neurotransmitter receptor hypothesis of antidepressant action. *J. Clin. Psychiatry, 45,* 37–44.

Stahl, S. M., & Meltzer; H. Y. (1978). A kinetic and pharmacologic analysis of 5-hydroxytryptamine transport by human platelets and platelet storage granules: Comparison with central serotonergic neurons. *J. Pharmacol. Exp. Ther., 205,* 118–132.

Stanley, M., & Mann, J. J. (1983). Increased serotonin-2 binding sites in frontal cortex of suicide victims. *Lancet, 1,* 214–216.

Stanley, M., Virgilio, J., & Gershon, S. (1982). Tritiated imipramine binding sites are decreased in the frontal cortex of suicides. *Science, 216,* 1337–1339.

Stark, P., & Hardison, C. D. (1985). A review of multicenter controlled studies of fluoxetine vs. imipramine and placebo in outpatients with major depressive disorder. *J. Clin. Psychiatry, 46,* 53–58.

Stockmeier, C. A., & Kellar, K. J. (1986). In vivo regulation of the serotonin-2 receptor in rat brain. *Life Sci., 38,* 117–127.

Stolz, J. F., Marsden, C. A., & Middlemiss, D. N. (1983). Effect of antidepressant treatment and subsequent withdrawal on 3H-5-hydroxytryptamine and 3H-spiperone binding in rat frontal cortex and serotonin receptor mediated behaviour. *Psychopharmacology, 80,* 150–155.

Sugrue, M. F. (1983a). Chronic antidepressant therapy and associated changes in central monoaminergic receptor functioning. *Pharmacol. Ther., 21,* 1–33.

Sugrue, M. F. (1983b). Do antidepressants possess a common mechanism of action? *Biochem. Pharmacol., 32,* 1811–1817.

Sulser, F. (1986). UPdate on neuroreceptor mechanisms and their implication for the pharmacotherapy of affective disorders. *J. Clin. Psychiatry, 47*(Suppl), 13–18.

Sulser, F. (1987). Serotonin-norepinephrine receptor interactions in the brain: Implications for the pharmacology and pathophysiology of affective disorders. *J. Clin. Psychiatry, 48,* 12–18.

Suranyi-Cadotte, B. E., Quirion, R., Nair, N. P., Lafaille, F., & Schwartz, G. (1985). Imipramine treatment differentially affects platelet 3H-imipramine binding and serotonin uptake in depressed patients. *Life Sci., 36,* 795–799.

Suranyi-Cadotte, B. E., Wood, P. L., Schwartz, G., & Nair, N. P. V. (1983). Altered platelet 3H-imipramine binding in schizoaffective and depressive disorders. *Biol. Psychiatry, 18,* 923–927.

Swade, C., & Coppen, A. (1981). Seasonal variation in biochemical factors related to depressive illness. *J. Affect. Disord., 2,* 249–255.

Takahashi, S., Takahashi, R., & Masamura, I. (1976). Measurement of 5-hydroxy-indole compounds during 5-HTP treatment in depressed patients. *Folia Psychiatr. Neurol. Jpn., 30,* 463–474.

Tang, S., & Morris, J. (1985). Variation in human platelet 3H-imipramine binding. *Psychiatry Res., 16,* 141–146.

Thompson, T. L., & Thomas, M. R. (1986). Depression: Medical interface with psychiatry and treatment advances. *J. Clin. Psychiatry, 47,* 31–36.

Thomson, J., Rankin, H., Ashcroft, G. W., Yates, C. M., McQueen, J. K., & Cummings, S. W. (1982). The treatment of depression in general practice: A comparison of L-tryptophan, amitriptyline, and a combination of L-tryptophan and amitriptyline with placebo. *Psychol. Med., 12,* 741–751.

Traskman, L., Asberg, M., Bertilsson, L., Cronholm, B., Mellstrom, B., Neckers, L. M., Sjoqvist, F., Thoren, P., & Tybring, G. (1979). Plasma levels of chlorimipramine and its desmethyl metabolite during treatment of depression. *Clin. Pharmacol. Ther., 26,* 600–610.

Traskman, L., Asberg, M., Bertilsson, L., & Sjostrand, L. (1981). Monoamine metabolites in CSF and suicidal behavior. *Arch. Gen. Psychiatry, 38,* 631–636.

Trimble, M., Chadwick, D., Reynolds, E., & Marsden, C. D. (1975). L-5-hydroxy-tryptophan and mood. *Lancet, 1,* 583.

Tuomisto, J. (1974). A new modification for studying 5-HT uptake by blood platelets: A re-evaluation of tricyclic antidepressants as uptake inhibitors. *J. Pharm. Pharmacol., 26,* 92–100.

Tuomisto, J., & Tukiainen, E. (1976). Decreased uptake of 5-hydroxytryptamine in blood platelets from depressed patients. *Nature, 266,* 596–598.

Tuomisto, J., Tukiainen, E., & Ahlfors, U. G. (1979). Decreased uptake of 5-hydroxytryptamine in blood platelets from patients with endogenous depression. *Psychopharmacology, 65,* 141–147.

Valzelli, L. (1984). Reflections on experimental and human pathology of aggression. *Prog. Neuropsychopharmacol. Biol. Psychiatry, 8,* 311–325.

van Hiele, L. J. (1980). L-5-hydroxytryptophan in depression: The first substitution therapy in psychiatry? *Neuropsychobiology, 6,* 230–240.

van Praag, H. M. (1981). Management of depression with serotonin precursors. *Biol. Psychiatry, 16,* 291–310.

van Praag, H. M. (1982a). Depression, suicide, and the metabolism of serotonin in the brain. *J. Affect. Disord., 4,* 275–290.

van Praag, H. M. (1982b). Serotonin precursors in the treatment of depression. In B. T. Ho, J. C. Schoolar, & E. Usdin (Eds.), *Advances in biochemical psychopharmacology: Serotonin in biological psychiatry,* Vol. 34 (pp. 259–286). New York: Raven Press.

van Praag, H. M. (1983). In search of the mode of action of antidepressants: 5-HTP/tyrosine mixtures in depressions. *Neuropharmacology, 22,* 433–440.

van Praag, H. M. (1984). Studies in the mechanism of action of serotonin precursors in depression. *Psychopharmacol. Bull., 20,* 599-602.

van Praag, H. M. (1986a). Indoleamines in depression and suicide. In J. M. van Ree & S. Matthysse (Eds.), *Progress in brain research,* Vol. 65 (pp. 59-71). Amsterdam: Elsevier.

van Praag, H. M. (1986b). Biological suicide research: Outcome and limitations. *Biol. Psychiatry, 21,* 1305-1323.

van Praag, H. M., & de Haan, S. (1981). Chemoprophylaxis of depressions: An attempt to compare lithium with 5-hydroxytryptophan. *Acta Psychiatr. Scand., 63,* 191-201.

van Praag, H. M., Flentge, F., Korf, J., Dols, L. C. W., & Schut, T. (1973b). The influence of probenecid on the metabolism of serotonin, dopamine and their precursors in man. *Psychopharmacologia, 33,* 141-151.

van Praag, H. M., Kahn, R., Asnis, G. M., Lemus, C. Z., & Brown, S. L. (1987a). Therapeutic indications for serotonin potentiating compounds: A hypothesis. *Biol. Psychiatry, 22,* 205-212.

van Praag, H. M., Kahn, R., Asnis, G. M., Wetzler, S., Brown, S. L., Bleich, A., & Korn, M. L. (1987c). Denosologization of biological psychiatry, or the specificity of 5-HT disturbances in psychiatric disorders. *J. Affect. Disord., 13,* 1-8.

van Praag, H. M., Kahn, R., Asnis, G. M., Wetzler, S., Brown, S. L., Bleich, A., & Korn, M. L. (1988). Beyond nosology in biological psychiatry. 5HT disturbances in mood-, aggression-, and anxiety-disorders. In M. Briley & J. Fillion (Eds.), *New concepts in depression* (pp. 96-119). New York: Macmillan.

van Praag, H. M., Korf, J., Lakke, J. P. W. F., & Schut, T. (1975). Dopamine metabolism in depression, psychoses and Parkinson's disease: The problem of the specificity of biological variables in behaviour disorders. *Psychol. Med., 5,* 138-146.

van Praag, H. M., Korf, J., & Puite, J. (1970). 5-Hydroxyindoleacetic acid levels in the cerebrospinal fluid of depressive patients treated with probenecid. *Nature, 225,* 1259-1260.

van Praag, H. M., Korf, J., & Schut, T. (1973a). Cerebral monoamines and depression. An investigation with the probenecid technique. *Arch. Gen. Psychiatry, 28,* 827-831.

van Praag, H. M., & Leijnse, B. (1963a). Die bedeutung der monoamineoxydasehemmung als antidepressives Prinzip I. *Psychopharmacologia, 4,* 1-14.

van Praag, H. M., & Leijnse, B. (1963b). Die bedeutung der monoamineoxydasehemmung als antidepressives Prinzip II. *Psychopharmacologia, 4,* 91-102.

van Praag, H. M., Lemus, C., & Kahn, R. (1987b). Hormonal probes of central serotonergic activity: Do they really exist? *Biol. Psychiatry, 22,* 86-98.

van Praag, H. M., van den Burg, W., Bos, E. R. H., & Dols, L. C. W. (1974). 5-Hydroxytryptophan in combination with clomipramine in 'therapy-resistant' depression. *Psychopharmacologia, 38,* 267-269.

Vetulani, J., Lebrecht, U., & Pilc, A. (1981). Enhancement of responsiveness of the central serotonergic system and serotonin-2 receptor density in rat frontal cortex by electroconvulsive shock treatment. *Eur. J. Pharmacol., 76,* 81-85.

Wagner, A., Aberg-Wistedt, A., Asberg, M., Bertilsson, L., Martensson, B., & Montero, D. (1987). Effects of antidepressant treatments on platelet tritiated imipramine binding in major depressive disorder. *Arch. Gen. Psychiatry, 44,* 870–877.

Walinder, J., Skott, A., Carlsson, A., Nagy, A., & Roos, B. E. (1976). Potentiation of antidepressant action of clomipramine by tryptophan. *Arch. Gen. Psychiatry, 33,* 1384–1389.

Wamsley, J. K., Byerley, W. F., McCabe, R. T., McConnell, E. J., Daeson, T. M., & Grosser, B. I. (1987). Receptor alterations associated with serotonergic agents: An autoradiographic analysis. *J. Clin. Psychiatry, 48,* 19–25.

Ward, N. G., Ang, J., & Pavinich, G. (1985). A comparison of the acute effects of dextroamphetamine and fenfluramine in depression. *Biol. Psychiatry, 20,* 1090–1097.

Westenberg, H. G. M., van Praag, H. M., de Jong, J. T. V. M., & Thyssen, J. H. H. (1982). Postsynaptic serotonergic activity in depressive patients: Evaluation of the neuroendocrine strategy. *Psychiatry Res., 7,* 361–375.

Whitaker, P. M., Warsh, J. J., Stancer, H. C., Persad, E., & Vint, C. K. (1984). Seasonal variation in platelet 3H-imipramine binding: Comparable values in control and depressed populations. *Psychiatry Res., 11,* 127–131.

Wiebe, R. H., Handmerger, S., & Hammon, D. B. (1977). Failure of 1-tryptophan to stimulate prolactin secretion in man. *J. Clin. Endocrinol. Metab., 45,* 1310–1312.

Willner, P. (1985). Antidepressants and serotonergic neurotransmission: An integrative review. *Psychopharmacology, 85,* 387–404.

Wirz-Justice, A. (1977). Theoretical and therapeutical potential of indoleamine precursors in affective disorders. *Neuropsychobiology, 3,* 199–233.

Wirz-Justice, A., & Puhringer, W. (1978). Seasonal incidence of an altered diurnal rhythm of platelet serotonin in unipolar depression. *J. Neural. Transm., 42,* 45–53.

Wood, P. L., Suranyi-Cadotte, B. E., Schwartz, G., & Nair, N. P. V. (1983a). Platelet 3H-imipramine binding and red blood cell choline in affective disorders: Indications of heterogenous pathogenesis. *Biol. Psychiatry, 18,* 715–719.

Wood, K., Swade, C., Abou-Saleh, M., Milln, P., & Coppen, A. (1983b). Drug plasma levels and platelet 5-HT uptake inhibition during long-term treatment with fluvoxamine or lithium in patients with affective disorders. *Br. J. Clin. Pharmacol., 15,* 365s–368s.

Woolf, P. D., & Lee, L. (1977). Effect of the serotonin precursor, tryptophan, on pituitary hormone secretion. *J. Clin. Endocrinol. Metab., 45,* 123–133.

Wurtman, R. J. (1982). Nutrients that modify brain function. *Sci. Am., 426,* 50–59.

Wurtman, R. J., Heft, F., & Melamed, E. (1981). Precursor control of neurotransmitter synthesis. *Pharmacol. Rev., 32,* 315–335.

Yuwiler, A., Brammer, G., Morley, J., Raleigh, M. J., Flannery, J. W., & Geller, B. (1981). Short-term and repetitive administration of oral tryptophan in normal men. *Arch. Gen. Psychiatry, 38,* 619–626.

Zis, A. P., & Goodwin, F. K. (1979). Novel antidepressants and the biogenic amine hypothesis of depression: The case for iprindole and mianserin. *Arch. Gen. Psychiatry, 36,* 1097–1107.

6

The Role of Serotonin in the Regulation of Anxiety

RENE S. KAHN
OREN KALUS
SCOTT WETZLER
HERMAN M. VAN PRAAG

Since 1948, when it was discovered in blood platelets, serotonin (5-HT) has gained increasing attention for its role in a variety of brain functions and mental disorders. Whereas van Praag and Korf (1971) demonstrated that a subgroup of depressed patients had decreased 5-HT metabolism, subsequent investigations have indicated that 5-HT dysfunction may be implicated in other psychiatric disorders as well. Since lowered 5-HT metabolism does not appear to be specific to one particular psychiatric disorder (such as depression), it may be that 5-HT dysfunction is related to a dimension of psychopathology that spans several diagnoses. One hypothesized dimension is aggression—either inwardly directed as in suicide, or outwardly directed toward others (van Praag, 1986). This chapter reviews research relating 5-HT to another dimension of psychopathology: anxiety.

In comparison with studies of 5-HT in depression, the role of 5-HT in anxiety has received considerably less attention. Most of the data supporting a connection between 5-HT and anxiety are based on animal studies. In contrast to the extensive research on the role of noradrenergic mechanisms in anxiety, 5-HT research in human subjects has only recently begun. Nonetheless, a substantial body of animal work and some exciting recent findings in humans warrant a closer examination of the 5-HT/anxiety relationship. One recent line of investigation of particular interest involves the role of hypersensitive serotonin receptors in the pathophysiology of panic disorder.

129

ANIMAL EXPERIMENTS

Methodological Issues

A major methodological problem in animal laboratory studies of anxiety (as well as affect) is that the emotion must be inferred exclusively from external behavior. Researchers have responded to this dilemma by defining particular behaviors (that are easily recognizable and reproducible under experimental conditions) as likely representatives of anxiety states.

Two standard paradigms frequently used to operationalize the construct of anxiety in animals are: (1) exposure to novel stimuli, and (2) introduction of a conflict situation. The former paradigm (novel environment) involves placing the animal in a large, ceilingless, brightly lit box. In this situation, animals tend to show decreased exploratory behavior (Crawley & Goodwin, 1980) and decreased social interaction (File, 1985), both of which are regarded as indicative of anxiety.

The conflict paradigm is based on a conditioned emotional response (CER) model (Estes & Skinner, 1941). In this model, the animal is conditioned to press a bar in order to obtain a reward (generally food). Later a signal (e.g., a light) is introduced, coupled to a punishment (e.g., electric shock), which also follows bar pressing. The animal faced with a conflict situation (between reward and punishment) decreases its bar pressing. The so-called behavioral suppression of bar pressing is taken to be the result of anxiety. Two widely used anxiety models developed by Geller and Seifter (1967) and by Vogel et al. (1971) are modifications of this basic CER paradigm (food being the reward in the Geller and Seifter model and liquid in Vogel's water-lick model).

Another feature of these models is that release from behavioral suppression is assumed to be related to anxiety reduction, and the quantity of release, a measure of the anxiolytic effect. Support for these inferences comes from the consistent observation of release from behavioral suppression by established anxiolytics, such as the benzodiazepines (BZs), barbiturates, and alcohol (Lal & Emmett-Oglesby, 1983).

One restriction of these models, though, is that they do not adequately measure increased anxiety. An additional problem is the difficulty in distinguishing a separate and unrelated generalized motor inhibition from anxiety-induced motor inhibition. Thus, although suitable for assessing anxiolytic effects, these models are inadequate for assessing increased anxiety. A recent modification of the novel environment model appears to overcome this limitation by reliably measuring the effects of both anxiolytic and anxiogenic drugs (Handley & Mithani, 1984; Pellow et al., 1985; Pellow & File, 1986). In the so-called "X-maze anxiety model" involving a maze with open and enclosed arms, general motor inhibition is expressed as a decrease in entries to both open *and* enclosed arms, while increased anxiety (without generalized motor inhibition) results in decreased entries only to the open arms of the X-maze. Anxiolytic effects appear as increased entries to the open arms of the maze (Montgomery, 1955).

Although we did not discuss all animal anxiety paradigms, most animal anxiety studies involve these basic experimental paradigms, and awareness of their general strengths and limitations should be kept in mind.

Manipulation of the 5-HT System

Decrease of 5-HT Function

5-HT antagonists. Various strategies have been used to decrease or increase 5-HT activity. One of the techniques used to examine the effects of diminishing 5-HT function has been the use of 5-HT antagonists.

Table 6-1 lists some of the nonspecific $5\text{-}HT_1/5\text{-}HT_2$ antagonists, such as methysergide, cinanserin, cyproheptadine, and metergoline (Sills et al., 1984; Hoyer et al., 1985), that have been used in animal anxiety studies. More recent anxiety studies have examined the effects of more selective agents, such as the selective $5\text{-}HT_2$ antagonist ritanserin and the selective $5\text{-}HT_3$ antagonists GR38242F and BRL43694—but only a small number of studies using these agents have been done. Despite the large number of studies with 5-HT antagonists, the findings have generally been inconclusive. The most consistent finding, that decreased 5-HT function results in diminished anxiety, has been obtained with studies using methysergide (in the Geller and Seifter model). In contrast, studies using cyproheptadine failed to show anxiety reduction, and the metergoline and cinanserin findings have been contradictory (though only a small number of studies were done).

The selective $5\text{-}HT_2$ antagonist ritanserin did not reduce anxiety in a food-motivated punishment model (Colpaert et al., 1985), nor did it have anxiolytic effects in a social interaction model (Gardner, 1986). It did, however, have anxiolytic effects in the X-maze model (Critchley and Handley, 1987).

The selective $5\text{-}HT_3$ antagonists GR38032F and BRL 43694 had anxiolytic effects in rats (in the novel environment model) (Costall et al., 1987; Jones et al., 1987), as well as in monkeys (Jones et al., 1987). Piper et al. (1987) also found that these agents had anxiolytic effects in rats in the novel environment model but no effects on rats in the Geller and Seifter model, and only weak anxiolytic effects in monkeys.

Interpretation of these findings is hampered by the fact that most of the agents used are not purely selective for 5-HT. Both methysergide and metergoline have pronounced dopamine (DA) agonistic effects (except in

TABLE 6-1
5-HT Antagonists in Animal Anxiety Studies

Author	Drug	Dose (mg/kg)	Model	Effect
Graeff, 1970	Methysergide	0.3	CER	Release of suppression
Winter, 1972	Methysergide	3–10	G + S	Release of suppression
Stein, 1975	Methysergide	10	G + S	Release of suppression
Graeff, 1974	Methysergide	3–10	G + S	Release of suppression
Cook, 1975	Methysergide	1–10	G + S	Release of suppression
Petersen, 1981	Methysergide	0.3–3	Waterlick	Release of suppression
Kilts, 1981	Methysergide	1–18	Waterlick	Release of suppression
Gardner, 1985	Methysergide	2–20	Waterlick	Release of suppression
Geller, 1974	Cinanserin	60	G + S	Release of suppression
Winter, 1972	Cinanserin	3–15	G + S	No effect
Sepinwall, 1978	Cinanserin	60	G + S	No effect
Cook, 1975	Cinanserin	15	G + S	Release of suppression
Kilts, 1981	Cinanserin	56	Waterlick	Release of suppression
Petersen, 1981	Cinanserin	10–60	Waterlick	No effect
Petersen, 1981	Cyproheptadine	1–10	Waterlick	No effect
Kilts, 1981	Cyproheptadine	1–18	Waterlick	No effect
Gardner, 1985	Cyproheptadine	10	CER	No effect
Leone, 1983	Metergoline	0.3–3	CER	Release of suppression
Gardner, 1985	Metergoline	10, 20	CER	No effect
Commissaris, 1982	Metergoline	0.25–2	Waterlick	No effect
Colpaert, 1985	Ritanserin	0.005–5	G + S	No effect
Gardner, 1986	Ritanserin	0.025–5	NE	No effect
File, 1987	Ritanserin	0.025–5	Xmaze	Increased entries
Costall, 1987	GR38032F	0.005–10	NE	Release of inhibition
Costall, 1987	BRL43694	0.001–1.0	NE	Release of inhibition
Jones, 1987	GR38032F	0.01, 0.1	NE	Release of inhibition
Piper, 1987	GR38032F	0.005–5	NE	Release of inhibition
Piper, 1987	BRL43694	0.005–5	NE	Release of inhibition
Piper, 1987	GR38032F	0.005–5	G + S	No effect
Piper, 1987	BRL43694	0.005–5	G + S	No effect

CER: Conditioned emotional response model (Esters & Skinner, 1958)
G + S: Geller and Seifter model (Geller & Seifter, 1967) and related models
Waterlick: Water-lick model (Vogel et al., 1971)
NE: Novel environment model (File, 1985) and related models
Xmaze: X-maze anxiety model (Montgomery, 1955)

doses under 0.1 mg/kg, which have not been used in the animal experiments) (Krulich et al., 1981). Similarly, cyproheptadine has effects on histamine and choline receptors (Remy et al., 1977). Cinanserin was considered to be selective for 5-HT by Geller et al. (1974) because its effects could be reversed by administration of 5-hydroxytryptophan (5-HTP, the precursor of 5-HT). However, the fact that 5-HTP gains access not just to 5-HT neurons, but also to catecholamine (CA) neurons, casts doubt on

TABLE 6-2
Parachlorophenylalanine (100–400 mg) in Animal Anxiety Studies

Author	Model	Effect	Comment
Robichaud, 1969	G + S	Release of suppression	
Geller, 1970	G + S	Release of suppression	Reversed by 5-HTP
Wise, 1972	G + S	Release of suppression	
Blakely, 1973	G + S	No effect	
Stein, 1973	G + S	Release of suppression	Reversed by 5-HTP
Tye, 1977	G + S	Release of suppression	Reversed by 5-HTP, not DOPA
Shephard, 1982	G + S	Release of suppression	Reversed by 5-MeODMT
Engel, 1984	G + S	Release of suppression	Reversed by 5-HTP, 8-OHDPAT
Kilts, 1981	Waterlick	Release of suppression	
Petersen, 1981	Waterlick	Release of suppression	
Ellison, 1977	NE	Release of inhibition	
File, 1977	NE	Release of inhibition	

G + S:	Geller and Seifter (Geller & Seifter, 1970) and related models
Waterlick:	Water-lick model (Vogel et al., 1971)
NE:	Novel environment (File, 1985) and related models
5-HTP:	5-hydroxytryptophan
DOPA:	Deoxyphenylalanine
5-MeODMT:	5-methoxydimethyltryptamine
8-OHDPAT:	8-hydroxy-N,N-dipropylamino tetralin

cinanserin's 5-HT selectivity as well. In both neurotransmitter systems 5-HTP is transformed into 5-HT, which acts as a false transmitter in the CA system, causing a compensatory increase in CA metabolism. The net functional effect is probably increased CA function (van Praag, 1983).

In summary, studies using 5-HT antagonists have provided inconsistent results. This may be attributable to differences among investigators using similar substances but different models, and to the nonselectivity of most of the compounds used. However, preliminary results with more selective 5-HT antagonists suggest that they are anxiolytic (presumably as a consequence of diminishing 5-HT activity).

Inhibition of 5-HT synthesis. Another method of experimentally diminishing 5-HT function is the use of 5-HT synthesis inhibitors, such as parachlorophenylalanine (pCPA).

As Table 6-2 indicates, studies involving pCPA provide more consistent findings than studies using 5-HT-antagonists. pCPA decreases 5-HT availability by about 90% [though it also has a slight effect (depending on the dose) on the availability of noradrenaline (NA)]. Administration of pCPA consistently causes release from behavioral suppression in animal anxiety models. This effect is abolished by the administration of 5-HTP (Geller & Blum, 1970; Stein et al., 1973; Tye et al., 1979; Engel et al., 1984), as well as by the 5HT$_{1a}$ agonists 5-methoxy dimethyl tryptamine (5-MeODMT) (Shephard et al., 1982) and 8-hydroxydepropylamino-tetralin (8-OHDPAT) (Engel et al., 1984). Augmentation of DA and NA function through administration of DOPA, the precursor of both DA and NA, does not reverse the pCPA effect (Tye et al., 1979), suggesting that catecholamines are not involved in pCPA's anxiolytic effects.

An objection might be raised that pCPA's anxiolytic effects are mediated by behavioral mechanisms other than anxiety reduction—since pCPA directly increases food intake (hyperphagia) (Blundell, 1984) and drinking (Barofski et al., 1980). Because conflict-based anxiety models depend on food and water as positive reinforcers, one might argue that pCPA's effects are secondary to direct stimulation of food intake and not to decreased anxiety. It seems more likely that pCPA is anxiolytic, since it also produces effects in the novel environment model, which does not depend on food or water reward.

Destruction of 5-HT Neurons.   Yet another method of reducing 5-HT function involves the use of agents toxic to 5-HT neurons. Both 5,7-dihydroxytryptamine (DHT) and 5,6-DHT eliminate 5-HT neurons in specific brain regions. In several studies, localized destruction of 5-HT–containing regions resulted in diminished anxiety responses. Injection of DHT in the ventral tegmentum caused marked release from behavioral suppression (in the Geller and Seifter model) 11 days after administration (Tye et al., 1977). A similar effect was found following intraventricular DHT administration in the water-lick model (Lippa et al., 1979). DHT lesioning of the dorsal raphe (in a novel environment model) resulted in anxiety reduction 12 days later, in contrast to median raphe lesionings, which did not (File et al. 1979). The latter findings suggest functional specificity for different 5-HT anatomical regions, and possibly a greater involvement of the dorsal raphe systems in anxiety mechanisms. Anxiolytic effects were also observed 14 days after lateral septum lesioning. In contrast, no anxiety reduction was found after destruction of CA neurons with 6-hydroxydopamine (6-OHDA) (in a novel environment model), suggesting that CA systems were not involved (Clarke & File, 1982).

Assessment of DHT's effects at times other than the ones used in the above studies has led to varying findings. No anxiety reduction was seen 21 days after intraventricular DHT lesioning in a conflict model (Thiebot et al., 1982), or three to five days after intraventricular administration in a water-lick model (Commissaris et al., 1981). However, several studies did show anxiety reduction at 10 to 14 days after DHT administration.

Conceivably, these disparities might be related to differential temporal 5-HT availability—but further investigation is needed to clarify this issue.

In summary, one may conclude that 5-HT destruction results in anxiety reduction in certain 5-HT regions at certain times, but does not have this effect in other regions or in the same region at different times.

Increase of 5-HT Function

Since diminishing 5-HT function (at least in some regions) results in anxiety reduction, one might predict that increasing 5-HT availability would cause the opposite effect. Empirical findings in animal studies have failed to prove or disprove this prediction, largely because of methodological limitations. The results of several studies with a variety of 5-HT agonists leave little doubt that increasing 5-HT function in animals does cause behavioral suppression. For example, Graeff and Schoenfeld (1970), using the 5-HT agonist α-methyl-tryptamine in the basic CER paradigm, reported inhibition of both punished and unpunished responding in pigeons. Similar results were found by Stein et al. (1973) and by Winter (1972) in rats given the same agent, as well as with other 5-HT agonists, such as m-chloro-phenylpiperazine (MCPP), fenfluramine (Kilts et al., 1982), and 5-MeODMT (Shephard et al., 1982). A problem of differentiating the cause of the behavioral inhibition arises, though, because increased 5-HT function is also associated with generalized motor inhibition. Consequently, in these models, 5-HT–induced anxiogenic effects cannot be differentiated from the general effects of 5-HT on motor behavior.

The X-maze model, as described earlier, does appear able to differentiate the two (Montgomery, 1955), and in this model, the 5-HT agonists 8-OHDPAT and 5-MeODMT did in fact selectively decrease open-arm entries of rats, indicating that anxiogenesis had occurred (Critchley & Handley, 1987).

Benzodiazepines (BZs), 5-HT, and Anxiety

Since BZs are clearly effective anxiety-reducing agents in humans and cause release from behavioral suppression in animals, it would be of interest to determine their effects on central 5-HT. Demonstrating a link between the two would lend additional support to the hypothesis of 5-HT involvement in anxiety. A number of investigations addressing this question have been conducted.

BZ and 5-HT Turnover

BZs both decrease 5-HT turnover (Chase et al., 1970; Wise et al., 1972; Lidbrink et al., 1974; Lippmann & Pugsley, 1974; Jenner et al., 1975; Pratt et al., 1979, 1985; Saner & Pletcher, 1979; Soubrie et al., 1983) and cause reduction in single-unit electrical activity of the 5-HT–containing raphe nuclei (Trulson et al., 1982; Laurent et al., 1983). Whether or not these BZ effects on 5-HT are related to their anxiolytic properties is unclear. Some investigators, such as Wise et al. (1972) have reported that anxiety reduction after several days of treatment with BZs did in fact correlate with decreased 5-HT turnover. This relationship was confirmed in a 25-day study using 5 mg/kg oxazepam (Velluci & File, 1979). However, Lister and File (1983), using a higher dose of oxazepam (10 mg/kg), could not replicate these earlier findings. McElroy et al., (1986), using chlordiazepoxide (CDP), also failed to find such a correlation.

Though a causal relationship between diminished 5-HT function (as deduced from decreased 5-HT turnover) and BZ-induced anxiety reduction is suggested, further definitive work is needed.

BZs and Manipulation of 5-HT Systems

Other studies examining BZ effects on 5-HT have been conducted in which 5-HT function was manipulated in a variety of ways in conjunction with BZ administration. Two basic hypotheses concerning the possible role of 5-HT in BZ's anxiolytic effects were addressed: (1) If BZ's anxiolytic effects are mediated through reduction of 5-HT activity, then 5-HT agonists should block this. (2) An intact 5-HT system is necessary for BZs to achieve their anxiolytic effect. In support of the first hypothesis, Wise et al. (1972) found that (in a Geller and Seifter model) intraventricular administration of 5-HT prevented oxazepam-induced release from behavioral suppression. Another study reported that prior dorsal raphe destruction of 5-HT neurons by 5,7-DHT blocked the anxiolytic effects of CDP (Thiebot et al., 1982). However, other studies failed to confirm these findings. Thiebot et al. (1984) found that 5,7-DHT administered systemically did not block the effect of CDP. Similar inconsistencies were found with pCPA. Although pCPA prevented CDP's release of behavioral suppression in a water-lick model, the results were variable (Cook & Sepinwall, 1975). Also, it appeared that the behavioral (anxiolytic) effects of combining BZs with 5-HT antagonists (Kilts et al., 1982) or 5-HT agonists (Shephard et al., 1982) did not differ from the effects of BZs administered alone.

No simple or readily apparent explanation can account for these contradictory findings. Additionally, methodological problems and inconsistent research practices cloud the issue even more. Researchers have been unable to replicate their findings upon changing doses of BZs or routes of administration. Also, many of these studies significantly differed in the way 5-HT systems were manipulated and so may not be comparable. Different routes of administration and types of agents were used. The 5-HT function was increased through intraventricular and systemic administration of 5-HT itself, as well as of different 5-HT agonists. Decreased 5-HT function was accomplished through use of DHT, pCPA, and 5-HT antagonists. Animal anxiety behavior models also significantly varied across studies.

In summary, though many studies investigating the neurochemical effects of BZs on 5-HT consistently report decreased 5-HT turnover and activity, a direct causal relationship between decreased 5-HT function and the anxiolytic effects of BZs is far from established.

Summary of Animal Findings

1. In a majority of the studies cited, diminishing 5-HT function resulted in decreased anxiety (particularly where pCPA was used), but the effects were often site-specific and time-dependent.

2. Increasing 5-HT function may result in anxiety (in the form of behavioral inhibition).

3. Though BZs decrease 5-HT turnover, it has not been established that this mechanism is responsible for their anxiolytic effects.

4. Methodological deficiencies and inconsistencies, including differences in research design, assessment of anxiety, and pharmacological agents used, have contributed to the ambiguous conclusions regarding the relationship of 5-HT and anxiety.

HUMAN EXPERIMENTS

Anxiety in Humans

Anxiety is an almost ubiquitous component of mental illness, present both as a symptom (in nonanxiety disorders) and as distinct syndromes (i.e., in the anxiety disorders). Though present in its purest form in the so-called anxiety disorders, it is also found in depression, schizophrenia, and personality disorders.

The revised third edition of the *DSM-III-R,* 1988 distinguishes among four major types of anxiety disorders: panic disorder with or without agoraphobia (PD); other phobias, such as social phobia and simple phobias; generalized anxiety disorder (GAD); and obsessive compulsive disorder (OCD). We will focus on research involving 5-HT function in OCD, PD, and GAD, since comparatively little work has been done on simple and social phobias.

5-HT and Anxiety in Humans

Applied Strategies

A variety of methods have been used to assess different aspects of 5-HT function in human anxiety studies. These have included studies measuring

5-HT metabolism, challenge studies with 5-HT agonists, and treatment studies with agents altering 5-HT availability.

Though measurement of the 5-HT metabolite 5-hydroxyindoleacetic acid (5-HIAA) in cerebrospinal fluid (CSF) is perhaps the most informative method for assessing central 5-HT metabolism, it has been done in only a few anxiety studies.

Another method, the so-called challenge paradigm, is particularly well suited to assessment of central 5-HT receptor sensitivity, but it is only valid if the challenge agents have high selectivity for the 5-HT receptor (van Praag et al., 1986). m-chlorophenylpiperazine (mCPP), a putatively selective 5-HT, agonist, appears to meet this criterion, and has been used in a number of studies. Measurement of hormonal and behavioral effects following the administration of a 5-HT$_1$ agonist permits an assessment of the state of the central 5-HT receptor system. Several challenge studies have been conducted with PD and OCD patients.

Finally, treatment studies in anxiety disorders with drugs selective for 5-HT systems have also been useful in exploring the relationship between 5-HT and anxiety in humans (van Praag et al., 1987).

Panic Disorder

Treatment studies.   A number of treatment studies using 5-HT agents in PD suggest that indirect 5-HT agonists are effective antipanic agents. Table 6-3 summarizes the results of some of these studies. One study, for example, compared the effects of 1-5-HTP (150 mg/day with 150 mg/day of the peripheral decarboxylase inhibitor carbidopa) and clomipramine (150 mg/day) in an eight-week placebo-controlled design ($n = 57$). Both compounds displayed antianxiety and antipanic effects (Kahn et al., 1987). Attributing their effectiveness solely to 5-HT mechanisms is problematic since 5-HTP has effects on NA systems and clomipramine's main metabolite, desmethylclomipramine, possesses NA reuptake blocking properties. Thus their therapeutic effects might be mediated through NA systems. Since the antipanic effects of clomipramine were equivalent to those of fluvoxamine, a selective 5-HT reuptake inhibitor, in a six-week double-blind study comprising 50 patients (Den Boer et al., 1987), it is likely that clomipramine's effects are also mediated through the 5-HT system. Moreover, when comparing fluvoxamine with the selective NA reuptake inhibitor maprotiline in 44 PD patients in a six-week study, Den Boer and Westenberg (1988) found fluvoxamine to be effective in reducing panic attacks, in contrast to maprotiline. Evans et al. (1986), comparing zimelidine (also a selective 5-HT reuptake inhibitor) and imipramine in a placebo-controlled study, found zimelidine, but not imipramine, to have antipanic effects. The inefficacy of imipramine in this study is somewhat

TABLE 6-3
5-HT Agonists in Panic Disorder

Author	Drug	Compared With	No. Pts.	No. Weeks	Dose (mg)	Effect
Evans, 1986	ZIM	Placebo	25	6	150	ZIM effective
	IMI				150	
Kahn, 1987	5-HTP*	Placebo	57	8	150	5-HTP effective
	CMI*				225	CMI effective
Den Boer, 1987	FLU*	CMI	50	8	150/225	Both effective
Den Boer, 1988	FLU*	MAP	44	6	150/150	FLU effective
Evans, 1981	ZIM	Open	6	5	300	Effective
Koczkas, 1981	ZIM	Open	13	5	300	Effective
Kahn, 1984	5-HTP*	Open	10	12	300	Effective
Mavissakalian, 1986	TRA	Open	11	10	300	Effective
Gorman, 1987	FLX*	Open	20	18	80	Effective

*Reported initial deterioration in patients on this drug.

5-HTP:	5-hydroxytryptophan	IMI:	Imipramine
CMI:	Clomipramine	TRA:	Trazodone
FLU:	Fluvoxamine	FLX:	Fluoxetine
ZIM:	Zimeldine	MAP:	Maprotiline

All comparative studies are parallel.

surprising (Liebowitz, 1985) and might be related to the small number of patients in the placebo group ($n = 4$). Open pilot studies using other 5-HT agonists, such as 5-HTP (Kahn & Westenberg, 1985), zimelidine (Evans & Moore, 1981; Koczkas et al., 1981), and trazodone (Mavissakalian, 1986), lend further support to the efficacy of 5-HT agonists in panic disorder. Though some questions remain about the selectivity of certain 5-HT agonists, there seems to be uniform agreement that they are effective in diminishing both the frequency and severity of panic attacks, as well as in diminishing agoraphobic symptoms (presumably as a result of decreased panic).

An interesting and somewhat puzzling phenomenon found in treatment studies involving indirect 5-HT agonists is the so-called "biphasic response," in which improvement in symptoms follows an initial period of symptom exacerbation. First observed in a 12-week, open pilot study of PD patients ($n = 10$) treated with 150–300 mg 1-5-HTP in combination with 150 mg carbidopa, 50% of the patients reported initial increased anxiety. They reported increased severity and frequency of panic attacks, as well as aggravation or induction of depressed mood during the initial 10 to 14 days of treatment. This initial deterioration, however, appeared to be transient; continuation of treatment for two to four weeks eventually resulted in clinical improvement (compared with pretreatment status) (Kahn & Westenberg, 1985), in terms both of generalized anxiety and of severity and frequency of the panic attacks. These preliminary findings were confirmed in a larger 5-HTP–clomipramine study ($n = 57$) in which the initial worsening of anxiety symptoms occurred in about 50% of patients receiving 5-HTP and in about 30% of patients receiving clomipramine. In fact, four out of five dropouts in the 5-HTP group and three out of four in the clomipramine group did so within the first two weeks (because of increased anxiety, panic, and depression) (Kahn et al., 1987). It is unlikely that this effect involves NA systems since it has also been reported using the selective 5-HT reuptake inhibitors fluvoxamine (Den Boer et al., 1987) and fluoxetine (Gorman et al., 1988).

This biphasic effect appears to be unique to PD, since it has not been reported in the multitude of studies using indirect 5-HT agonists in depressed patients. We have hypothesized that it is due to hypersensitive receptor function in PD patients (to be discussed more fully later in this chapter).

In summary, 5-HT agonists appear to be therapeutic in PD, although some patients experience an initial worsening of their symptoms.

Challenge Studies. Further evidence that indirect 5-HT agonists may initially increase anxiety in PD patients is provided by the mCPP challenge test. When given intravenously (0.1 mg/kg), mCPP induced anxiety and panic in both PD patients and normal controls (Charney et al., 1987). This effect appears to be dose related since doses of mCPP that are expected to lead to lower blood levels (i.e., 0.5 mg/kg p.o.) do not induce anxiety in normal subjects (Mueller et al., 1985, 1986; Zohar & Insel, 1987; Kahn et al., 1988a, 1990). Interestingly, a low oral dose of mCPP (0.25 mg/kg) increased anxiety and panic in PD patients in comparison with normal controls and with patients with major depression (Kahn et al., 1988a) (Figure 6-1). The different effects of mCPP might be attributable to differences in 5-HT receptor sensitivity. We have hypothesized that low (oral) doses of mCPP increase anxiety in PD patients and not in normal controls because of 5-HT receptor hypersensitivity in PD. High (intravenous) doses, in contrast, induce anxiety in both groups because of massive overstimulation of 5-HT receptors, thereby obliterating receptor-sensitivity differences.

Hormonal effects of mCPP appear to corroborate this hypothesis. While a low oral dose of mCPP (0.25 mg/kg) induced augmented cortisol (Figure 6-2) release in PD patients as compared with normal controls and depressed patients (Kahn et al., 1988b, 1988c), higher doses (e.g., 0.1 mg/kg mCPP intravenously) induced similar cortisol and prolactin responses in PD patients and normal controls (Charney et al., 1987).

Other investigators have contested the notion that 5-HT function differs between PD and normal controls. Using the tryptophan/prolactin test, (Charney & Heninger, 1986) found no differences in prolactin response

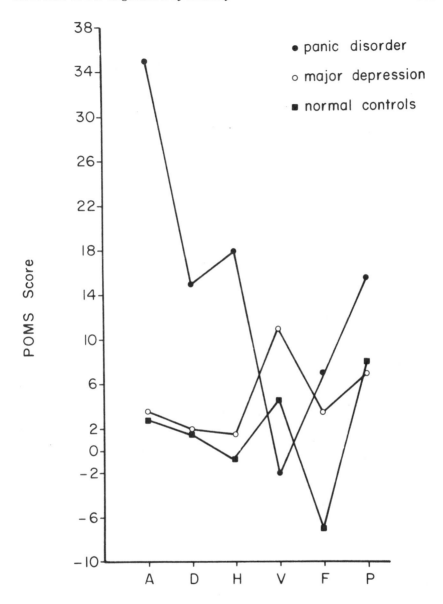

Figure 6-1. Placebo-corrected peak minus baseline values (i.e., peak baseline on mCPP minus peak baseline on placebo) on the Profiles of Mood States (POMS) in 10 patients with panic disorder, 10 patients with major depression, and 11 normal controls. Subjects received 0.25 mg/kg mCPP and placebo in a double-blind design. Behavioral responses were rated at 30 minute intervals from 9 A.M. until 1:30 P.M. using an abbreviated version of a self-rating scale, the POMS. Baseline was defined as the time when the capsules were administered, and peak was defined as the highest value on the remain in 210 minutes. Comparing the three groups on a multivariate profile analysis (using the Greenhouse-Geisser correction) indicated a significant group by behavioral dimension interaction ($p < 0.02$), with higher anxiety, depression, hostility, and physical symptoms response in the PD group as compared with both normal controls and depressed patients. The depressed group did not differ significantly in behavioral response from the normal controls. A = anxiety; D = depression; H = hostility; V = vigour; F = fatigue; P = physical symptoms (Kahn et al., 1988a).

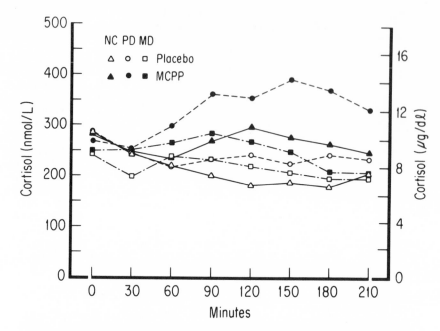

Figure 6-2. Cortisol response over time to placebo and 0.25 mg/kg mCPP p.o. in 20 normal controls (triangles), 20 patients with panic disorder (PD; circles), and 10 patients with major depression (MD; squares). Solid symbols represent response on mCPP, and open symbols represent response on placebo. Tablets were administered at time (0), after a one-hour adaptation period. Cortisol response on mCPP as compared with placebo was significantly higher in the PD group than in the normal controls ($p < 0.001$) and higher in the PD group than in the MD group ($p < 0.001$). MD patients had a similar cortisol response to that of normal controls (Kahn et al., 1988c).

between PD patients and normal controls. Tryptophan, however, may not be an appropriate 5-HT challenge agent because it can affect catecholamines as well as 5-HT. It does so by competing with tyrosine (the precursor of DA and NA) for the same carrier mechanism needed for brain entry (Wurtman, 1982), thereby reducing tyrosine influx into the brain. Diminished brain tyrosine levels, in turn, could lead to decreased catecholamine levels. Consequently, assessment of prolactin release after high intravenous doses of tryptophan might reflect DA function rather than 5-HT function (van Praag et al., 1987).

Obsessive Compulsive Disorder

Evidence from challenge and treatment studies suggests that 5-HT is involved in obsessive compulsive disorder (OCD), though the nature of this

TABLE 6-4
5-HT Agonists in Obsessive Compulsive Disorder

Author	Drug	Compared With	No. Pts.	No. Weeks	Dose (mg)	Effect
Thoren, 1980	CMI NOR	Placebo	35	5	150 150	CMI effective
Marks, 1980	CMI	Placebo	40	4	225	CMI effective
Montgomery, 1980	CMI	Placebo, Crossover	14	4	75	CMI effective
Ananth, 1981	CMI	AMI	20	4	300	CMI effective
Insel, 1983	CMI CLO	Placebo	13	4 + 6	300 30	CMI effective
Insel, 1985	ZIM DMI	Placebo, CMI	13	5	300 300	CMI effective
Zohar, 1987	CMI	DMI	10	6	300	CMI effective
Yaryuria, 1977	TRY	Open	7	6 mo.	3–9 g	Effective
Kahn, 1984	ZIM	Open	6	3 mo.	300	Effective
Fontaine, 1986	FLX	Open	8	9	80	Effective
Price, 1987	FLU	Open	9	4	300	Effective

CMI: Clomipramine   DMI: Desipramine
NOR: Nortriptyline   TRY: Tryptophan
CLO: Clorgylline   FLX: Fluoxetine
AMI: Amitriptyline   FLU: Fluvoxamine
ZIM: Zimeldine
All comparative studies are parallel unless stated differently.

involvement is unclear. Two studies measuring baseline CSF 5-HIAA in OCD patients yielded contradictory findings. Asberg et al. (1982) found that a preponderance of OCD females had low CSF 5-HIAA (as was found in melancholic females). The average values, however, were no different from normals. In contrast, Insel et al. (1985) found higher CSF 5-HIAA in OCD patients (males and females) compared with normals. One possible explanation for the discrepant findings is the different sex distributions and the small sample size ($n = 8$) in the study by Insel et al.

Clearer evidence for the role of 5-HT dysfunction in OCD comes from the increasing number of treatment studies reporting successful treatment of OCD with 5-HT agents (see Table 6-4).

Several placebo-controlled studies involving clomipramine (a 5-HT reuptake inhibitor) demonstrated both antiobsessional and anticompulsive effects. In contrast, other tricyclic antidepressants with lesser or no effects on 5-HT reuptake, such as desmethylimipramine (Zohar & Insel, 1987), nortriptyline (Thoren et al., 1980), and amitriptyline (Ananth et al., 1981), have been found ineffective in treating OCD. Two studies showed a relationship between clinical improvement and clomipramine levels, and no relationship to the levels of clomipramine's noradrenergic metabolite (Stern et al., 1980; Insel et al., 1983). This would suggest that clomipramine's therapeutic effects are related to its 5-HT agonistic properties (vide supra) and not to its noradrenergic properties. In addition, improvement correlated with reduction of CSF 5-HIAA concentration (Thoren et al., 1980). Further evidence of 5-HT involvement in OCD is provided by open studies demonstrating the effectiveness of the 5-HT agonists tryptophan (Yaryuria-Tobias & Bhagavan, 1977), zimelidine (Kahn et al., 1984), fluoxetine (Fontaine & Chouinard, 1986), and fluvoxamine (Price et al., 1987) in OCD.

Challenge studies with mCPP in OCD have provided intriguing and, at the same time, puzzling findings. In one study (Zohar et al., 1987), mCPP administration in OCD patients resulted in increased anxiety and obsessions (as compared with normal controls), suggesting the presence of 5-HT receptor hypersensitivity. Yet cortisol response was blunted, and prolactin response was no different from that of normals, indicating the 5-HT receptor hypersensitivity was not involved in 5-HT-mediated hormonal responses. On rechallenge with mCPP following three and a half months of clomipramine treatment, the induction of anxiety and obsessions was absent (Zohar et al., 1988), suggesting that downregulation of 5-HT receptors had occurred. However, other investigators (Charney et al., 1988) failed to find exacerbation of OCD symptoms with mCPP challenge (0.1 mg/kg intravenously) or with tryptophan challenge (7 g intravenously). In contrast to the study by Zohar et al. (1987), Charney et al. found blunted prolactin response in female OCD patients as compared with normal controls, but no differences in cortisol response between the two groups. Thus, although the present data indicate a role for 5-HT in OCD, the exact nature of this relationship is far from clear.

Generalized Anxiety Disorder

Evidence that 5-HT function may be involved in GAD has been obtained from several treatment studies involving 5-HT agents. Two new drugs, buspirone and ritanserin, both having pronounced effects on 5-HT systems, have been shown to be effective in GAD. In most investigations, buspirone has proved to be as anxiolytic as the BZs (Table 6-5).

Buspirone appears to exert its effects through the 5-HT_{1a} receptor, for which it has a high affinity. It also binds to DA_2 sites, but the latter is probably less clinically significant because this binding is 16 times weaker (Peroutka, 1985). Buspirone has been noted to have agonistic and antagonistic effects on 5-HT_{1a} receptors, but its net effect is probably to decrease 5-HT function, since administration of buspirone decreases raphe cell activity (Van der Maelen & Wildeman, 1984).

Preliminary results involving the selective 5-HT_2 antagonist ritanserin show that it also is effective in GAD (Leysen et al., 1985). Administered for two weeks in a 10-mg/day dose in a placebo-controlled study ($n = 83$), it

TABLE 6-5
Buspirone in Anxiety

Author	Diagnosis	Drug	No. Pts.	Dose (mg/day)	No. Weeks	Result
Goldberg, 1979	Anxiety Neurosis	Buspirone (B)	18	20 (mean)	4	B = D > P
		Diazepam (D)	20	19 (mean)		
		Placebo (P)	18	20 (mean)		
Wheatley, 1982	Anxiety of four weeks' duration	Buspirone (B)	43	30 (max)	4	B = D > P
		Diazepam (D)	46	30 (max)		
		Placebo (P)	42	30 (max)		
Goldberg, 1982	GAD	Buspirone (B)	18	30 (max)	4	B = D > P
		Diazepam (D)	18	30 (max)		
		Placebo (P)	18	30 (max)		
Goldberg, 1982	GAD	Buspirone (B)	98	16 (mean)	4	B = C
		Clorazepate (C)	31	20 (mean)		
Rickels, 1982	GAD	Buspirone (B)	81	40 (max)	4	B = D > P
		Diazepam (D)	81	40 (max)		
		Placebo (P)	78	40 (max)		
Cohn, 1986	GAD	Buspirone (B)	20	50 (max)	4	B = A = L
		Alprazolam (A)	20	5 (max)		
		Lorazepam (L)	20	10 (max)		
Cohn, 1986	GAD	Buspirone (B)	255	60 (max)	4	B = C
		Chlorazepate (C)	81	90 (max)		
Ross, 1987	GAD	Buspirone (B)	10	40 (max)	4	B = D = P
		Diazepam (D)	9	40 (max)		
		Placebo (P)	11	40 (max)		
Olajide, 1987	GAD	Buspirone (B)	⎱ 30 (crossover)	30 (max)	3	D > B = P
		Diazepam (D)	⎰	30 (max)	3	
		Placebo (P)		30 (max)	3	

A: Alprazolam   C: Clorazepate   P: Placebo
B: Buspirone   D: Diazepam   GAD: Generalized anxiety disorder

was found to be more effective than placebo and as effective as lorazepam (Ceulemans et al., 1985a) in a group of GAD patients. Another study ($n = 191$) comparing ritanserin (10 mg/day) with placebo and diazepam (10 mg/day) found ritanserin (after three weeks of treatment) to be more effective than diazepam or placebo (Ceulemans et al., 1985b). Its therapeutic effect may be dose related, since a lower (5 mg/day) dose of ritanserin appeared to be ineffective (Ceulemans et al., 1985a).

Anxiety in Depressive Disorders

A relation between 5-HT and anxiety in major depression is hinted at by the twin findings that (1) anxiety is often a prominent component of mood disorders, and (2) 5-HT has been implicated in the pathogenesis of depression. Only a few studies, however, have investigated this directly. Both Banki (1977) and Rydin et al. (1982) found an inverse correlation between CSF 5-HIAA and anxiety in depressed patients. Redmond et al. (1986) also found such a correlation, though it was less pronounced than the relationship between anxiety and 3-methoxy-4-hydroxy-phenyl-glycol (MHPG, the main metabolite of NA). Clearly, more studies will be needed to investigate both the role of 5-HT and the role of other neurotransmitter systems in depressive/anxiety states.

Summary of Human Findings

Though much of the data on the role of 5-HT in human anxiety are preliminary, and at times are inconsistent and contradictory, some broad observations and generalizations may be ventured:

1. Indirect 5-HT agonists are effective in OCD and PD.
2. Preliminary evidence suggests 5-HT antagonists are effective in GAD.
3. Indirect 5-HT agonists exert a biphasic effect in PD, characterized by initial worsening and subsequent improvement.
4. The presence of hypersensitive postsynaptic 5-HT receptors in PD is suggested by augmented hormonal and behavioral responses of PD patients to the 5-HT postsynaptic agonist mCPP.
5. Challenge with 5-HT agonists in OCD patients provides contradictory evidence; increased (behavioral) and decreased (hormonal) 5-HT responsivity.
6. An inverse relationship between CSF 5-HIAA levels and anxiety has been reported in patients with major depression.

DISCUSSION

The State of 5-HT Receptors and Anxiety

From the preceding review of animal and human anxiety studies, it seems apparent that no single or simple theory of 5-HT in anxiety can account for all the findings. Yet a number of seemingly contradictory findings may be explained by alterations in the functioning of postsynaptic 5-HT receptors. We have hypothesized that in panic disorder, postsynaptic 5-HT receptors may be hypersensitive, and that increased 5-HT function is causally related to panic/anxiety (Kahn & van Praag, 1988).

This hypothesis is consistent with a number of the findings previously described. For example, the initial deterioration in the treatment response of PD patients to 5-HT agonists would be expected if the 5-HT receptor system were hypersensitive. The subsequent anxiety reduction follows as a consequence of compensatory downregulation of 5-HT receptors. Hypersensitivity of postsynaptic 5-HT receptors would also explain the increased anxiety response and augmented cortisol response of PD patients in comparison with normal controls and major depressives when they are challenged with (low oral doses of) mCPP. Higher (intravenous) doses of mCPP induce equivalent levels of anxiety in normal subjects and PD patients as a result of overstimulation of 5-HT systems. They obscure differences in receptor sensitivity between normals and patients.

This hypothesis also accounts for the low CSF 5-HIAA found in anxious depressives. Compensatory downregulation of 5-HT metabolism would be an adaptive response to initially hypersensitive 5-HT receptor systems.

Further investigation of the validity of the 5-HT receptor hypersensitivity theory in anxiety will depend on appropriate experimental methodology. For example, before they are used as challenge agents in patients, 5-HT agonists need to be carefully tested in normal subjects to validate their 5-HT specificity and dose–effect relationships (van Praag et al., 1987). Second, minimal effective doses should be determined to avoid overstimulating 5-HT receptors. Following these guidelines will clarify the often contradictory and inconsistent findings previously reported.

As with any hypothesis, certain precautions are warranted. First, much of the data on which this hypothesis rests are preliminary and require confirmation and replication. Moreover, despite its ability seemingly to reconcile a wide range of findings, the hypersensitivity hypothesis is likely to be an oversimplification. That there are at least six different 5-HT receptor systems in the brain (some of which are both pre- and postsynaptically located) is only one indication of the complexity of 5-HT systems. Finally, the hypersensitivity hypothesis cannot account for all types of anxiety disorders. Nevertheless, the hypothesis has heuristic value and can serve to point toward additional avenues of investigation.

5-HT and Other Psychopathology

5-HT dysfunction has been associated with forms of psychopathology other than anxiety, including depressive disorders (van Praag & Korf,

1971), suicidal behavior (van Praag, 1986), and outwardly directed aggression (Valzelli, 1984). The presence of 5-HT disturbances in these disorders may shed additional light on the role of 5-HT in anxiety. Clinically, mood, anxiety, and aggression disorders tend to cluster. A clinical association between anxiety and depression is a well-recognized phenomenon. PD and OCD, for example, are frequently accompanied by major depression (Breier et al., 1984; Gittleson, 1966a), and depressed patients have an increased incidence of panic attacks (Breier et al., 1985), generalized anxiety (Roth et al., 1972), and obsessive compulsive symptoms (Gittleson, 1966b). Similarly, depression, suicide, and outwardly directed aggression are linked inasmuch as depression is a common precursor to suicidal behavior and depressed patients exhibit more outwardly directed aggression (Weissman et al., 1973). That suicidal and aggressive behavior are related is suggested by the finding that suicide rates are increased in individuals with histories of violent behavior (West, 1965).

The relation between 5-HT disturbances and these psychopathological disorders (including anxiety) can only be speculated about at this time. Is each disorder independently related to particular disturbances of the central 5-HT system, or is a particular 5-HT disturbance linked to a particular psychopathological trait common to all the disorders? These are just two of the many questions that come to mind. Clarification of these issues will depend, at the very least, on the availability of behavioral measurement instruments with high resolving power. Current assessment methodology is wanting in this respect and improved techniques are urgently needed.

5-HT and Other Theories of Anxiety

5-HT, NA, and Anxiety

Increased NA function has also been proposed as a pathogenic factor in panic attacks (Redmond & Huang, 1979; Charney & Redmond, 1983) since a single dose of yohimbine (an alpha$_2$ antagonist) induces more anxiety and panic and a greater MHPG increase in PD patients that in normal controls (Charney et al., 1984). In addition, plasma MHPG levels decrease during a successful treatment program with many different antipanic medications, such as imipramine and alprazolam (Charney et al., 1985a, 1985b; Carr et al., 1986).

How can one reconcile the role of 5-HT in the pathogenesis of anxiety with the evidence of noradrenergic involvement as well? Several possible explanations may be considered. For example, certain anxiety states might be related to a predominant dysfunction of one neurotransmitter system, while other anxiety states might be related to disturbances in the other neurotransmitter system. Alternatively, since 5-HT and NA systems have extensive connecting pathways, a disturbance in one may cause secondary or complementary effects in the other. 5-HT neurons, for example, project from the dorsal raphe to the locus coeruleus (LC, the main nucleus of NA-containing neurons) as shown by autoradiographic (Descarries & Leger, 1978), immunocytochemical (Pickel et al., 1978), and histochemical methods (Leger et al., 1979). Destruction of the mesencephalic part of the raphe system reportedly causes an increase in NA turnover within the LC (Pujol et al., 1978). Furthermore, stimulation of dorsal raphe nuclei blocks the increase in LC firing typically observed after administration of noxious stimuli. Moreover, this inhibitory effect of dorsal raphe stimulation on the LC is abolished or diminished by pretreatment with pCPA, DHT, and methysergide (Segal, 1979). Also, direct application of 5-HT on the LC suppresses its firing (Segal, 1979). Conversely, increased NA function causes increased 5-HT activity in the raphe nuclei (Baraban & Aghajanian, 1980; Marwaha & Aghajanian, 1982). Based on these 5-HT/NA interactions, one possible conclusion is that NA's anxiogenic effects are mediated through enhancement of 5-HT function.

The preceding examples suggest that no simple dysfunction in any one neurotransmitter system can account for anxiety production, and that complex interactions between multiple neurotransmitters are likely to be involved. This becomes further apparent in examining (in the next section) the role of another neurochemical system, GABA, which is also implicated in anxiety mechanisms.

5-HT, GABA, and Anxiety

The discovery of BZ receptors and the increased understanding of their role in the clinical efficacy of BZs has led some investigators to postulate a BZ-GABA (γ-aminobutyic acid) hypothesis of anxiety production (Paul et al., 1981). The basic premise of this hypothesis is that BZs decrease anxiety by facilitating GABA function. According to this hypothesis, BZs exert their anxiolytic effect by activating GABA's inhibitory effects on neuronal excitability (through the facilitation of cellular influx of Cl-ions, resulting in increased neuronal polarity) (Costa et al., 1975). Evidence in support of this hypothesis comes from studies in which administration of BZ receptor antagonists induces anxietylike behavior in monkeys (Ninan et al., 1982) and in humans (Dorrow et al., 1983).

GABA's role in anxiety should also be viewed in the context of its interaction with other neurotransmitters. For example, recent evidence indicates that the GABA and 5-HT systems are highly intertwined, both anatomically and functionally. We have already reviewed evidence relating BZ's anxiolytic action to 5-HT function. Other findings include: (1) certain neurons of the raphe nuclei contain both 5-HT and GABA (Belin et al., 1983;

Nanopoulos et al., 1982); (2) systemic administration of GABA agonists decreases 5-HT synthesis and 5-HT transmission (probably by inhibition of raphe neuronal activity) (Nishikawa & Scatton, 1983, 1985a); (3) local infusion of GABA in the raphe nuclei causes decreased 5-HT activity in their projection area (Nishikawa & Scatton, 1985b); (4) GABA agonists and antagonists injected in the median raphe respectively cause decreased and increased 5-HT turnover (Forchetti & Meek, 1981); and (5) in vivo voltammetry shows that GABA inhibits striatal 5-HT transmission (Scatton et al., 1984).

In summary, these findings suggest that BZs may exert their anxiolytic effects by indirectly decreasing 5-HT function (through their facilitation of GABA). This possible intriguing link between GABA and 5-HT requires further investigation.

CONCLUSION

This chapter has reviewed the animal and human findings concerning the relationship between 5-HT function and anxiety. An overly broad and preliminary generalization suggests that some anxiety states can be linked to increased 5-HT activity. We have proposed a more specific hypothesis of anxiety regulation—that some anxiety states (namely panic disorder) may be generated by hypersensitive postsynaptic 5-HT receptors. An attractive feature of this hypothesis is that it can account for a number of clinical findings, including the biphasic treatment response of PD patients to indirect 5-HT agonists and their anxiogenic response to 5-HT agonist challenge. Considering the complexity of anxiety regulation and the potential interactions among different neurotransmitters, we expect that generalizations about one single system necessarily will be too simple. Whatever role 5-HT may play in the regulation of anxiety, the recent introduction of 5-HT-selective anxiolytics has ushered in a new era of anxiety treatment and research.

REFERENCES

American Psychiatric Association (1987). Diagnostic and statistical manual of Mental disorders. (3rd ed.—Revised). Washington, DC: American Psychiatric Association.

Ananth, J., Pecknold, J. C., & van der Steen, N. (1981). Double-blind comparative study of clomipramine and amitryptiline in Obsessive Compulsive Neurosis. *Prog. Neuropsychopharm, 5*, 257–264.

Asberg, M., Thoren, P., & Bertilsson, L. (1982). Clomipramine treatment of obsessive disorder-biochemical and clinical aspects. *Psychopharmacol. Bull., 18*, 13–21.

Banki, C. M. (1977). Correlation of anxiety and related symptoms with cerebrospinal fluid, 5-hydroxyindoleacetic acid in depressed women. *J. Neural. Transm., 41*, 135–143.

Baraban, F. M., & Aghajanian, G. K. (1980). Suppression of firing activity of 5HT neurons in the dorsal raphe by alpha-adrenoceptor antagonist. *Neuropharmacology, 19*, 355–363.

Barofski, A. L., Grier, H. C., & Pradkan, T. K. (1980). Evidence for regulation of water intake by median raphe 5HT neurons. *Physiol. Behav., 24*, 951–955.

Belin, M. F., Nanopoulos, D., Didier, M., et al. (1983). Immunohistochemical evidence for the presence of gamma-aminobutyric acid and serotonin in one nerve cell. A study on the raphe nuclei of the rat using antibodies to glutamate decarboxylase and serotonin. *Brain Res., 275*, 329–339.

Blakely, T. A., & Parker, L. F. (1973). The effects of parachlorophenylalanine on experimentally induced conflict behavior. *Pharmacol. Biochem. Behav., 1*, 609–613.

Blundell, J. E. (1984). Serotonin and appetite. *Neuropharmacology, 23*(12B), 1537–1551.

Breier, A., Charney, D. S., & Heninger, G. R. (1984). Major depression in patients with agoraphobia and panic disorder. *Arch. Gen. Psychiatry, 41*, 1129–1135.

Breier, A., Charney, D. S., & Heninger, G. R. (1985). The diagnostic validity of anxiety disorders and their relationship to depressive illness. *Am. J. Psychiatry, 142*, 787–797.

Carr, D. B., Sheehan, D. V., Surman, O. S., Coleman, J. H., Greenblatt, D. J., Heninger, G. R., Jones, K. J., Levine, P. H., & Watkins, D. W. (1986). Neuroendocrine correlates of lactate-induced anxiety and their response to chronic alprazolam therapy. *Am. J. Psychiatry, 143*(4), 483–494.

Ceulemans, D. L. S., Hoppenbrouwers, M. L. J. A., Gelders, Y. G., & Reyntjens, A. J. M. (1985a). The influence of ritanserin, a serotonin antagonist, in anxiety disorders: A double-blind placebo-controlled study versus lorazepam. *Pharmacopsychiatry, 18*, 303–305.

Ceulemans, D. L. S., Hoppenbrouwers, M. L., Gelders, Y., et al. (1985b). The effect of benzodiazepine withdrawal on the therapeutic efficacy of a serotonin antagonist in anxiety disorders. IVth World Congress of Biological Psychiatry, Philadelphia, Pa.

Charney, D. S., Goodman, W. K., Price, L. H., Woods, S. W., Rasmussen, S. A., & Heninger, G. R. (1988). Serotonin function in obsessive-compulsive disorder: A comparison of the effects of tryptophan and m-chlorophenylpiperazine in patients and healthy subjects. *Arch. Gen. Psychiatry, 45*, 177–185.

Charney, D. S., Heninger, G. R., & Breier, A. (1984). Noradrenergic function in panic anxiety. Effects of yohimbine in healthy subjects and patients with agoraphobia and panic disorder. *Arch. Gen. Psychiatry, 41*, 751–763.

Charney, D. S., & Heninger, G. R. (1985a). Noradernergic function and the mechanism of action of antianxiety treatment I. The effect of long-term alprazolam treatment. *Arch. Gen. Psychiatry, 42*, 458–467.

Charney, D. S., & Heninger, G. R. (1985b). Noradrenergic function and the mechanism of action of antianxiety treatment II. The effect of long-term imipramine treatment. *Arch. Gen. Psychiatry, 42*, 473–481.

Charney, D. S., & Heninger, G. R. (1986). Serotonergic function in panic disorders. *Arch. Gen. Psychiatry, 43*, 1059–1065.

Charney, D. S., & Redmond, D. E., Jr. (1983). Neurobiological mechanisms in human anxiety. Evidence supporting central noradrenergic hyperactivity. *Neuropharmacology, 22*, 1531–1536.

Charney, D. S., Woods, S. W., Goodman, W. K., et al. (1987). Serotonin function in anxiety: II. Effects of the serotonin agonist mCPP in panic disorder patients and healthy subjects. *Psychopharmacology, 92*, 14–24.

Chase, T. N., Katz, R. I., & Kopin, I. J. (1970). Effect of diazepam on fate of intracisternally injected serotonin-c^{14}. *Neuropharmacology, 9*, 103–108.

Clarke, A., & File, S. E. (1982). Selective neurotoxin lesions of the lateral septum: Changes in social and aggressive behaviours. *Pharmacol. Biochem. Behav., 17*, 623–628.

Cohn, J. B., Bowden, C. L., Fisher, J. G., et al. (1986). Double/blind comparison of buspirone and clorazepate in anxious outpatient *Am. J. Med., 80* (3b), 10–16.

Cohn, J. B., & Wilcox, C. (1986). Low-sedation potential of buspirone compared with alprazolam and lorazepam in the treatment of anxious patients: A double-blind study. *J. Clin. Psychiatry, 47*, 409–412.

Colpaert, F. C., Meert, T. F., Niemegeers, C. J. E., & Janssen, P. A. J. (1985). Behavioral and 5HT antagonist effects of ritanserin: A pure and selective antagonist of LSD discrimination in the rat. *Psychopharmacology, 86*, 45–54.

Commissaris, R. L., & Rech, R. H. (1982). Interactions of metergoline with diazepam, quipazine and hallucinogenic drugs on a conflict behavior in the rat. *Psychopharmacology, 76*, 782.

Commissaris, R. L., Lyness, W. H., & Rech, R. H. (1981). The effects of d-Lysergic acid diethylamide (LSD), 2,5-dimethoxy-4-methylamphetamine (DOM), pentobarbital and methaqualone on punished responding in control and 5,7-dihydroxytryptamine-treated rats. *Pharmacol. Biochem. Behav., 14*, 617–623.

Cook, L., & Sepinwall, J. (1975). Behavioral analysis of the effects and mechanism of action of benzodiazepines. In E. Costa & P. Greengard (Eds.), *Mechanism of action of benzodiazepines* (pp. 1–28). New York: Raven Press.

Costa, E., Guidotti, A., & Mao, C. C. (1975). New concepts on the mechanism of action of benzodiazepines. *Life Sci., 17*, 167–186.

Costall, B., Domeney, A. M., Gerrard, P. A., et al. (1987). Effects of the 5HT receptor antagonist GR 38032F, ICS205-930 and BRL43694 in tests for anxiolytic activity. *Br. J. Pharmac., 90*, 195P.

Crawley, J., & Goodwin, F. K. (1980). Preliminary report of a simple animal behavior model for the anxiolytic effects of benzodiazepines. *Pharmac. Biochem. Behav., 13*, 167–170.

Critchley, M. A. E., & Handley, S. L. (1987). Effects in the X-maze anxiety model of agents acting at the 5HT1 and 5HT2 receptors. *Psychopharmacology, 93*, 502–506.

Den Boer, J. A., & Westenberg, H. G. M. (1988). Effect of a serotonin and noradrenalin uptake inhibitor in panic disorders: A double-blind comparative study with fluvoxamine and maprotiline. *Int. Clin. Psychopharm., 3*, 59–74.

Den Boer, J. A., Westenberg, H. G. M., Kamerbeek, W. D. J., et al. (1987). Effect of serotonin uptake inhibitors in anxiety disorders: A double-blind comparison of clomipramine and fluvoxamine. *Int. Clin. Psychopharm., 2*, 21-32.

Descarries, L., & Leger, L. (1978). Serotonin nerve terminals in the locus coeruleus of the adult rat. In S. Garattini, J. F. Pujol, & R. Samanin (Eds.), *Interactions between putative neurotransmitters in the brain* (pp. 355-367). New York: Raven Press.

Dorrow, R., Horowski, R., Paschelke, G., & Amin, M. (1983). Severe anxiety induced by FG 7142, a beta-carboline ligand for benzodiazepine receptors. *Lancet, 92*, 98-99.

Ellison, G. D. (1977). Animal models of psychopathology. The low-norepinephrine and low-serotonin rat. *Am. Psychol., 32*, 1036-1045.

Engel, J. A., Hjorth, S., Svensson, K., et al. (1984). Anticonflict effect of the putative serotonin receptor agonist 8-hydroxy-2-(DI-n-Propylamino)tetraline (8-OH-DPAT). *Eur. J. Pharmacol., 105*, 365-368.

Estes, W. K., & Skinner, B. F. (1941). Some quantitative properties of anxiety. *J. Exp. Psychol., 29*, 390-400.

Evans, L., Kenardy, J., Schneider, P., et al. (1986). Effect of a selective serotonin uptake inhibitor in agoraphobia with panic attacks. *Acta Psychiat. Scan., 73*, 49-53.

Evans, L., & Moore, G. (1981). The treatment of phobic anxiety by zimelidine. *Acta Psychiat. Scan., 63*(Suppl 290), 342-345.

File, S. E. (1985). Animal models for predicting clinical efficacy of anxiolytic drugs: Social behaviour. *Neuropsychobiology, 13*, 55-62.

File, S. E., & Hyde, J. R. (1977). The effects of p-chlorophenylalanine and ethanolamine-O-sulphate in an animal test of anxiety. *J. Pharm. Pharmac., 29*, 735-738.

File, S. E. Hyde, J. R. G., & Macleod, N. K. (1979). 5,7-Dihydroxytryptamine lesions of dorsal and median raphe nuclei and performance in the social interaction test of anxiety and in a home-cage aggression test. *J. Affect. Disord., 1*, 115-122.

Fontaine, R., & Chouinard, G. (1986). An open clinical trial of fluoxetine in the treatment of obsessive compulsive disorder. *J. Clin. Psychopharmacol., 6*, 98-101.

Forchetti, C. M., & Meek, J. L. (1981). Evidence for a tonic GABAergic control of serotonin neurons in the median raphe nucleus. *Brain Res., 206*, 208-212.

Gardner, C. R. (1985). *Neuropharmacology of serotonin* (A. R. Green, Ed.) (pp. 281-325). Oxford: Oxford University Press.

Gardner, C. R. (1986). Recent developments in 5HT-related pharmacology of animal models of anxiety. *Pharmacol. Biochem. Behav., 24*, 1479-1485.

Geller, I., & Blum, K. (1970). The effects of 5-HTP on para-chlorophenylalanine (p-CPA) attenuation of "conflict" behavior. *Eur. J. Pharmacol., 9*, 319-324.

Geller, I., Hartmann, R. J., Croy, D. J., et al. (1974). Attenuation of conflict behavior with cinanserin, a serotonin antagonist: Reversal of the effect with 5-hydroxytryptophan and -methyltryptamine. *Res. Comm. Chem. Pathol. Phamacol., 7*, 165-175.

Geller, I., & Seifter, J. (1960). The effects of meprobamate, d-amphetamine and promazine on experimentally-induced conflict in the rat. *Psychopharmacologia, 1,* 482-492.

Gerson, S. C., & Baldessarini, R. J. (1980). Motor effects of serotonin in the central nervous system. *Life Sci., 27,* 1435-1451.

Gittleson, N. (1966a). The depressive psychosis in the obsessional neurotic. *Br. J. Psychiatry, 112,* 883-887.

Gittleson, N. (1966b). The fate of obsessions in depressive psychosis. *Br. J. Psychiatry, 112,* 705-708.

Goldberg, H. L., & Finnerty, R. J. (1979). The comparative efficacy of buspirone and diazepam in the treatment of anxiety. *Am. J. Psychiatry, 136,* 1184-1187.

Goldberg, H. L., & Finnerty, R. (1982). Comparison of buspirone in two separate studies (1982). *J. Clin. Psychiatry, 43,* 87-92.

Gorman, J. M., Liebowitz, M. R., Fyer, A. J., et al. (1988). An open trial of fluoxetine in the treatment of panic attacks. *J. Clin. Psychopharmacol., 7,* 329-332.

Graeff, F. G., (1974). Tryptamine antagonists and punished behavior. *J. Pharmacol. Exp. Ther., 189,* 344-350.

Graeff, F. G., & Schoenfeld, R. I. (1970). Tryptaminergic mechanisms in punished and nonpunished behavior. *J. Pharmacol. Exp. Ther., 173*(2), 277-283.

Handley, S. L., & Mithani, S. (1984). Effects of L-adrenocepter agonists and antagonists in a maze-exploration model of "fear-motivated" behavior. *Naunyn-Schmiedeberg's Arch. Pharmacol., 327,* 1-5.

Hoyer, D., Engel, G., & Kalkman, H. O. (1985). Molecular pharmacology of 5-HT, and 5-HT$_2$ recognition sites in rat and pig brain membranes: Radioligand binding sites with [3H]5-HT, [3H] 8-OH-DPAT, (-) [125I] Iodocyanopindolol, [3H] Mesulergine and [3H] Kotanserin. *Eur. J. Pharmacol., 118,* 13-23.

Insel, T. R., Mueller, E. A., Alterman, I., et al. (1985). Obsessive-compulsive disorder and serotonin: Is there a connection? *Biol. Psychiatry, 20,* 1174-1188.

Insel, T. R., Murphy, D. L., Cohen, R. M., et al. (1983). Obsessive compulsive disorder: A double blind trial of clomipramine and clorgyline. *Arch. Gen. Psychiatry, 40,* 605-612.

Jenner, P., Chadwick, D., Reynolds, E. H., et al. (1975). Altered 5-HT metabolism with clonazepam, diazepam and diphenylhydantoin. *J. Pharm. Pharmac., 27,* 707.

Jones, B. J., Oakley, N. R., & Tyers, M. B. (1987). The anxiolytic activity of GR38032F, a 5HT3 antagonist, in the rat and cynomolgus monkey. *Br. J. Pharmac., 90,* 88P.

Kahn, R. S., & van Praag, H. M. (1988). A Serotonin hypothesis of panic disorders. *Human Psychopharmacology, 3,* 285-288.

Kahn, R. S., Westenberg, H. G. M., & Jolles, J. (1984). Zimelidine treatment of obsessive-compulsive disorder. *Acta. Psychiat. Scand., 69,* 259-261.

Kahn, R. S., & Westenberg, H. G. M. (1985). 1-5-Hydroxytryptophan in the treatment of anxiety disorders. *J. Affect. Disord., 8,* 197-200.

Kahn, R. S., Westenberg, H. G. M., Verhoeven, W. M. A., et al. (1987). Effect of a serotonin precursor and uptake inhibitor in anxiety disorders; a double-blind comparison of 5-hydroxytryptophan, clomipramine and placebo. *Int. Clin. Psychopharm., 2*, 33–45.

Kahn, R. S., Wetzler, S., Asnis, G. M., et al. (1990). The effects of M-chlorophenylpiperazine in normal subjects: A dose response study. *Psychopharmacology., 100*, 339–334.

Kahn, R. S., Wetzler, S., Asnis, G. M., et al. (1988b). Neuroendocrine evidence for 5HT receptor hypersensitivity in patients with panic disorder. *Psychopharmacology, 96*, 360–364.

Kahn, R. S., Wetzler, S., Asnis, G. M., et al. (1988c). Serotonin receptor sensitivity in panic disorder and major depression, submitted.

Kahn, R. S., Wetzler, S., van Praag, H. M., et al. (1988a). Behavioral indications of serotonergic supersensitivity in patients with panic disorder. *Psychiatry Res., 25*, 101–104.

Kilts, D. D., Commissaris, R. L., Cordon, J. J., et al. (1982). Lack of central 5-hydroxytryptamine influence on the anticonflict activity of diazepam. *Psychopharmacology, 78*, 156–164.

Kilts, C. D., Commissaris, R. L., & Rech, R. H. (1981). Comparison of anti-conflict drug effects in three experimental animal models of anxiety. *Psychopharmacology, 74*, 290–296.

Koczkas, S., Holmberg, G., & Wedin, L. (1981). A pilot study of the effect of the 5-HT-uptake inhibitor, zimelidine, on phobic anxiety. *Acta Psychiatr. Scand. Suppl., 290(63)*, 328–341.

Krulich, L., McCann, S. M., & Mayfield, M. A. (1981). On the mode of the prolactin release-inhibiting action of the serotonin receptor blockers metergoline, methysergide, and cyproheptadine. *Endocrinology, 108*(4), 1115–1124.

Lal, F., & Emmett-Oglesby, M. W. (1983). Behavioral analogues of anxiety. Animal models. *Neuropharmacology, 22*, 1423–1441.

Laurent, J. P., Mangold, M., Humbel, U., et al. (1983). Reduction by two benzodiazepines and pentobarbitone of the multiunit activity in substantia nigra, hippocampus, nucleus locus coeruleus and nucleus raphe dorsalis of encephale isole rats. *Neuropharmacology, 22*(4), 501–511.

Leger, L., Wiklund, L., Descarries, L., et al. (1979). Description of an indolaminergic cell component in the cat locus coeruleus: A fluorescence histochemical and radioautographic study. *Brain Res., 168*, 43–56.

Leone, C. M. L., de Aguiar, J. C., & Graeff, F. G. (1983). Role of 5-hydroxytryptamine in amphetamine effects on unpunished behavior. *Psychopharmacology, 80*, 78–82.

Leysen, J. E., Gommeren, W., & van Gompel, P. (1985). Receptor binding properties in vitro and in vivo of ritanserin: A very potent and long acting 5HT2 antagonist. *Mol. Pharmacol., 27*, 600–611.

Lidbrink, P., Corrodi, H., & Fuxe, K. (1974). Benzodiazepines and barbiturates: Turnover changes in central 5-hydroxytryptamine pathways. *Eur. J. Pharmacol., 26*, 35–40.

Liebowitz, M. R. (1985). Imipramine in the treatment of panic disorder and its complications. *Psychiat. Clin. N. Am., 8*, 37–47.

Lippa, A. S., Nash, P. A., & Greenblatt, E. N. (1979). Preclinical neuropsychopharmacological testing procedures for anxiolytic drugs. In S. Fielding &

H. Lal (Eds.), *Anxiolytics, industrial pharmacology* (pp. 3, 41). New York: Futura.

Lippmann, N., & Pugsley, T. A. (1974). Effects of benzoctamine and chlordiazepoxide on turnover and uptake of 5-hydroxytryptamine in the brain. *Br. J. Pharmac., 51*, 571-575.

Lister, R. G., & File, S. E. (1983). Changes in regional concentrations in the rat brain of 5-hydroxytryptamine and 5-hydroxyindoleacetic acid during the development of tolerance to the sedative action of chlordiazepoxide. *J. Pharm. Pharmacol., 35*, 601-603.

Marks, I. M., Stern, R. S., Mawson, D., et al. (1980). Clomipramine and exposure for obsessive-compulsive rituals. *Br. J. Psychiatry, 136*, 1-25.

Marwaha, J., & Aghajanian, G. K. (1982). Relative potencies of alpha-1 and alpha-2 antagonists in the locus coeruleus, dorsal raphe and dorsal lateral geniculate nuclei: An electrophysiological study. *J. Pharmac. Exp. Ther., 222*, 287-293.

Mavissakalian, M. (1986). Trazodone in the treatment of panic agoraphobia. New research program and abstracts. American Psychiatric Association, 139th annual meeting, Washington, DC.

McElroy, J. F., Feldman, R. S., & Meyer, J. S. (1986). A comparison between chlordiazepoxide and CL218,872, a synthetic non-benzodiazepine ligand for benzodiazepine receptors, on serotonin and catecholamine turnover in brain. *Psychopharmacology, 88*, 105-108.

Montgomery, K. C. (1955). The relation between fear induced by novel stimulation and exploratory behavior. *J. Comp. Physiol. Psychol., 48*, 254-260.

Montgomery, S. A. (1980). Clomipramine in obsessional neurosis: A placebo controlled trial. *Pharm. Med., 1*, 189-192.

Morgane, P. J., & Jacobs, M. S. (1979). Raphe projections to the locus coeruleus in the rat. *Brain Res. Bull., 4*, 519-534.

Mueller, E. A., Murphy, D. L., & Sunderland, T. (1986). Further studies of the putative serotonin agonist, m-chlorophenylpiperazine: Evidence for a serotonin receptor mediated mechanism of action in humans. *Psychopharmacology, 89*, 388-391.

Mueller, E. A., Sunderland, T., & Murphy, D. L. (1985). Neuroendocrine effects of m-CPP, a serotonin agonist, in humans. *J. Clin. Endocrinol. Metab., 61*(6), 1179-1184.

Nanopoulos, D., Belin, M. F., Maitre, M., et al. (1982). Immunocytochemical evidence for the existence of GABAergic neurons in the nucleus raphe dorsalis, possible existence of neurons containing serotonin and GABA. *Brain Res., 232*, 375-389.

Ninan, P. T., Insel, T. M., Cohen, R. M., et al. (1982). Benzodiazepine receptor-mediated experimental "anxiety" in primates. *Science, 218*, 1332-1334.

Nishikawa, T., & Scatton, B. (1983). Evidence for a GABAergic inhibitory influence on serotonergic neurons originating from the dorsal raphe. *Brain Res., 279*, 325-329.

Nishikawa, T., & Scatton, B. (1985a). Inhibitory influence of GABA on central serotonergic transmission. Involvement of the habenulo-raphe pathways in the GABAergic inhibition of ascending cerebral serotonergic neurons. *Brain Res., 331*, 81-90.

Nishikawa, T., & Scatton, B. (1985b). Inhibitory influence of GABA on central serotonergic transmission. Raphe nuclei as the neuroanatomical site of the GABAergic inhibition of cerebral serotonergic neurons. *Brain Res., 331*, 91–103.

Noyes, R., Crowe, R. R., Harris, E. L., et al. (1986). Relationship between panic disorder and agoraphobia. *Arch. Gen. Psychiatry, 43*, 227–232.

Olajide, D., & Lader, M. (1987). A comparison of buspirone, diazepam and placebo in patients with chronic anxiety states. *J. Clin. Psychopharmacol., 7*, 148–152.

Paul, S. M., Marangos, P. J., & Skolnick, P. (1981). The benzodiazepine-GABA-chloride ionophore receptor complex: Common site of minor tranquilizer action. *Biol. Psychiatry, 16*, 213–229.

Pellow, S., Chopin, P., File, S. E., & Briley, M. (1985). Validation of open/closed arm entries in an elevated plus-maze as a measure of anxiety in the rat. *J. Neurosci. Methods, 14*, 149–167.

Pellow, S., & Fine, S. E. (1986). Anxiolytic and anxiogenic drug effects on exploratory activity in an elevated plus-maze: A novel test of anxiety in the rat. *Pharmacol. Biochem. Behavs., 24*, 525–529.

Peroutka, S. J. (1985). Selective interaction of novel anxiolytics with 5-hydroxy-tryptamine$_{1a}$ receptors. *Biol. Psychiatry, 20*, 971–979.

Petersen, E. N., & Lassen, J. B. (1981). A water lick conflict paradigm using drug experienced rats. *Psychopharmacology, 75*, 236–239.

Pickel, V. M., Tong, H. J., & Reis, D. J. (1978). Immunocytochemical evidence for serotonergic innervation of noradrenergic neurons in nucleus locus ceruleus. In S. Garattini, J. F. Pujol, & R. Samanin (Eds.), *Interactions between putative neurotransmitters in the brain* (pp. 369–382). New York: Raven Press.

Piper, D., Upton, N., Thomas, D., et al. (1987). The effects of the 5HT3 receptor antagonists BRL 43694 and GR 38042F in animal behavioral models of anxiety. *Br. J. Pharmac., 91*, 314P.

Pratt, J. A., Jenner, P., & Marsden, C. D. (1985). Comparison of the effects of benzodiazepines and other anticonvulsant drugs on synthesis and utilization of 5-HT in mouse brain. *Neuropharmacology, 24*, 59–68.

Pratt, J., Jenner, P., Reynods, E. H., et al. (1979). Clonazepam induces decreased serotoninergic activity in the mouse brain. *Neuropharmacology, 18*, 791–799.

Price, L. H., Goodman, W. K., Charney, D. S., et al. (1987). Treatment of severe obsessive compulsive disorder with fluvoxamine. *Am. J. Psychiatry, 144*, 1059–1061.

Pujol, J. F., Keane, P., McRae, A., Lewis, B. D., & Renaud, B. (1978). Biochemical evidence for serotonergic control of the locus ceruleus. In S. Garattini, J. F. Pujol, & R. Samanin (Eds.), *Interactions between putative neurotransmitters in the brain* (pp. 401–410). New York: Raven Press.

Redmond, D. E., Jr., & Huang, Y. H. (1979). Current concepts II. New evidence for a locus coeruleus-norepinephrine connection with anxiety. *Life Sci., 25*, 2149–2162.

Redmond, D. E., Katz, M. M., Maas, J. W., et al. (1986). Cerebrospinal fluid amine metabolites: Relationships with behavioral measurements in depressed, manic and healthy control subjects. *Arch. Gen. Psychiatry, 43*, 938–947.

Remy, D. C., Rittle, K. E., Hunt, C. A., et al. (1977). (+)- and (−)-3-Methoxycyproheptadine. A comparative evaluation of the antiserotonin, antihistaminic, anticholinergic, and orexigenic properties with cyproheptadine. *J. Med. Chem., 20,* 1681–1684.

Rickels, K., Weisman, K., Norstad, N., et al. (1982). Buspirone and diazepam in anxiety: A controlled study. *J. Clin. Psychiatry, 43,* 81–86.

Robichaud, R. C., & Sledge, K. L. (1969). The effects of p-chlorophenylalanine on experimentally induced conflict in the rat. *Life Sci., 8,* 965–969.

Ross, C. A., & Matas, M. (1987). A clinical trial of buspirone and diazepam in the treatment of generalized anxiety disorder. *Can. J. Psychiatry, 32,* 351–355.

Roth, M., Gurney, C., Garside, R. F., et al. (1972). The relationship between anxiety states and depressive illness, part I. *Brit. J. Psychiatry, 121,* 147–161.

Rydin, E., Schalling, D., & Asberg, M. (1982). Rorschach ratings in depressed and suicidal patients with low CSF 5-HIAA. *Psychiatry Res., 7,* 229–243.

Saner, A., & Pletcher, A. (1979). Effect of diazepam on cerebral 5-Hydroxytryptamine synthesis. *Eur. J. Pharmacol., 55,* 315–318.

Scatton, B., Serrano, A., Rivot, J. P., et al. (1984). Inhibitory GABAergic influence on striatal serotonergic transmission exerted in the dorsal raphe as revealed by in vivo voltammetry. *Brain Res., 305,* 343–352.

Segal, M. (1979). Serotonergic innervation of the locus coeruleus from the dorsal raphe and its action on responses to noxious stimuli. *J. Physiol, 286,* 401–415.

Sepinwall, J., & Cook, L. (1978). Behavioral pharmacology of antianxiety drugs. In L. L. Iversen, S. D. Iversen, & S. H. Snyder (Eds.), *Biology of mood and antianxiety drugs. Handbook of psychopharmacology* (pp. 345–393). New York: Plenum.

Shephard, R. A., Buxton, D. A., & Broadhurst, P. L. (1982). Drug interactions do not support reduction in serotonin turnover as the mechanism of action of benzodiazepines. *Neuropharmacology, 21,* 1027–1032.

Sills, M. A., Wolfe, B. B., & Frazer, A. (1984). Determination of selective and nonselective compounds for the 5-HT$_1$ receptor subtypes in rat frontal cortex. *J. Pharmacol. Exp. Ther., 231,* 480–487.

Soubrie, P., Blas, C., Ferron, A., et al. (1983). Chlordiazepoxide reduces in vivo serotonin release in the basal ganglia of encephale isole but not anesthetized cats: Evidence for a dorsal raphe site of action. *J. Pharmacol. Exp. Ther., 226,* 526–532.

Stein, L., Belluzi, J. D., & Wise, D. (1977). Benzodiazepines: Behavioral and neurochemical mechanisms. *Am. J. Psychiatry, 134,* 665–669.

Stein, L., Wise, C. D., & Belluzzi, J. D. (1975). Effects of benzodiazepines on central serotonergic mechanisms. In E. Costa (Ed.), *Mechanism of action of benzodiazepines.* New York: Greengard Raven Press.

Stein, L., Wise, C. D., & Berger, B. D. (1973). Antianxiety action of benzodiazepines: Decrease in activity of serotonin neurones in the punishment system. In S. Garratini, E. Mussini, & I. O. Randall (Ed.), *The benzodiazepines* (pp. 299–326). New York: Raven Press.

Stern, R. S., Marks, I. M., & Mawson, D. (1980). Clomipramine and exposure for compulsive rituals: Plasma levels, side effects, and outcome. *Br. J. Psychiatry, 136,* 161–166.

Taylor, D. P., Eison, M. S., Riblet, L. A., et al. (1985). Pharmacological and clinical effects of buspirone. *Pharmacol. Biochem. Behav., 23,* 687–694.

Thiebot, M. H., Hamon, M., & Soubrie, P. (1982). Attenuation of induced-anxiety in rats by chlordiazepoxide: Role of raphe dorsalis benzodiazepine binding sites and serotoninergic neurons. *Neuroscience, 7,* 2287–2294.

Thiebot, M. H., Soubrie, P., Hamon, M., et al. (1984). Evidence against the involvement of serotonergic neurons in the anti-punishment activity of diazepam in the rat. *Psychopharmacology, 82,* 355–359.

Thoren, P., Asberg, M., Bertilsson, L., et al. (1980). Clomipramine treatment of obsessive compulsive disorder: II. Biochemical aspects. *Arch. Gen. Psychiatry, 37,* 1289–1295.

Thoren, P., Asberg, M., Cronholm, B., et al. (1980). Clomipramine treatment of obsessive compulsive disorder: I. A. controlled clinical trial. *Arch. Gen. Psychiatry, 37,* 1281–1289.

Trulson, M. E., & Arasteh, K. (1985). Buspirone decreases the activity of 5-hydroxytryptamine-containing dorsal raphe neurons in-vitro. *J. Pharm. Pharmacol., 38,* 380–382.

Trulson, M. E., Preussler, D. W., Howell, G. A., et al. (1982). Raphe unit activity in freely moving cats: Effects of benzodiazepines. *Neuropharmacology, 21,* 1045–1050.

Tye, N. C., Everitt, B. J., & Iversen, S. D. (1977). 5-Hydroxytryptamine and punishment. *Nature, 268,* 741–742.

Tye, N. C., Iversen, S. D., & Green, A. R. (1979). The effects of benzodiazepines and serotonergic manipulations on punished responding. *Neuropharmacology, 18,* 689–695.

Valzelli, L. (1984). Reflections on experimental and human pathology of aggression. *Prog. Neuro-Psychopharmacol. Biol. Psychiat., 8,* 311–325.

Van der Maelen, C. P., & Wildeman, R. C. (1984). Iontophoretic and systemic administration of the non-benzodiazepine anxiolytic drug buspirone causes inhibition of serotonergic dorsal raphe neurons in rats. *Fed. Proc., 43,* 947.

van Praag, H. M. (1983). In search of the mode of action of antidepressants: 5HT/tyrosine mixtures in depressions. *Neuropharmacology, 22,* 433–440.

van Praag, H. M. (1986). Biological suicide research: Outcome and limitations. *Biol. Psychiatry, 21,* 1305–1323.

van Praag, H. M., Kahn, R. S., Brown, S., et al. (1987). Therapeutic indications for 5HT potentiating compounds. *Biol. Psychiatry, 22,* 205–212.

van Praag, H. M., & Korf, J. (1971). Endogenous depressions with and without disturbances in the 5hydroxytryptamine metabolism: A biochemical classification? *Psychopharmacologia, 19,* 148–152.

van Praag, H. M., Lemus, C. Z., & Kahn, R. S. (1986). Peripheral hormones: A window on the central MA? *Psychopharm. Bull., 22,* 565–570.

van Praag, H. M., Lemus, C. Z., & Kahn, R. S. (1987). Hormonal probes of central serotonergic activity: Do they really exist? *Biol. Psychiatry, 22,* 86–98.

Vellucci, S. V., & File, S. E. (1979). Chlordiazepoxide loses its anxiolytic action with long-term treatment. *Psychopharmacology, 62,* 61–65.

Vogel, J. R., Beer, B., & Clody, D. E. (1971). A simple and reliable conflict procedure for testing antianxiety agents. *Psychopharmacology, 21*, 1–7.

Weissman, M., Fox, K., & Klerman, J. L. (1973). Hostility and depression associated with suicide attempts. *Am. J. Psychiatry, 130*, 450–455.

West, D. J. (1965). *Murder followed by suicide*. London: Heinemann.

Wetzler, S. (1986). Methodological issues for the differentiation of anxiety and depression. *Clin. Neuropharmacol., 9*, 248–250.

Wheatley, D. (1982). Buspirone: Multicenter efficacy study. *J. Clin. Psychiatry, 43*, 92–94.

Winter, J. C. (1972). Comparison of chlordiazepoxide, methysergide and cinanserin as modifiers of punished behavior and as antagonists of N,N-dimethyltryptamine. *Arch. Int. Pharmacodyn., 197*, 147–152.

Wise, C. D., Berger, B. D., & Stein, L. (1972). Benzodiazepines: Anxiety-reducing activity by reduction of serotonin turnover in the brain. *Science, 17*, 181.

Wurtman, R. J. (1982). Nutrients that modify brain functions. *Sci. Am., 246*, 42–51.

Yaryura-Tobias, J. S., & Bhagavan, H. N. (1977). L-Tryptophan in obsessive compulsive disorders. *Am. J. Psychiatry, 134*, 1298–1299.

Zohar, J., & Insel, T. R. (1987). Obsessive compulsive disorder: Psychobiological approaches to diagnosis, treatment and pathophysiology. *Biol. Psychiatry, 22*, 667–687.

Zohar, J., Insel, T. R., Zohar-Kadouch, R. C., et al. (1988). Serotonergic responsivity in obsessive-compulsive disorder: Effects of chronic clomipramine treatment. *Arch. Gen. Psychiatry, 45*, 167–172.

Zohar, J., Mueller, E. A., Insel, T. R., et al. (1987). Serotonergic responsivity in obsessive-compulsive disorder: Comparison of patients and health controls. *Arch. Gen. Psychiatry, 44*, 946–951.

7

Is There a Specific Role for Serotonin in Obsessive Compulsive Disorder?

JOSEPH ZOHAR
RACHEL C. ZOHAR-KADOUCH

PREVALENCE OF OCD

The lifetime prevalence of obsessive compulsive disorder (OCD) in the general population, although traditionally thought to be 0.05% (Woodruff & Pitts, 1969), has recently been reported to be as high as 1.3% to 2% in the United States (Robins et al., 1984) and 3% in Edmonton, Canada (Bland et al., 1988). If the lifetime prevalence of OCD in the general population is so high, why is it that we do not see these patients more often? Patients with OCD tend to be very secretive about their symptoms, and many of them do not seek help unless they develop complications, the most common of which is depression. Moreover, they may not reveal the presence of obsessive compulsive symptoms unless direct, specific questions about obsessions and compulsions are asked by a clinician who is familiar with the clinical characteristics of OCD.

CLINICAL CHARACTERISTICS OF OCD

Patients with OCD complain of persistent, unwanted thoughts or impulses (obsessions and/or repetitive, ritualistic behaviors, which they feel driven to perform, or compulsions). Although both obsessions and compulsions are present in a variety of psychiatric disorders, as well as in normal mental life, OCD is distinguished by three cardinal features. First, the symptoms are ego-dystonic; that is, the individual realizes that they are excessive or unreasonable and attempts to ignore or suppress them. Second, the obsessions and/or the compulsions cause marked distress, consume a significant amount of time, and lead to significant interference in functioning. Third, the individual recognizes that these preoccupations and/or rituals are the product of his or her own mind and are not imposed from without, as in delusions of thought insertion.

OCD presents in several forms (Insel, 1984). "Washers" are obsessed with dirt or contamination (Rachman & Hodgson, 1980; Akhtar et al., 1975). They usually avoid door knobs, light switches, telephones, money, and other "contaminated objects" so that they will not need to spend hours washing their hands.

"Checkers" are obsessed with doubt, usually involving a fear of harming or offending others or a need for symmetry. Typically, they fear that the stove has not been turned off, the doors have not been locked, or that a bump on the road is a body. They will then have to check repetitively to reassure themselves that this is not the case. Unfortunately, their checking, instead of resolving the uncertainty, often contributes to an even greater doubt.

Approximately 25% of patients with OCD have pure obsessions without compulsive rituals (Akhtar et al., 1975; Welner et al., 1976). These patients have repetitive intrusive thoughts or impulses, usually aggressive (e.g., "I cannot ride the subway since I am afraid that I might push somebody"), or sexual and always embarrassing.

Primary obsessional slowness is a rare, yet very disabling, form of this syndrome (Rachman, 1974). Although slowness results from most rituals, occasionally it becomes the predominant symptom. These patients will spend hours each day on the most simple acts of personal hygiene. Many become housebound, and if they are able to reach a doctor's office, they may require several hours of checking before they are able to leave.

The revised third edition of the *Diagnostic and Statistical Manual of Mental Disorders* (DSM-III-R) defines the most recent criteria required for diagnosis of OCD (see Table 7-1). By DSM-III-R criteria, in contrast to those delineated in the older DSM-III, another Axis I disorder may coexist with OCD. However, the content of the obsession must be unrelated to the second disorder if OCD is diagnosed. Thus, guilty thoughts in the presence of a major depressive disorder or thoughts about food in the presence of an eating disorder should not be considered as symptoms of OCD.

OCD, previously referred to variously as obsessional neurosis, compulsion neurosis, or obsessional disorder, is frequently confused with compulsive personality disorder. Compulsive personality disorder refers to persons afflicted with excessive perfectionism, orderliness, and rigidity that are ego-syntonic; that is, the person does not attempt to ignore or suppress them. In contrast, the symptoms of OCD are ego-dystonic. Moreover, epidemiological evidence reveals that a substantial number of patients with OCD do not exhibit premorbid compulsive traits (Rasmussen & Tsuang, 1984).

TABLE 7-1
DSM-III-R Diagnostic Criteria for Obsessive-Compulsive Disorder

A. Either obsessions or compulsions:

Obsessions: (1), (2), (3), and (4):

    (1) recurrent and persistent ideas, thoughts, impulses, or images that are experienced, at least initially, as intrusive and senseless, e.g., a parent's having repeated impulses to kill a loved child, a religious person's having recurrent blasphemous thoughts

    (2) the person attempts to ignore or suppress such thoughts or impulses or to neutralize them with some other thought or action

    (3) the person recognizes that the obsessions are the product of his or her own mind, not imposed from without (as in thought insertion)

    (4) if another Axis I disorder is present, the content of the obsession is unrelated to it, e.g., the ideas, thoughts, impulses, or images are not about food in the presence of an Eating Disorder, about drugs in the presence of a Psychoactive Substance Use Disorder, or guilty thoughts in the presence of a Major Depression

Compulsions: (1), (2), and (3):

    (1) repetitive, purposeful, and intentional behaviors that are performed in response to an obsession, or according to certain rules or in a stereotyped fashion

    (2) the behavior is designed to neutralize or to prevent discomfort or some dreaded event or situation; however, either the activity is not connected in a realistic way with what it is designed to neutralize or prevent, or it is clearly excessive

    (3) the person recognizes that his or her behavior is excessive or unreasonable (this may not be true for young children; it may no longer be true for people whose obsessions have evolved into overvalued ideas)

B. The obsessions or compulsions cause marked distress, are time-consuming (take more than an hour a day), or significantly interfere with the person's normal routine, occupational functioning, or usual social activities or relationships with others.

Reprinted with permission from the *Diagnostic and Statistical Manual of Mental Disorders, Third Edition, Revised.* Copyright 1987 American Psychiatric Association.

Other behaviors in which people engage excessively and with a sense of compulsion, such as pathological gambling, overeating, alcohol or drug abuse, and hypersexuality, are also distinguished from the true compulsions of OCD since, to some degree, they are experienced as pleasurable, whereas compulsions are inherently not pleasurable.

OCD AND SEROTONERGIC FUNCTION

One way to examine whether patients with OCD have a psychobiological abnormality involving serotonergic function is to compare drug-free OCD patients with matched controls on several indices of serotonergic function.

This approach has been utilized in studies of platelet ^{3}H-imipramine binding, cerebrospinal fluid (CSF) 5-hydroxyindoleacetic acid (5-HIAA) concentration, and behavioral and endocrinological responses to pharmacological challenge with a selective serotonin agonist.

High-affinity ^{3}H–imipramine binding sites in human platelets closely resemble those binding sites in human brain (Rehavi et al., 1984) and are closely associated with the presynaptic uptake site for ^{3}H-serotonin (Paul et al., 1981). Hence they may serve as a model for the study of central serotonergic neurons (Lingjaerde, 1984). The maximal binding of ^{3}H–imipramine (B_{max}) was found to be significantly lower (B_{max} values, adolescents—OCD vs. controls = 292 ± 186 vs. 587 ± 150 fmole/mg protein; adults—OCD vs. controls = 334 ± 129 fmole/mg protein, $p < 0.01$, Student's t test) for eight adolescent and 10 adult patients with OCD compared with 18 age- and sex-matched controls. (Weizman et al., 1986), although these results were not found in a previous study (Insel et al., 1985). In this study ^{3}H–imipramine binding to platelets was reported to be unchanged, although there was a trend toward reduced ^{3}H-imipramine binding sites in the OCD patients. However, much of this trend was attributable to two patients with very low binding values. These patients were the only ones included who had received clomipramine in the past (more than three months before the study). Removing them and their two matched controls from the sample abolishes the difference between the remaining 10 OCD patients and their 10 matched controls (OCD B_{max} = 634.4 ± 81.3 fmol protein vs. normal B_{max} = 634.4 ± 157.8 fmol/mg protein).

CSF concentration of 5-HIAA (the primary serotonin metabolite) has been used as an indicator of central serotonin turnover (Jimmerson & Berrettini, 1985). Significantly higher (30% higher, $p < .001$, Mann-Whitney U test) CSF 5-HIAA concentrations, corrected for height and weight, have been noted in a small cohort ($n = 8$) of patients with OCD compared with 5-HIAA values of 23 controls (Insel et al., 1985). It should be noted that in a previous larger study, a nonsignificant 19% increase in CSF 5-HIAA levels of 24 pretreatment hospitalized patients with OCD was found as compared with 37 paid healthy volunteers (Thoren et al., 1980a).

Higher levels of CSF 5-HIAA in patients with OCD are of theoretical interest, since violent and impulsive patients, who appear to be phenomenologically opposite to patients with OCD, show significantly lower CSF HIAA levels compared with normal controls (van Praag, 1983; Linnoila et al., 1983; Virkkunen et al., 1987).

To investigate serotonin function in OCD further, we compared behavioral and endocrine effects following activation of the serotonergic system by administration of a serotonin agonist in untreated patients with OCD and in healthy controls (Zohar et al., 1987a). Traditional drugs such as tryptophan or 5-hydroxytryptophan that are known to affect serotonergic metabolism and action are not entirely specific for the serotonergic system (Fernstrom & Wurtman, 1974; Saavedra & Axelrod, 1974), or are associated with severe adverse effects (Engelman et al., 1974). Moreover, several selective serotonin uptake inhibitors, such as zimelidine and citalopram, have recently been declared unsafe for clinical use, while some direct postsynaptic receptor agonists, such as dimethyltryptamine (Meltzer et al., 1982), are not useful because of their hallucinogenic properties. We therefore elected to study the novel serotonin receptor agonist m-chlorophenylpiperazine (mCPP) (Samanin et al., 1979; Fuller et al., 1980), a synthetic, nonindole, aryl-substituted piperazine derivative that rapidly penetrates the blood-brain barrier (Engelman et al., 1974). mCPP is a metabolite of the antidepressant trazodone (Caccia et al., 1981), and thus might be expected to be safe and well tolerated in humans. In preclinical biochemical studies, mCPP showed potent displacement of ^{3}H-serotonin from membrane homogenate in vitro (Fuller et al., 1981; Invernizzi et al., 1981), and caused decreased central serotonin synthesis and turnover in vivo (Samanin et al., 1980; Fuller et al., 1981), interpreted as a feedback effect following postsynaptic receptor stimulation. In animal studies, mCPP produces typical changes in serotonin-mediated behaviors, such as decreased food consumption (Samanin et al., 1979; Mennini et al., 1980) and decreased locomotion (Vetulani et al., 1982). Neuroendocrine changes associated with mCPP include increased prolactin, cortisol, and corticotropin levels (Maj & Lewandowska, 1980; Aloi et al., 1984). mCPP also produces physiological reactions such as hyperthermia (Aloi et al., 1984). All of these changes are to be expected of a postsynaptic serotonin receptor agonist, are reversed by the administration of the serotonin receptor antagonist metergoline, and are responsive to presumed alterations in serotonin receptor sensitivity (Samanin et al., 1979; Maj & Lewandowska, 1980; Aloi et al., 1984).

Using mCPP as a serotonin probe, we investigated (1) whether patients with OCD would differ from healthy controls in their behavioral and endocrine response to challenge by mCPP, and (2) whether mCPP would affect the symptoms of OCD.

All studies consisted of oral, single-dose drug or placebo administered under double-blind, random-assignment conditions on separate days. Oral, as compared with intravenous, administration of mCPP was chosen on the basis of concurrent studies in normal subjects comparing mCPP 0.5 mg/kg administered orally with 0.1 mg/kg administered intravenously (Murphy et al., 1989). Oral administration of 0.5 mg/kg of mCPP produced plateau-phase plasma mCPP concentrations, and peak elevations of prolactin and cortisol that were essentially identical to those found after smaller doses of mCPP (0.1 mg/kg) administered intravenously over 90 seconds. In contrast, differential route of administration produced striking differences in the subjective effects of mCPP. After intravenous administration of mCPP (0.1 mg/kg), subjects experienced significant increases in anxiety, depressive affect, feelings of derealization, and a sense of impaired cognitive capacity, whereas larger doses of oral mCPP (0.5 mg/kg) produced smaller or negligible changes on all of these measures in this cohort of normal volunteers. Additionally, somatic side effects were more pronounced after intravenous mCPP. Since we wanted to minimize possible physical and psychological side effects while maximizing hormonal changes, we chose the oral route of administration.

The 0.5 mg/kg dose was chosen on the basis of concurrent studies in normal subjects with doses of mCPP between 0.25 and 2.5 mg/kg. In contrast to the 0.5 mg/kg dose, which was generally very well tolerated and produced consistent increases in prolactin and cortisol levels and temperature, doses of 1.0 mg/kg and greater produced transient nausea or vomiting in six of 13 subjects, and also produced transient perceptual distortions, feelings of derealization, crying spells, anxiety, or dysphoria in several subjects (Mueller et al., 1985).

Figure 7-1 shows the effect of a single dose of 0.5 mg/kg of mCPP, administered orally under double-blind, placebo-controlled, random-assignment conditions, to nine patients before treatment and after four months of treatment, and administered once to 14 control subjects. Relative to healthy controls, the untreated patients with OCD became significantly more anxious, depressed, and dysphoric, and showed greater increases in altered self-reality (e.g., feeling "out of touch," "mistrustful," "having unusual thoughts," "unreal or strange") (F[1,19] > 5.5, $p < 0.05$; *post hoc* Student's *t* tests, all $p < 0.05$). The placebo responses, as well as the physical effects, were very mild in both groups and did not significantly differ between the patients and the controls.

This finding suggests that untreated patients with OCD are more responsive to the behavioral effects of mCPP than normal controls. However, it does not indicate whether mCPP affects the symptoms of OCD. Subsequently, to test this effect, each patient was asked to complete (with the help of an experienced psychiatrist) two specific rating scales aimed at assessing changes in obsessions and compulsions. One of the scales was a modified form of the Comprehensive Psychiatric Rating Scale—Obsessive Compulsive Subscale (CPRS-OC) developed by Thoren and co-workers (1980); the modified CPRS-OC-5 includes only those five items (rated 0 to 3) that reflect OC symptoms (compulsive thoughts, rituals, indecision, lassitude, and concentration difficulties) and excludes three items (sadness, inner tension, and worrying over trifles) that are not specific to OCD. The other scale was the National Institute of Mental Health's Global Scales, in-

EFFECTS OF CMI TREATMENT ON PEAK CHANGES IN NIMH SELF-RATING SCORES (Δm CPP–Δ PLACEBO)

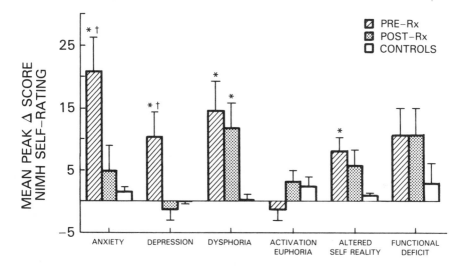

Figure 7-1. Peak changes in NIMH self-rating scores (ðmCPP-ðPlacebo) in OCD patients before and during treatment with clomipramine and controls. Peak behavioral changes of patients with obsessive compulsive disorder before treatment (shaded bars, $n = 9$), after four months of clomipramine treatment (dotted bars, $n = 9$), and controls (open bars, $n = 14$) after single-dose metachlorophenylpiperazine administration (0.5 mg/kg) under randomized double-masked conditions. NIMH indicates National Institute of Mental Health. Anxiety—feels anxious, restless, worried, frightened. Depression—feels sad, depressed, hopeless, worthless. Dysphoria—feels irritable, angry, uncomfortable mentally. Activation-euphoria—feels elated, more talkative, especially energetic, has racing thoughts. Altered self-reality—feels out of touch, mistrustful or suspicious, unreal or strange, has unusual thoughts, hears voices, sees things others do not. Functional difficulty—has difficulty concentrating and functioning, feels slowed down. Asterisk indicates $p \leq 0.05$, Student's t test on peak changes, patients versus controls. Dagger indicates $p < 0.5$, t test of paired data on peak changes, patients before clomipramine treatment versus patients during clomipramine treatment in each subject.

cluding those for OC symptoms, anxiety, and depression, rated from 1 to 15 (Murphy et al., 1980). All the ratings were done before and at 90, 180, and 210 minutes after drug or placebo administration.

Following mCPP but not placebo, untreated patients with OCD experienced a transient but marked exacerbation of their OC symptoms (Figure 7-2). The peak behavioral response was generally observed in the first three hours following mCPP administration and the duration of this exacerbation ranged from several hours (50% of patients) to 48 hours (20% of patients). Moreover, following mCPP but not placebo, five patients spontaneously described emergence of new obsessions or reoccurrence of obsessions that had not been present for several months.

As oral administration of mCPP, 0.5 mg/kg, has also been associated with anxiogenic effects and induction of panic attacks in patients with panic disorders (Klein et al., submitted), it is not clear whether mCPP increases OC symptoms selectively or whether there may be a nonspecific exacerbation of diverse psychopathology by this drug. Certainly, mCPP affected several symptoms other than obsessions in our patients with OCD, and thus one might assume that this drug may be increasing anxiety or dysphoria, with an exacerbation of OC symptoms occurring as a secondary phenomenon. This assumption would be strengthened if patients with OCD were hypersensitive to other anxiogenic compounds. However, several recent studies with anxiogenic agents, such as lactate (Gorman et al., 1985), yohimbine (Rasmussen et al., 1987), and caffeine (Zohar et al., 1987b), have shown no increase in either anxiety or OC symptoms in patients with OCD, suggesting that these patients do not have a hypersensitivity to provocative agents that exacerbate anxiety disorders. Moreover, so far mCPP is the only agent that has been reported to be associated with exacerbation of obsessive compulsive symptoms (Zohar et al., 1987a), suggesting that it may actually increase these symptoms selectively.

In contrast to the behavioral hypersensitivity, equivalent and significant increases in prolactin were observed in both groups. (See Figure 7-3.) Peak plasma cortisol concentrations after mCPP were lower in the patients than the controls; the patients also tended to have lower baseline cortisol values than the controls. (See Figure 7-4.)

The lack of a differentially increased secretion of "stress hormones" such as prolactin and cortisol (Mills & Chir, 1980), in the presence of an apparently very stressful experience in patients with OCD, is a puzzling phenomenon. One possible interpretation is that the effect of mCPP on behavior is mediated by a different mechanism than the effect of mCPP on endocrine regulation. The lack of difference in baseline levels of prolactin or cortisol between patients and controls is consistent with this interpretation, which implies that in patients with OCD, only those elements of the serotonin system that mediate the OC symptoms are affected. A second possible interpretation is that the effects of mCPP bypass the normal stress-control mechanisms that regulate the increased secretion of prolactin and cortisol. A third interpretation is that the patients with OCD are hormonally hy-

Effects of CMI Treatment on Peak Change from Baseline after Placebo and mCPP

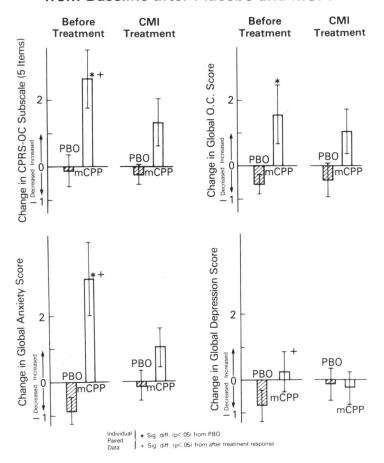

Figure 7-2. Peak change from baseline after placebo and mCPP before and during treatment with clomipramine. Peak changes (mean ± SEM) from baseline on behavioral ratings before and after four months of clomipramine treatment. Placebo and metachlorophenylpiperazine (mCPP) were administrated orally under double-masked, random-assignment conditions to the same nine patients with obsessive compulsive (OC) disorder. CPRS-OC-5 indicates Comprehensive Psychiatric Rating Scale—Obsessive Compulsive five-item subscale; other scales are National Institute of Mental Health Global Scales. Asterisk indicates $p < 0.05$, t test of paired data comparing peak change after mCPP with peak change after placebo in each subject; plus sign indicates $p < 0.05$, t test of paired data comparing peak changes after mCPP before clomipramine treatment with peak change after mCPP during clomipramine treatment in each subject.

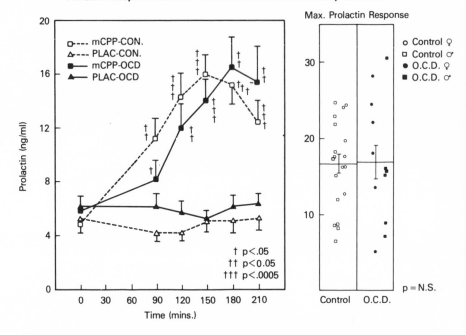

Prolactin Response to mCPP in OCD Patients and Healthy Controls

Figure 7-3. Mean prolactin time–response curve (± SEM) (left) and distribution of maximal response (right) after metachlorophenylpiperazine (mCPP) administered orally under double-masked, random-assignment conditions to patients with obsessive compulsive disorder (OCD) ($n = 12$) and healthy controls (Con) ($n = 19$). Plac indicates placebo. In figure at right, squares indicate men, circles indicate women, open figures indicate controls, and closed figures indicate patients with OCD (no significant differences). Dagger indicates $p < 0.05$; double dagger, $p < 0.005$; and triple dagger $p < 0.0005$, t test of paired data comparing change after mCPP to change after Plac for either patients with OCD or healthy controls ([1,25] = 38.2, p,0.0001)

poresponsive. This interpretation is hinted at by reduced cortisol responses to mCPP in these patients as compared with patients with panic disorder, who exhibit increased cortisol response to 0.25 mg/kg of orally administered mCPP (Kahn et al., 1988).

OCD AND CLOMIPRAMINE

If OCD is associated with abnormal serotonergic function, one would expect that drugs that alter serotonergic function might be therapeutically effective in the treatment of OCD. Indeed, as early as 1968, Renynghe de Voxrie reported that the tricyclic antidepressant clomipramine (CMI), a po-

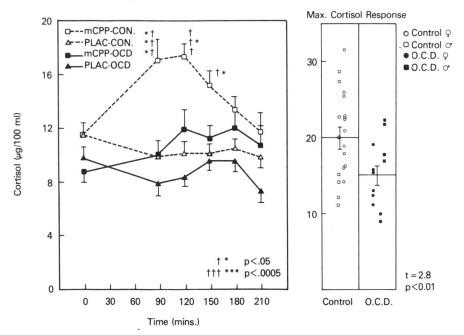

Cortisol Response to mCPP in OCD Patients and Healthy Controls

Figure 7-4. Mean cortisol time–response curve ($\pm$ SEM) (left) and distribution of maximal cortisol response (right) after metachlorophenylpiperazine (mCPP) administered orally under double-masked, random-assignment conditions to patients with obsessive compulsive disorder (OCD) ($n = 12$) and healthy controls (Con) ($n = 20$). Plac indicates placebo. In figure at right, squares indicate men; circles, women; open figures, controls, and closed figures, patients with OCD ($t = 2.8$, $p < 0.01$). Dagger indicates $p < 0.05$; triple daggers $p < 0.0005$, t test of paired data comparing change after mCPP with change after Plac for healthy controls ([1,24] = 13.23, p,0.001 for controls; F not significant for patients); asterisk, $p < 0.05$; and triple asterisks, $p < 0.0005$, Student's t test comparing change after mCPP in patients with OCD.

tent serotonin reuptake blocker, reduced obsessional symptoms in 10 of 15 obsessive patients (Renynghe de Voxrie, 1968). During the 1970s, a series of confirmatory but uncontrolled studies extended this initial observation to other patients with primary OCD (Yaryura-Tobias & Neziroglu, 1975; Rack, 1977; Ananth et al., 1979).

More recently, a group of carefully controlled double-blind studies using CMI have been published. In four studies (Marks et al., 1980; Montgomery, 1980; Thoren et al., 1980; Flament et al., 1985), CMI was shown to be more effective than placebo in reducing OCD symptomatology. Preliminary results from a recent double-blind, placebo-controlled, multicenter study, which included more than 500 patients with OCD, also demonstrate the superiority of CMI over placebo in the treatment of patients with OCD (De-Veaugh-Geiss, 1988).

However, it is conceivable that the therapeutic effect of CMI in OCD does not reflect a specific antiobsessional effect and that CMI is simply an effective antidepressant for a specific subgroup of patients (those with OCD) who frequently became depressed. To address this question, the therapeutic efficacy of CMI in OCD has been compared with the therapeutic efficacy of several other, less serotonergic tricyclic antidepressants. Thoren et al. (1980) reported that CMI was slightly more effective than nortriptyline, although this difference did not reach statistical significance. Ananth et al. (1981) reported that CMI, but not amitriptyline, produced significant amelioration of obsessions, depression, and anxiety. Volavka et al. (1985) reported CMI to be slightly more antiobsessional than imipramine at 12 weeks, but probably not at six weeks, of treatment, although differences in the baseline scores and in the symptom clusters between the two drug groups complicate the interpretation of these results.

Taken together, these studies suggest that CMI is probably more potent in the treatment of OCD than several other excellent tricyclic antidepressants, including nortriptyline, amitriptyline, and imipramine. This apparent specificity of CMI for reducing OCD symptoms is strikingly different from the roughly equivalent results given by CMI and the other tricyclic antidepressants in the treatment of depression and panic disorder, and thus deserving of more meticulous study. Since all previous studies comparing CMI with other tricyclics were parallel studies in which some of the patients had a secondary depression together with OCD, we decided to conduct a crossover study in which direct (versus parallel) comparison of CMI with other tricyclic antidepressants would be carried out in a cohort of nondepressed patients with OCD (Zohar & Insel, 1987c). This double-blind, random-assignment, crossover study compared the effects of CMI with those of desipramine (DMI). DMI was chosen as the comparison drug because it predominantly inhibits noradrenergic synaptic uptake, in contrast to CMI, which has potent effects on serotonin uptake (vide infra).

The distribution of maximum percent change from pretreatment baseline after treatment with CMI and DMI in patients with OCD ($n = 10$ for both conditions) is shown in Figure 7-5. The results demonstrate that (1) CMI is significantly more potent than DMI in reducing OC symptoms, and (2) DMI, an excellent antidepressant, lacks significant antiobsessional effects in this cohort of nondepressed patients with OCD. These CMI/DMI differences were not attributable to the order in which the drugs were given (they were given according to a counterbalanced design) and could not be related

Percentage Change of O.C. Symptomatology in CMI and DMI Treated Patients

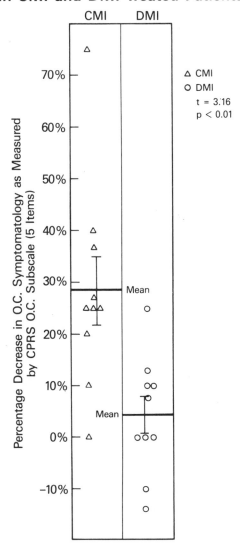

Figure 7-5. Distribution of maximum percent change from pretreatment baseline on clomipramine (CMI) and desipramine (DMI) in obsessive compulsive (OC) patients ($n = 10$ for both trials) (as measured by the Comprehensive Psychiatric Rating Scale—Obsessive Compulsive Subscale (CPRS-OC) developed by Thoren et al. (1980) and modified by us to score only five items specific for OCD symptoms (i.e., rituals, compulsive thoughts, indecision, worrying over trifles, and lassitude) (Zohar & Insel, 1987)

to intergroup diagnostic differences, as part of the analysis used the subjects as their own controls. Plasma levels for DMI and CMI were roughly equivalent and were all within the therapeutic range for antidepressant effects.

It should be emphasized that the differences in improvement of OC ratings, although clearly significant, were not large. After six weeks of CMI treatment, only a 28% improvement in obsessional symptoms was noted. Eight of the patients in this study (including the patient with 0% improvement) entered an open-label six-month trial with CMI, leading to an eventual overall rate improvements of 40 to 90%. In each case, the symptoms remained to some extent, but were easier to resist and no longer interfered with functioning. Other studies (Volavka et al., 1985; Insel & Zohar, 1987) have also reported that CMI's antiobsessional effects have a relatively long time course, with small but significant reductions at four to six weeks, becoming more marked after 12 weeks.

CLOMIPRAMINE AND SEROTONIN

Compared with other tricyclics, CMI is an extremely potent inhibitor of serotonin reuptake (Ross & Renyi, 1977). The main metabolite of CMI, desmethylclomipramine (DCMI), which is present at about twice the concentration of CMI in human plasma, also has high affinity for the ^{3}H–imipramine binding site, believed to be the serotonin transporter site (Paul et al., 1980). By way of comparison, the affinity of desipramine (DMI), the main metabolite of imipramine, for the ^{3}H–imipramine binding site, is an order of magnitude less than the affinity of DCMI (Paul et al., 1980).

Several lines of evidence suggest that CMI's antiobsessional effects may be due to its effects on serotonin reuptake. Two studies have reported a significant correlation between plasma levels of CMI, but not of DCMI (which has a powerful inhibitory effect on the reuptake of both norepinephrine and serotonin), and clinical improvement in OCD (Stern et al., 1980; Insel et al., 1983). Thoren et al. (1980a) reported that the clinical response of patients with OCD treated with CMI was positively correlated ($r = .75$) with decrease in CSF concentrations of 5-HIAA, but not with 3-methoxy-4-hydroxyphenethylene glycol (MHPG), the main noradrenergic metabolite, or homovanillic acid (HVA), the main dopaminergic metabolite. Similarly, Flament et al. (1985) reported a significant correlation ($r = .62$ to .68) between clinical improvement and decrease in platelet serotonin in children with OCD treated with CMI.

Finally, to investigate possible changes in brain serotonergic responsivity during treatment with CMI, we administered mCPP and placebo under double-blind conditions to nine patients with OCD, before and after treatment with CMI (Zohar et al., 1988). Unlike our previous observations of a marked transient increase in obsessional symptoms and anxiety following mCPP in untreated OCD patients, readministration of mCPP after four months of treatment with CMI did not significantly increase obsessional symptoms and anxiety (Figures 7-1 and 7-2).

Thus, additionally, the ability of CMI to reduce OC symptoms in patients with OCD, the significant correlation shown between improvement in OCD symptoms during treatment with CMI and decreased CSF 5-HIAA (Thoren et al., 1980a), and the significant positive correlation seen between clinical improvement and decrease in platelet serotonin in children with OCD treated with CMI (Flament et al., 1985) are all consistent with the hypothesis that the therapeutic effects of CMI in patients with OCD may be associated with the development of serotonin receptor subsensitivity or downregulation.

THE SEROTONIN HYPOTHESIS OF OCD

The classical "serotonergic hypothesis" of OCD (Yaryura-Tobias et al., 1977) suggests that OCD may be due to a deficiency in serotonin, as patients appear to have a favorable response to the serotonin reuptake blocker CMI. Additional support for the serotonin deficiency hypothesis has come from reports of reduced whole-blood serotonin in patients with OCD (Yaryura-Tobias et al., 1977) and from uncontrolled trials of the serotonin precursor L-tryptophan, which has been reported to reduce obsessional symptoms (Yaryura-Tobias & Bhagavan, 1977) and to augment the antiobsessional effect of CMI (Rasmussen, 1984). Based on this hypothesis, one might expect that administration of a serotonin agonist like mCPP to patients with OCD would reduce obsessive compulsive symptoms, at least briefly. However, mCPP has been observed to increase rather than to decrease obsessive compulsive symptoms in these patients (Zohar et al., 1987a). Moreover, beneficial CMI treatment in patients with OCD was associated with decreased serotonergic responsivity compared with the same patients' responses to the same serotonergic challenge before treatment (Zohar et al., 1988).

Such findings are consistent with the hypothesis that increased serotonergic responsiveness, rather than serotonin deficiency, is associated with the psychopathologic characteristics of OCD. This formulation of the "serotonergic hypothesis" for OCD would also be consistent with the relatively long period needed for CMI to become effective in this disorder (Insel & Zohar, 1987). However, if hyperresponsivity of the serotonergic system, rather than serotonin deficiency, is associated with the psychopathological characteristics of OCD, we might also expect to see worsening of OCD symptoms during the initial phase of treatment with serotonin reuptake blockers, as these medications initially cause an increase of serotonin content in the synaptic cleft before downregulation of the receptors. A recent reanalysis of daily ratings of patients from an earlier inpatient study (Insel et al., 1983) has provided preliminary support for the notion that many patients with OCD experience a mild exacerbation of their symptoms during the first three to five days of CMI treatment (Zohar, Insel, Murphy, unpublished findings, 1987).

CLINICAL IMPLICATIONS

Based on the serotonergic hypothesis of OCD discussed above, one would expect that other medications with potent serotonin reuptake inhibition properties would also be effective in the treatment of OCD. Indeed, several recent studies have reported that nontricyclic selective serotonin reuptake blockers such as zimelidine (Prasad, 1984; Kahn et al., 1984; Fontaine & Chouinard, 1985; but also see Insel et al., 1985) are effective antiobsessional agents. However, zimelidine has been recently declared unsafe for clinical use and so cannot be used for the treatment of OCD. Very recently, two selective serotonin reuptake blockers, the bicyclic fluoxetine (Turner et al., 1985) and the unicyclic fluvoxamine (Price et al., 1987; Perse et al., 1987; Goodmann et al., 1989), have been shown to be effective in OCD in double-blind pilot studies. Pending further studies, it appears that fluoxetine and fluvoxamine might be alternatives to CMI in the treatment of OCD.

Additionally, case reports have described augmentation of CMI's antiobsessional effects with the serotonin precursor L-tryptophan (Rasmussen, 1984) and with lithium (Rasmussen, 1984; Stern & Jenike, 1983; Eisenberg & Asnis, 1985). In preclinical studies, lithium was found to increase electrophysiological measures of serotonergic functioning in animals during chronic tricyclic treatment (Blier & de Montigny, 1985).

As the data concerning CMI's efficacy in OCD have expanded (Zohar & Insel, 1987a), the importance of determining the necessary duration of treatment with CMI has become increasingly important. To examine the length of treatment necessary with CMI, a prospective placebo-controlled, double-blind, discontinuation study was carried out (Pato et al., 1988). The study included 21 patients with OCD who manifested sustained improvement during five to 27 months of treatment with CMI. Of 18 patients who completed the study, 16 patients experienced profound worsening of OCD symptoms after discontinuation of CMI. This worsening became statistically significant four weeks after CMI discontinuation, and appeared unrelated to CMI treatment duration prior to discontinuation or to the type of obsessive compulsive symptoms originally present. Reinstitution of CMI, in an open fashion, at the completion of the discontinuation study, showed that these patients then returned to their prestudy levels of improvement. A possible implication of this study is that prolonged CMI administration is warranted for the majority of patients with OCD. However, further studies are needed to evaluate whether treatment for more than the period examined (the mean was 10.7 ± 5 months) would allow for discontinuation without recurrence of symptoms.

CONCLUSION

Several lines of evidence indicate that there is a specific role for abnormal serotonin metabolism in OCD. The most impressive evidence is that, so far, OCD is the only psychiatric disorder in which only drugs that inhibit synaptic serotonin uptake (i.e., clomipramine, fluvoxamine, and fluoxetine) have been reported to be therapeutically effective (Zohar & Insel, 1987d). By contrast, selective norepinephrine uptake blockers such as desipramine and nortriptyline, or nonselective inhibitors such as imipramine and amitriptyline, appear ineffective for patients with OCD.

The antiobsessional effects of CMI have been hypothesized to be mediated through the serotonergic system, since the clinical response of OCD patients treated with CMI is positively correlated with decreased CSF 5-HIAA (but not with MHPG or HVA) and with decreased platelet serotonin. Moreover, a significant correlation between plasma levels of CMI (but not of its primary metabolite DCMI, which has a powerful inhibitory effect on the reuptake of both norepinephrine and serotonin) and clinical improvement were reported.

Therapeutic responses linked to serotonergic changes do not, however, necessarily implicate a primary serotonergic abnormality in patients with OCD. Studies of drug-free OCD patients with matched controls on several indices of serotonergic function such as serotonergic content and ^{3}H–imipramine binding in blood platelets and 5-HIAA in CSF present little or conflicting evidence for a consistent psychobiological abnormality in the serotonergic function of patients with OCD.

On the other hand, administration of mCPP, a novel serotonin agonist, is associated with increased behavioral sensitivity in patients with OCD relative to controls, and with a transient but marked exacerbation of their OC symptoms. Treatment with CMI in those patients alters this sensitivity to mCPP. These findings are consistent with the hypothesis that increased serotonergic responsiveness in central serotonin receptors may be associated with the psychopathologic characteristics of OCD.

While serotonin seems to play a special role in the psychobiology of

OCD, the focus on a single neurotransmitter (or a single receptor) is undoubtedly an oversimplification of this intriguing disorder. The task ahead is to understand the relationship of this single variable, serotonin metabolism, to the multitude of neurobiological, anatomical, and psychological variables that contribute to this disorder.

REFERENCES

Akhtar, S., Wig, N. H., Verma, V. K., & Pershad, L. (1975). A phenomenological analysis of symptoms in obsessive compulsive neurosis. *Br. J. Psychiatry, 127* 342–348.

Aloi, J. A., Insel, T. R., Mueller, E. A., & Murphy, D. L. (1984). Neuroendocrine and behavioral effects of m-chlorophenylpiperazine administration in rhesus monkeys. *Life Sci., 34* 1325–1331.

American Psychiatric Association (1987). *Diagnostic and statistical manual of mental disorders* (3rd ed.—Revised). Washington, DC: American Psychiatric Association.

Ananth, J., Pecknad, J. C., Vandersteen, N., et al. (1981). Double blind comparative study of clomipramine and amitryptyline in obsessive neurosis. *Prog. Neuropsychopharmacol. Bio. Psych., 5*, 257–269.

Ananth, J., Solyom, L., Bryntyick, S. & Krishnappa, Y. (1979). Clorimipramine therapy for obsessive compulsive neurosis. *Am. J. Psychiatry, 136*, 700–701.

Bland, R. C., Orn, H., & Newman, S. C. (1988). Lifetime prevalence of psychiatric disorders in Edmonton. *Actapsychiatr. Scand.*, (suppl. 338) 24–32.

Blier, P., & de Montigny, C. (1985). Short-term lithium administration enhances serotonergic neurotransmission electrophysiological evidence in the rat CNS. *Eur. J. Pharmacol. 113*, 69–79.

Caccia, S., Ballabio, M., & Samanin, R. J. (1981). m-Chlorophenylpiperazine, a central 5-hydroxytryptamine agonist, is a metabolite of trazodone. *Pharm. Pharmacol., 33*, 477–478.

DeVeaugh-Geiss, J. (1988). A multicenter trial of Anafranil in obsessive compulsive disorder. *Proceedings of 141st Annual Meeting*, American Psychiatric Association, Montreal, pp. 259–260.

Eisenberg, J., & Asnis, C. (1985). Lithium as an adjunct treatment in obsessive compulsive disorder (letter). *Am. J. Psychiatry, 142*, 663.

Engelman, K., Lovenberg, W., & Sjoerdsma, A. (1974). Inhibition of serotonin by parachlorophenylalanine in patients with carcinoid syndrome. *N. Engl. J. Med., 277*, 1103–1108.

Fernstrom, S., & Wurtman, R. J. (1974). Nutrition and the brain. *Sci. Am., 230*, 85–96.

Flament, M. F., Rapoport, J. L., Berg, C. J., Sceery, W., Kilts, C., Mellstrom, B., & Linnoila, M. (1985). Clomipramine treatment of childhood obsessive compulsive disorder: A double blind controlled study *Arch. Gen. Psych., 42*, 977–983.

Fontaine, R., & Chouinard, G. (1985). Antiobsessive effect of fluoxetine. *Am. J. Psychiatry, 142*, 989.

Fuller, R. W., Mason, N. R., & Molloy, B. P. (1980). Structural relationships in the inhibition of 3H-serotonin binding to rat membranes in vitro by l-phenylpiperazines. *Biochem. Pharmacol., 29*, 833–835.

Fuller, R. W., Snoddy, H. D., Mason, N. R., & Owen, J. E., (1981). Disposition and pharmacological effects of m-chlorophenylpiperazine in rats. *Neuropharmacology, 20*, 155–162.

Goodmann, W. K., Price, L. H, Rasmussen, S. A., Delgado, P. L., Heninger, G. R., & Charney, D. S. (1989). Efficacy of fluvoxamine in obsessive compulsive disorder: A double-blind comparison with placebo. *Arch. Gen. Psychiatry, 46*, 36–44.

Gorman, J. M., Liebowitz, M. R., Fyer, A. J., Davies, S. O., & Klein, D. F. (1985). Lactate infusions in obsessive compulsive disorder. *Am. J. Psychiatry, 142*, 864–866.

Insel, T. R. (1984). Obsessive-compulsive disorder: The clinical picture. In T. R. Insel (Ed.), *New findings in obsessive-compulsive disorder*. Washington, DC: American Psychiatric Press, Inc.

Insel, T. R., Murphy, D. L., Cohen, R. M., Alterman, I., Kilts, C., & Linnoila, M. (1983). Obsessive-compulsive disorder—A double blind trial of clomipramine and clorgyline. *Arch. Gen. Psychiatry, 40*, 605–612.

Insel, T. R., Mueller, E.A., Alterman, I., Linnoila, M., & Murphy, D. L. (1985). Obsessive-compulsive disorder and serotonin: Is there a connection? *Biol. Psychiatry, 20*, 1174–1185.

Insel, T. R., & Zohar, J. (1987). Psychopharmacologic approaches to obsessive compulsive disorder. In H. Y. Meltzer (Ed.), *Psychopharmacology: The third generation of progress* (pp. 1205–1210). New York: Raven Press.

Invernizzi, R., Cotecchia, S., DeBlasi, A., Mennini, T., Pataccini, R., & Saminin, R. (1981). Effects of m-chlorophenylpiperazine, on receptor binding and brain metabolism of monoamines in rats. *Neurochem. Int., 3*, 239–244.

Jimmerson, D. C., & Berretini, W. (1985). Cerebrospinal fluid metabolite studies in depression: Research update. In H. Beckman & P. Riederer (Eds.), *Pathochemical markers in major psychoses* (pp. 129–143). Berlin: Springer Verlag.

Kahn, R. S., Asnis, G. M., Wetzler, S., & van Praag, H. M. (1988). Neuroendocrine evidence for serotonin receptor hypersensitivity in panic disorder, *Psychopharmacology, 96*, 360–364.

Kahn, R. S., Westenberg, H. G. M., & Jolles, J. (1984). Zimelidine treatment of obsessive compulsive disorder. *Acta Psychiatr. Scand., 69*, 259–261.

Klein, E., Zohar, J., Geraci, M. F., Murphy, D. L., & Uhde, T. W. (submitted for publication). Anxiogenic effects of m-CPP in patients with panic disorder: Comparison to caffeine's anxiogenic effects.

Lingjaerde, O. (1984). Blood platelets as a model system for studying the biochemistry of depression. In E. Usdin, M. Asberg, L. Bertilsson, et al. (Eds.), *Frontiers in biochemical and pharmacological research in depression: Advances in biochemical psychopharmacology*. New York: Raven Press.

Linnoila, M., Virkkunen, M., Scheinin, M., Nuutila, A., Rimon, R., & Goodwin, F. K. (1983). Low cerebrospinal fluid 5-HIAA concentration differentiates impulsive from non-impulsive violent behavior. *Life Sci., 33*, 2609–2614.

Maj, J., & Lewandowska, A. (1980). Central serotoninmimetic action of phenylpiperazine. *Pol. J. Pharmacol. Pharm., 32*, 495–504.

Marks, I. M., Stern, R., Mawson, D., Cobb, J., & McDonald, R. (1980). Clomipramine and exposure for obsessive compulsive rituals. *Br. J. Psychiatry, 136*, 1–25.

Meltzer, H,. Wiita, B., Tricou, B. J., Simonovic, M., Fang, V., & Manov, G. (1982). Effect of serotonin precursors and serotonin agonists on plasma hormone levels. In B. T. Ho, J. C. Schoolar, & E. Usdin (Eds.), *Serotonin in biological psychiatry* (p. 117). New York: Raven Press.

Mennini, T., Poggasi, E., Caccia, S., Bendotti, C., Borsini, F., & Saminin, R., (1980). In U. Z. Littauer, Y. Dudai, & I. Silman (Eds.), *Neurotransmitters and their receptors* (pp. 101–108). New York: Wiley.

Mills, F. G., & Chir, B. (1980). The endocrinology of stress. *Aviat. Space Environ. Med., 56*, 642–650.

Montgomery, S. A. (1980). Clomipramine in obsessional neurosis: A placebo-controlled trial. *Pharmaceut. Med., 1*, 189–192.

Mueller, E. A., Murphy, D. L., & Sunderland, T. (1985). Neuroendocrine effects of m-chlorophenylpiperazine, a serotonin agonist in humans. *J. Clin. Endocrinol. Metab., 61*, 1–6.

Murphy, D. L., Mueller, E. A., Hill, J. L., Tolliver, T., & Jacobson, F. M. (1989). Comparative anxiogenic, neuroendocrine, and other physiologic effects of m-Chlorophenylpiperazine, given intravenously or orally to healthy volunteers. *Psychopharmacology, 98*, 275–282.

Murphy, D. L., Pickar, D., & Alterman, I. (1980). Methods for the quantitative assessment of depressive and manic behavior. In E. I. Burdock, A. Sudilovsky, & S. Guershon (Eds.), *The behavior of psychiatric patients* (pp. 355–391). New York: Marcel Dekker.

Pato, M. T., Zohar-Kadouch, R. C., Zohar, J., & Murphy, D. L. (1988). Return of symptoms after discontinuation of clomipramine in patients with obsessive-compulsive disorder. *Am. J. Psychiatry, 145*, 1521–1525.

Paul, S. N., Rehavi, M., Hulihan, B., Skolnick, P., & Goodwin, F. K. (1980). A rapid and sensitive radioreceptor assay for tertiary amine tricyclic antidepressants. *Commun. Psychopharmacol., 4*, 487–494.

Paul, S. N., Rehavi, N., Rice, K. C., et al. (1981). Does high affinity 3H-imipramine binding label serotonin reuptake sites in brain and platelet? *Life Sci., 28*, 2753–2760.

Perse, T. V., Greist, J. H., Jefferson, J. W., Rosenfeld, R., & Dar R. (1987). Fluvoxamine treatment of obsessive compulsive disorder. *Am. J. Psychiatry, 144*, 1059–1061.

Prasad, A. (1984). Obsessive-compulsive disorder and trazodone (letter to editor), *Am. J. Psychiatry, 141*, 612–613.

Price, L. H., Goodman, W. K., Charney, D. S., Rasmussen, S. A., & Heninger, G. R. (1987). Treatment of severe obsessive compulsive disorder with fluvoxamine. *Am. J. Psychiatry, 144*, 1059–1061.

Rachman, S. J. (1974). Primary obsessional slowness. *Behav. Res. Ther., 11*, 463–471.

Rachman, S. J., & Hodgson, R. J. (1980). *Conventional treatment and prognosis: Obsession and compulsion* (pp. 97–105). Englewood Cliffs, NJ: Prentice-Hall.

Rack, P. H. (1977). Clinical experience in the treatment of obsessional states. *J. Int. Med. Res., 5*, 81–90.

Rasmussen, S. A. (1984). Lithium and tryptophan augmentation in clomipramine-resistant obsessive-compulsive disorder. *Am. J. Psychiatry, 141*, 1283–1285.

Rasmussen, S. A., Goodman, W. K., Woods, S. W., Heninger, G. R., & Charney, D. S. (1987). Effects of yohimbine in obsessive compulsive disorder. *Psychopharmacology*. 93, 308–313.

Rasmussen, S. A., & Tsuang, M. T. (1984). The epidemiology of obsessive-compulsive disorder. *J. Clin. Psychiatry, 45*, 450–457.

Renynghe de Voxrie, G. E. (1968). Anafranil (G 34586) in obsessive neurosis. *Acta Neurolog. Belg., 68*, 787–792.

Rehavi, M., Paul, S. M., & Skolnick, P. (1984). High affinity binding sites for tricyclic antidepressant in brain and platelets. In P. J. Marangos, I. C. Campbell, & R. M. Cohen (Eds.), *Brainreceptor methodologies, Part B*. Orlando, FL: Academic Press.

Robins, L. N., Heltzer, V. E., Weissman, M. M., Orvaschel, H., Gruenberg, E., Burke, J. D., & Regier, D. A. (1984). Lifetime prevalence of psychiatric disorder in three communities. *Arch. Gen. Psychiatry, 41*, 949–967.

Ross, S. B., & Renyi, A. L. (1977). Inhibition of the neuronal uptake of 5-hydroxytryptamine and noradrenaline in rat brain by (Z) and (E)-3-(4-bromophenyl)-N,N-dimethyl-3(3-pyridil) allylamines and their secondary analogues. *Neuropharmacology, 16*, 57–63.

Saavedra, J. & Axelrod, J. (1974). Brain tryptamine and the effect of drugs. *Adv. Biochem. Psychopharmacol., 10*, 135–139.

Saminin, R., Caccia, S., Bendotti, C., Borsini, F., Borroni, E., Invernizzi, R., Pataccini, R., & Mennini, T. (1980). Further studies on the mechanism of the serotonin dependent anorexia in rats. *Psychopharmacology, 68*, 99–104.

Saminin, R., Mennini, T., & Ferraris, A. (1979). m-Chlorophenylpiperazine, a central serotonin agonist causing powerful anorexia in rats. *Naunyn. Schmiedebergs Arch. Pharmacol., 308*, 159–163.

Stern, T. A., & Jenike, M. A. (1983). Treatment of obsessive-compulsive disorder with lithium carbonate. *Psychosomatics, 24*, 674–683.

Stern, R. S., Marks, I. M., Wright, J., & Luscombe, D. K. (1980). Clomipramine: Plasma levels, side effects and outcome in obsessive compulsive neurosis. *Postgrad. Med. J., 56*, 134–139.

Thoren, P., Åsberg, M., Bertilsson, L., Mellstrom, B., Sjoqvist, F., & Traskman, L. (1980a): Clomipramine treatment of obsessive compulsive disorder II. Biochemical aspects. *Arch. Gen. Psychiatry, 37*, 1289–1294.

Thoren, P., Åsberg, M., Cronholm, B., Jornestedt, L., & Traskman, L. (1980). Clomipramine treatment of obsessive-compulsive disorder I. A controlled clinical trial. *Arch. Gen. Psychiatry, 37*, 1281–1285.

Turner, S. M., Jacob, R. G., Beidel, D. C., & Himmelhock, J. (1985). Fluoxetine treatment of obsessive-compulsive disorder. *J. Clin. Psychopharmaco., 5*, 207–212.

van Praag, H. M. (1983). CSF 5-HIAA and suicide in non-depressed schizophrenic. *Lancet, ii,* 977-978.

Vetulani, J., Sansone, M., Bednarczyk, B., & Hano, J. (1982). Different effects of 3-chlorophenylpiperazine on locomotor activity and acquisition of conditioned avoidance response in different strains of mice. *Naunyn. Schmiedebergs Arch. Pharmacol., 319,* 271-274.

Virkkunen, M., Nuutila, A., Goodwin, F., & Linnoila, M. (1987). Cerebrospinal fluid monoamine metabolite levels in male arsonists. *Arch. Gen. Psychiatry, 44,* 241-247.

Volavka, J., Neziroglu, F., & Yaryura-Tobias, J. A. (1985). Clomipramine and imipramine in obsessive-compulsive disorder. *Psychiat. Res., 14,* 83-91.

Weizman, A., Carmi, M., Hermesh, H., et al. (1986). High affinity imipramine binding and serotonin uptake in platelets of eight adolescent and ten adult obsessive-compulsive patients. *Am. J. Psychiatry, 143,* 335-339.

Welner, A., Reich, T., Robins, E., Fishman, R., & van Doren, T. (1976). Obsessive compulsive neurosis. *Com. Psychiatry, 17,* 527-539.

Woodruff, R., & Pitts, F. (1969). Monozygotic twins with obsessional illness. *Am. J. Psychiatry, 120,* 1075-1080.

Yaryura-Tobias, J. A., & Bhagavan, H. N. (1977). L-Tryptophan in obsessive-compulsive disorders. *Am. J. Psychiatry, 234,* 1298-1299.

Yaryura-Tobias, J. A., & Neziroglu, F. (1975). The action of clomipramine in obsessive compulsive neurosis: A pilot study. *Curr. Ther. Res., 17,* 111-116.

Yaryura-Tobias, J. A., Bebirian, R. J., Neziroglu, F., & Bhagavan, H. N. (1977). Obsessive/compulsive disorders as a serotonin defect. *Res. Comm. Psychol. Psychiatry Behav., 2,* 279-286.

Zohar, J., & Insel, T. R. (1987c). Obsessive-compulsive disorder. Psychobiological approaches to diagnosis, treatment, and pathophysiology. *Biol. Psychiatry, 22,* 667-687.

Zohar, J., & Insel, T. R. (1987d). Drug treatment of obsessive-compulsive disorder. *J. Affect. Disorder, 13,* 193-202.

Zohar, J., Insel, T. R., Zohar-Kadouch, R. C., Hill, J. L., & Murphy, D. L. (1988). Serotonergic responsivity in obsessive-compulsive disorder. Effects of chronic clomipramine treatment. *Arch. Gen. Psychiatry, 45,* 167-172.

Zohar, J., Klein, E. M., Mueller, E. A., Insel, T. R., Uhde, T. W., & Murphy, D. L. (1987b). 5HT obsessive compulsive disorder and anxiety. *Proceedings,* American Psychiatric Association, 140th Annual Meeting, Chicago, p. 175.

Zohar, J., Mueller, E. A., Insel, T. R., Zohar-Kadouch, R. C., & Murphy, D. L. (1987a). Serotonergic responsivity in obsessive-compulsive disorder. Comparison of patients and healthy controls. *Arch. Gen. Psychiatry, 44,* 946-951.

8

A Serotonergic Theory
of Schizophrenia*

AVRAHAM BLEICH
SERENA-LYNN BROWN
HERMAN M. VAN PRAAG

This chapter suggests a reexamination of the role of serotonin (5-hydroxy-tryptamine, or 5-HT) in schizophrenia, based upon data from recent psychopharmacological and biological studies of this disorder. We will first review the bases of the dopaminergic and 5-HTergic theories of schizophrenia. We will then discuss central 5-HT measures (postmortem brain studies, cerebrospinal fluid [CSF] metabolite studies, and neuroendocrine challenge measures), peripheral 5-HT measures (platelet and whole-blood 5-HT levels, platelet 5-HT uptake, and platelet ^{3}H-imipramine binding), and treatment studies utilizing 5-HT precursors, 5-HT depleting agents, and 5-HT antagonists. We will review consistencies and inconsistencies in the literature and propose a new way of viewing the possible linkage between abnormal 5-HT function and a subset of schizophrenics, suggesting future directions for research and examination in this area.

THE DOPAMINE HYPOTHESIS OF SCHIZOPHRENIA

Biological research on the pathogenesis of schizophrenia has been dominated by the "dopamine (DA) hypothesis" for more than two decades. The original proponents of this hypothesis suggested that schizophrenia was caused by a primary disturbance of DA transmission or metabolism resulting in an increase in DAergic function (van Praag, 1967; Meltzer & Stahl, 1976; Snyder, 1976). The following data were cited in support of this hypothesis: (1) A number of antipsychotic (neuroleptic) drugs had been

*Adapted with permission from *Schizophrenia Bulletin*, Bleich, A., Brown, S. L., Kahn, R., Van Praag, H. M. (1988). The Role of Serotonin in Schizophrenia. *Schizophrenia Bulletin*, *14*, 297–315.

183

shown to be DA antagonists, with antipsychotic potency directly correlated with DA receptor binding and blockade (Miller et al., 1974; Meltzer & Stahl, 1976). (2) Clinical similarities had been observed and noted between amphetamine psychosis and paranoid schizophrenia. It had further been shown that amphetamines caused the release of presynaptic DA and norepinephrine (NE), and that antipsychotics could attenuate the acute symptoms of amphetamine psychosis (Snyder, 1973; Angrist et al., 1974). (3) More recently, positron emission tomography has shown increased binding of (3-N-(11C)methyl)spiperone to DA D_2 receptors in the caudate nuclei of both antipsychotic-treated and untreated schizophrenics, thus suggesting an increase in DA receptor number in this disease, unrelated to antipsychotic treatment (Wong et al., 1986).

As pharmacological research techniques have become more sophisticated, it has been shown that certain antipsychotics (e.g., chlorpromazine, thioridazine, and clozapine) have a high affinity for 5-HTergic as well as DAergic receptors (Reynolds et al., 1983; Altar et al., 1986). At the same time, it has become increasingly apparent that antipsychotic treatment of schizophrenia is only partially effective. While conventional antipsychotics diminish the psychotic, productive symptoms, negative symptomatology is hardly affected. It is not surprising, then, that in the search for novel treatments for this disorder, questions have been raised about the role of DAergic versus other transmitter mechanisms in the pathogenesis of schizophrenia, and about whether different subsets of schizophrenic symptomatology might be under the influence of different receptor systems.

CROW'S HYPOTHESIS: A DOPAMINERGIC AND A NONDOPAMINERGIC FORM OF SCHIZOPHRENIA?

Early in this decade, Crow (1980a, 1980b) proposed that schizophrenia can be divided into two syndromal dimensions. The type I syndrome is thought to reflect an increase in DAergic function, and to respond well to antipsychotics. This syndrome consists primarily of positive symptoms, with a predominance of hallucinations, delusions, thought disorder, and bizarre behavior. The type II syndrome is thought to be associated with structural abnormalities in the brain (cortical atrophy or ventricular enlargement), chronic course, and a limited response to antipsychotics. This syndrome consists primarily of negative symptoms, such as social and emotional withdrawal, apathy and loss of drive, restricted and blunted affective responsivity, narrowing of ideation, and poverty of speech.

The comprehensiveness of Crow's hypothesis is helpful in conceptualizing an integration of some of the biological and psychological dimensions of this illness, and thus is of significant heuristic value. On the other hand, such a far-ranging theory is vulnerable to many problems, including verification of its various components and the interrelationships among them. For example, the relationship between enlarged ventricles and negative symptoms, proposed by Crow (1980a, 1980b) and by others (Andreasen et al., 1982; Pearlson et al., 1984), does not appear to be as direct as initially hypothesized (Weinberger, 1984; Losconzy et al., 1986a). In fact, Crow et al. (1986) have subsequently proposed, based upon recent postmortem brain studies conducted by their group, that the temporal lobe may be in fact the primary site of structural brain abnormalities in schizophrenics.

Clinically, the concept of negative symptomatology requires clarification. Carpenter et al. (1985) have pointed out that there are at least several lists by different authors purporting to define negative symptoms. They also provide their own definition of primary negative symptoms, or deficit symptoms, which they consider to be core features of the disease, and differentiate these from secondary negative symptoms, which can be the consequence of other psychopathological components of the disease process, such as depression or emotional and social withdrawal resulting from psychotic decompensation. They suggest that negative symptoms could also be associated with antipsychotic-induced side effects (e.g., akinesia and sedation), or prolonged exposure to an understimulating environment (e.g., chronic institutionalization).

Various psychopharmacological interventions might then be targeted at individual and separate components of such a putative negative symptom complex, thus explaining how quite different psychopharmacological agents, sometimes with opposing actions (e.g., antipsychotics, amphetamines, levodopa, propranolol, alprazolam, and monoamine oxidase inhibitors) have been reported to ameliorate negative symptoms (Carpenter et al., 1985; Meltzer et al., 1986; Bucci, 1987).

Even with the problems noted, Crow's two-syndrome hypothesis has important implications for the crucial issue of heterogeneity in schizophrenia. Recently, it has been demonstrated that several newer, more selective and/or potent 5-HT antagonists can be efficacious in the treatment of schizophrenia, especially the negative syndrome (Ceulemans et al., 1985a, 1985b; Gelders et al., 1985a, 1985b). Therefore, particularly in view of the lack of complete efficacy of DA antagonists in this syndrome, Crow's two-syndrome paradigm may provide a valuable new way of reexamining the possible role of 5-HT in schizophrenia.

THE 5-HT HYPOTHESIS OF SCHIZOPHRENIA

5-HTergic theories of schizophrenia originated several decades ago with the observation that the hallucinogenic drug LSD was a peripheral 5-HT antagonist. This led Gaddum (1954) and Woolley and Shaw (1954) to suggest that schizophrenia might be related to a deficiency of 5-HT.

A "transmethylation" theory of schizophrenia, suggesting that normally occurring biogenic amines, including certain indoleamines, might be converted to methylated amines with hallucinogenic properties, thus accounting for some forms of schizophrenia, was then proposed (Kaplan et al., 1974; Gillin et al., 1976a).

However, this theory has been disproved, as no differences have been found in the concentration of these methylated indoleamines in the urine (Carpenter et al., 1975; Gillin et al., 1976a), whole blood and plasma (Axelsson & Nordgren, 1974; Lipinsky et al., 1974) or CSF (Corbett et al., 1978) of schizophrenic patients in comparison with normal controls. In addition, the type of psychosis induced by transmethylated indoleamines and other hallucinogens such as LSD primarily involves perceptual disturbances, and thus represents only one narrow dimension of schizophrenic psychopathology (Szara, 1967; Snyder, 1972), thereby putting the very foundation of the transmethylation theory in question.

Nevertheless, new data have emerged suggesting other pathways for the possible involvement of 5-HT in schizophrenia, justifying the reexamination of its role in this psychiatric disorder.

CENTRAL 5-HT MEASURES

Postmortem Studies

Progress in the direct assessment of possible abnormalities in the 5-HT system has been somewhat limited because the only direct means of assaying central 5-HT function in schizophrenia has been the analysis of levels of 5-HT, its primary metabolite 5-hydroxyindoleacetic acid (5-HIAA), and its precursor tryptophan, all reflecting 5-HT metabolism and, therefore considered to be presynaptic parameters. The measurement of 5-HT (generally 5-HT_2) receptor density in postmortem brain samples of schizophrenics has been the only direct postsynaptic parameter available for investigation.

Few studies of this kind have been completed, and the limited data are difficult to interpret because of differences in type of control group, cause of death, drug-free interval before death, age, food intake, time elapsing between death and autopsy, regions of brain sampled, dissection techniques, and laboratory techniques in the different studies.

Five studies have examined 5-HT or 5-HIAA levels in postmortem brain specimens of chronic schizophrenics compared with normal controls. Crow et al. (1979) have shown increased 5-HT in the putamen of nine chronic schizophrenics (medication histories unknown) as compared with normal controls who died of similar causes. Farely et al. (1980) reported increases in both 5-HT and 5-HIAA in the globus pallidus and nucleus accumbens, and increases in 5-HT alone in the medial olfactory area and the lateral hypothalamus of chronic paranoid schizophrenics, as compared with normal controls. Korpi et al. (1986) found significantly elevated 5-HT concentrations in the basal ganglia and significantly elevated 5-HIAA concentrations in the occipital cortexes of 30 chronic schizophrenics with or without suicide as the cause of death, as compared with normal controls without psychiatric or neurological disorders. No differences in hypothalamic 5-HT concentration were reported between schizophrenics who did or did not commit suicide.

However, Winblad et al. (1979) found the opposite; that is, decreased mean 5-HT levels in hypothalamus, medulla oblongata, and hippocampus of postmortem brain specimens of 12 schizophrenics on antipsychotics at the time of death, half of whom had previously been lobotomized. In addition, Joseph et al. (1979) found no significant difference in 5-HT, 5-HIAA, or tryptophan concentrations in the putamen, hippocampus, or temporal cortex of 15 individuals retrospectively diagnosed as schizophrenics, both on and off antipsychotics, as compared with normal control specimens taken from a general hospital morgue.

Postmortem studies of cortical 5-HT receptor binding in schizophrenic brain specimens have generally utilized one of two radioligands, ^{3}H-LSD or ^{3}H-ketanserin, and results have been variable. Bennett et al. (1979) reported reduced ^{3}H-LSD binding in frontal cortex from 21 schizophrenics, some of whom had been heavily dosed with antipsychotics prior to death. On the other hand, Whitaker et al. (1981) found no differences in ^{3}H-LSD binding in the frontal cortex of 13 chronic schizophrenics compared with normal controls. They also reported that there was a significant increase in cortical ^{3}H-LSD binding for five of these schizophrenics, drug-free for one year before death, compared with the normal controls.

Mita et al. (1986) reported decreased ^{3}H-ketanserine binding sites in the prefrontal cortex of nine schizophrenics, with no differences shown between those on and not on antipsychotics. However, Reynolds et al. (1983) found no significant differences in ^{3}H-ketanserine binding in the frontal cortex of 11 schizophrenics (medication history unknown) as compared with controls.

In conclusion, it appears that postmortem brain studies of schizophrenics, while providing one of the few means of directly assessing 5-HT function in the brain (by examining 5-HT, 5-HIAA, and tryptophan concentrations, as well as 5-HT postsynaptic receptor binding parameters), have unfortunately yielded inconsistent and contradictory results. In all probability this is due to the shortcomings of this method, as discussed above.

TABLE 8-1
Cerebrospinal Fluid (CSF) 5-hydroxyindoleacetic Acid (5-HIAA):
Schizophrenic Patients vs. Controls

Investigators	Number of Schizophrenic Subjects	Condition	CSF 5-HIAA
Ashcroft et al., 1966	7	Unmedicated, baseline*	Low
Bowers et al., 1969	7	Unmedicated, baseline*	Low
Persson & Roos, 1969	40	Medicated, baseline*	NS†
Rimon et al., 1971	22	Unmedicated, baseline*	NS†
Bowers, 1974	17	Unmedicated, postprobenecid	NS†
Post et al., 1975	17	Unmedicated, postprobenecid	NS†
Gattaz et al., 1982	28	Unmedicated, baseline*	Low
Nybäck et al., 1983	26	Unmedicated, baseline*	NS†
Potkin et al., 1983	24	Unmedicated, baseline*	NS†

*Without probenecid. †No significant differences between groups.

CSF Studies

A common strategy for investigating central 5-HT metabolism in humans is measurement of the 5-HT metabolite 5-HIAA in CSF. Investigators have traditionally measured either baseline CSF 5-HIAA directly or after administration of probenecid, which inhibits the transport of 5-HIAA from the central nervous system (CNS), including the CSF, to the periphery. Probenecid-induced 5-HIAA accumulation in the CSF is considered a (crude) indicator of 5-HT metabolism in the CNS, and thus is considered to reflect presynaptic 5-HT parameters.

Data from studies examining CSF 5-HIAA in schizophrenic patients compared with control subjects have been inconsistent. Several studies (Ashcroft et al., 1966; Bowers et al. 1969; Gattaz et al., 1982) have found decreased CSF 5-HIAA levels in schizophrenics. However, the majority of investigators have not been able to demonstrate any differences in CSF 5-HIAA in schizophrenics as compared with controls (Persson & Roos, 1969; Rimon et al., 1971; Bowers, 1974; Post et al., 1975; Nyback et al., 1983; Potkin et al., 1983). Table 8-1 summarizes data on CSF 5-HIAA findings in schizophrenics versus controls.

More recently, researchers in this area have attempted to link CSF 5-HIAA concentration in schizophrenia to specific identifying characteristics. When schizophrenic patients are divided into two subpopulations, those with brain atrophy (increased sulcal width and/or enlarged brain ventricles, also expressed as an increase in ventricle-to-brain ratio, or VBR) and those without brain atrophy, a new trend emerges.

Three groups of investigators (Nyback et al., 1983; Potkin et al., 1983; Losonczy et al., 1986b) have reported data showing decreased CSF 5-HIAA in schizophrenics with brain atrophy as compared both with schizophrenics without brain atrophy and with normal controls. The total number of patients involved in these studies was 67; patients were drug-free at the time of the studies and both baseline (Nyback et al., 1983; Potkin et al., 1983) and post-probenecid CSF 5-HIAA levels (Losonczy et al., 1986b) were measured.

It should be noted, however, that the DA metabolite homovanillic acid (HVA) has also been shown to be decreased in the same population of schizophrenic patients, those with enlarged ventricles. Interestingly, CSF 5-HIAA correlates significantly with CSF HVA, and both correlate negatively with VBR. One possible explanation for such a correlation between these metabolites could be that they have similar transport mechanisms from the CSF (Van Kammen et al., 1986).

Another subdivision within the group of schizophrenic patients involves those who have attempted suicide versus those who have never attempted suicide. Van Praag (1983), Ninan et al. (1984), and Banki et al. (1984) have all shown a correlation between low CSF 5-HIAA and suicidal behavior, especially recent suicide attempts, in schizophrenics. However, Roy et al. (1985) were unable to replicate this finding. Interestingly, Levy et al. (1984) found that an increased VBR in chronic schizophrenics is significantly associated with a history of suicide attempts. Therefore, suicidality might be another possible factor linking decreased central 5-HT metabolism and type II schizophrenia.

Van Kammen et al. (1986) recently presented data from seven studies including more than 100 schizophrenic patients suggesting that CSF 5-HIAA concentration is not altered during antipsychotic treatment. This is somewhat surprising in view of the fact that antipsychotics might affect the 5-HTergic system both presynaptically and postsynaptically by inhibiting 5-HT uptake (Arora & Meltzer, 1983) and by blocking 5-HT receptors (Reynolds et al., 1983; Altar et al., 1986).

Finally, a few additional studies have shown an association between increased CSF 5-HIAA and a family history of schizophrenia (Sedvall & Wode-Helgodt, 1980) and the schizophrenic symptom of "mannerisms and posturing" (King et al., 1985) within the schizophrenic population. The meaning of these data is unclear as yet. Table 8-2 summarizes data on CSF 5-HIAA differences between schizophrenic subgroups.

In conclusion, it appears that:

1. Cortical atrophy or ventricular enlargement is significantly associated with decreased CSF 5-HIAA levels in schizophrenic patients. These data are consistent across all three studies completed at this time.

TABLE 8-2
Cerebrospinal Fluid (CSF) 5-hydroxyindoleacetic Acid (5-HIAA) in Schizophrenia: Subgroup Differences

Investigators	Number of Schizophrenic Subjects	Condition	CSF 5-HIAA
Sedvall & Wode-Helgodt, 1980	36	Unmedicated, baseline*	High in schizophrenic patients with family history of schizophrenia
Nybäck et al., 1983	26	Unmedicated, baseline*	Low in schizophrenic patients with cortical atrophy or ventricular enlargement
Potkin et al., 1983	24	Unmedicated, baseline*	Low in schizophrenic patients with cortical atrophy or ventricular enlargement
Van Praag, 1983	20	Unmedicated, postprobenecid	Low in schizophrenic patients with history of suicide attempts
Ninan et al., 1984	16	Unmedicated, baseline*	Low in schizophrenic patients with history of suicide attempts
Banki et al., 1984	15	Unmedicated, baseline*	Low in schizophrenic patients with history of suicide attempts
Roy et al., 1985	54	Unmedicated, baseline*	No significant difference between suicidal and nonsuicidal schizophrenic patients
King et al., 1985	21	Unmedicated, baseline*	High in schizophrenic patients with abnormal motor behavior
Losonczy et al., 1986	28	Unmedicated, postprobenecid	Low in schizophrenic patients with cortical atrophy or ventricular enlargement

*Without probenecid.

2. The association between decreased CSF 5-HIAA and suicidal behavior, already demonstrated in depression (van Praag, 1986), has also been found in schizophrenia.

3. Antipsychotic treatment does not appear to affect CSF 5-HIAA levels.

CHALLENGE STUDIES

The neuroendocrine challenge paradigm is a recently developed strategy for studying the functional state of central monoaminergic (MAergic) systems. Release of hormones known to be under MAergic (in this case, 5-HTergic) control, such as cortisol, prolactin, and growth hormone, is measured in peripheral blood after stimulation or inhibition of 5-HT receptors with either 5-HT agonists or antagonists. The magnitude of the hormonal response is thought to be a measure of the responsiveness of the 5-HT system. In a hypersensitive system, 5-HT agonists will induce an augmented release of such hormones, whereas in a hypoactive system, the reverse is expected to occur. If 5-HT antagonists are employed, the opposite results are anticipated (Murphy et al., 1986).

So far, only two 5-HT challenge studies, investigating prolactin and growth hormone (GH) response in schizophrenic patients during antipsychotic treatment, have been reported in the literature. Cowen et al. (1985) found higher prolactin peaks and diminished GH response in schizophrenics as compared with normal controls after administration of 6–10 g of intravenous tryptophan. Hoshino et al. (1985) administered a single oral dose of 3 mg/kg of 5-hydroxytryptophan (5-HTP), the immediate precursor of 5-HT, and found increased blood 5-HT and inconsistent results for prolactin and GH levels both at baseline and post–5-HTP in schizophrenics.

The variable and inconsistent results of these studies probably are attributable to the effect of the antipsychotic treatment and the very small number of patients studied. It should be also noted that neither tryptophan nor 5-HTP stimulates the 5-HT receptor directly; rather, both compounds cause indirect stimulation by increasing 5-HT synthesis and availability. In addition, both of these 5-HT precursors also have major effects on the DAergic and NAergic systems (to be discussed below).

The challenge paradigm appears to be a valid and important means for studying central neurotransmitter function, provided the 5-HT challenger is selective. Since such selective agents are now being developed, van Praag et al. (1987a, 1987b) have suggested that this paradigm should be more extensively employed in the study of the 5-HTergic system, examining medication-free patients and using selective 5-HT agents.

PLATELET STUDIES

Over the past decade, the human blood platelet, which is a neuroectodermal derivative, has emerged as a peripheral model for the study of the transport, storage, metabolism, and release of 5-HT by 5-HTergic nerve endings (Sneddon, 1973; Stahl, 1977). Because of biochemical and morphological similarities between blood platelets and CNS 5-HT synapses, and because of data suggesting that virtually all 5-HT in blood is associated with the platelets (Yuwiler et al., 1981), it has become an acceptable practice to utilize platelets as a minimally invasive means of studying 5-HT in the CNS.

Platelet and While-Blood 5-HT Levels

Eight groups of investigators, having studied approximately 250 chronic schizophrenic patients, all reported elevated platelet or whole-blood 5-HT levels (i.e., hyperserotonemia) in schizophrenics as compared with normal controls (Todrick et al., 1960; Torre et al., 1970; Garelis et al., 1975; DeLisi et al., 1981; Freedman et al., 1981; Jackman et al., 1983; Stahl et al., 1983; King et al., 1985; Muck-Seler et al., 1988). These increased platelet 5-HT levels were not found to be an artifact of age, sex, or medication, as no in vivo effect of antipsychotics on platelet 5-HT level was shown (DeLisi et al., 1981; Jackman et al., 1983; Stahl et al., 1983; Muck-Seler et al., 1988).

However, several other researchers have failed to replicate such findings (Feldstein et al., 1959; Joseph et al., 1977; Kolakowska & Molyneux, 1987).

DeLisi et al. (1981) found that high 5-HT levels in blood were significantly correlated with specific computed tomographic (CT) abnormalities (enlargement of cerebral ventricles, cortical atrophy, or both) in chronic schizophrenics. However, Jackman et al. (1983) were not able to replicate this finding. In other studies, a significant correlation has been shown between increased whole-blood and platelet 5-HT levels and the diagnoses of chronic undifferentiated or paranoid schizophrenia (Freedman et al., 1981), auditory hallucinations (Jackman et al., 1983), and abnormal motor behavior in chronic schizophrenics (King et al., 1985). Table 8-3 summarizes data on platelet and whole-blood 5-HT in schizophrenics versus controls.

Platelet 5-HT concentration is determined by several factors, including synthesis, uptake, storage, catabolism, and release of 5-HT. Platelets do not synthesize 5-HT; rather, it is synthesized by enterochromaffin cells in the intestine and is then taken up by platelets through active and passive processes (Sneddon, 1973). The elevated platelet 5-HT concentrations found in

TABLE 8-3

Platelet or Whole-Blood Serotonin: Schizophrenic Patients vs. Controls

Investigators	Number of Schizophrenic Subjects	Medicated	Platelet or Whole-Blood Serotonin Concentrations
Feldstein et al., 1959	22	+	NS*
Todrick et al., 1960	35	+	High
Garelis et al., 1975	16	+ and −	High only in unmedicated schizophrenic patients
Joseph et al., 1977	16	−	NS*
DeLisi et al., 1981	33	+ and −	High in schizophrenic patients with cortical atrophy or ventricular enlargement
Freedman et al., 1981	33	+	High in schizophrenic patients, particularly with chronic undifferentiated subtype
Jackman et al., 1983	41	+ and −	High in schizophrenic patients, particularly correlated with auditory hallucinations
Stahl et al., 1983	14	+ and −	High in schizophrenic patients
King et al., 1985	25	−	High in schizophrenic patients, particularly correlated with cerebrospinal fluid 5-hydroxindoleacetic acid and abnormal motor behavior
Kolakowska & Molyneux, 1987	62	+	NS*
Muck-Seler et al., 1988	55	+ and −	High in schizophrenic patients, particularly with a chronic course

*No significant differences between groups.

chronic schizophrenics cannot be explained by an abnormality in platelet 5-HT uptake, storage, or release (Jackman et al., 1983; Stahl et al., 1983).

Alternatively, the increased 5-HT content of platelets could be the consequence of decreased activity of platelet monoamine oxidase (MAO), the enzyme that deaminates 5-HT into 5-HIAA. Although lowered MAO activity has been reported in chronic schizophrenics (Potkin et al., 1978; Stahl et al., 1983), other investigators have not found this (Meltzer et al., 1982). Moreover, platelet MAO activity does not correlate with platelet 5-HT concentration in chronic schizophrenics (Joseph et al., 1977; Freedman et al., 1981). Finally, increased platelet 5-HT content could be a result of increased plasma availability of the 5-HT precursor tryptophan. This hypothesis appears unlikely, however, since tryptophan levels in fact have been shown to be lowered in the plasma of schizophrenic patients (Manowitz et al., 1973; Domino & Krause, 1974; Freedman et al., 1981).

In conclusion, there is reasonable agreement among investigators that chronic schizophrenics have elevated platelet and whole-blood 5-HT levels. Neither the cause nor the clinical significance of this finding is known at this time, nor is the relationship between 5-HT in platelets and 5-HT in synapses completely understood.

Platelet 5-HT Uptake

The human blood platelet possesses a high-affinity active transport system that is temperature dependent and is inhibited by ouabain (Sneddon, 1969). The kinetic parameters of this transport system are V_{max}, indicating the number of carrier molecules, and K_m, a measure of the affinity of the carrier molecules for 5-HT. This system has been studied in schizophrenics in order to determine whether active transport of 5-HT into the platelet is associated with the increased platelet 5-HT concentration that some investigators have shown in schizophrenia.

A number of studies conducted by Rotman's group (Modai et al., 1979; Rotman et al., 1979, 1980, 1982a, 1982b) have shown that platelet 5-HT uptake in schizophrenic patients is significantly reduced (in a manner related to a decrease in V_{max}) in comparison with normal controls. While some of the patients in these studies were taking antipsychotic medications, these investigators claim to have found no effect of antipsychotics on 5-HT uptake in in vitro studies of platelets of normal controls (Modai et al., 1979; Rotman et al., 1979). Decreased platelet 5-HT uptake in schizophrenics has been reported by other investigators in studies of antipsychotic-treated patients (Wood et al., 1983), drug-free patients (Kaplan & Mann, 1982), and both drug-free and antipsychotic-treated schizophrenics (Lingjaerde, 1983). In contrast, these findings could not be confirmed by other investigators (Meltzer et al., 1981; Arora & Meltzer, 1982, 1983; Jackman et al., 1983;

Stahl et al., 1983; Muck-Seler et al., 1988), who reported no significant differences in platelet 5-HT uptake or kinetic parameters (V_{max} and K_m) between (primarily) drug-free schizophrenic patients and normal controls.

Arora and Meltzer (1983) have investigated the effect of chlorpromazine on platelet 5-HT uptake in schizophrenic patients and normals. 5-HT uptake was studied before and after two to three weeks of treatment with chlorpromazine (200–600 mg/day). Administration of chlorpromazine was associated with a significant decrease in platelet uptake of 5-HT in most subjects in both groups. Decreased platelet 5-HT uptake in chronic schizophrenics on antipsychotics was also reported by Lingjaerde (1983) and by Stahl et al. (1983). However, Muck-Seler et al. (1988) found no effect of antipsychotics on platelet 5-HT uptake in chronic schizophrenic patients. Table 8-4 summarizes data on platelet 5-HT uptake studies.

In conclusion, it appears that:

1. Studies of 5-HT platelet uptake (considered to be a presynaptic parameter) in schizophrenic patients are inconsistent. Discrepancies between the investigated populations (e.g., in terms of chronicity, drug treatment, etc.), as well as variance of assay techniques, make it difficult to draw any conclusions from these data.

2. Antipsychotic medications probably decrease platelet 5-HT uptake in schizophrenic patients.

[3]H-Imipramine Binding Sites

Recently, high-affinity and saturable binding sites for ^{3}H-imipramine have been found on human platelets. These sites appear to be specific for tricyclic antidepressants and their active metabolites (Langer et al., 1981), and seem to have a functional relationship to the 5-HT uptake or transport site, probably modulating inhibition of 5-HT uptake (Paul et al., 1980).

While Rotman et al. (1982b) reported decreased ^{3}H-imipramine binding and 5-HT uptake in platelets of schizophrenic patients, Wood et al. (1983), Gentsch et al. (1985), Weizman et al. (1987), and Kanof et al. (1987) could not find any significant difference in ^{3}H-imipramine binding between schizophrenics and normal controls. Thus, it seems likely that the ^{3}H-imipramine binding site is intact in schizophrenia.

TREATMENT STUDIES

If 5-HT plays a role in the pathogenesis of schizophrenia, clinical treatments using selective 5-HT agonists or antagonists should affect schizophrenic symptomatology and might shed some light on the nature of this relationship.

TABLE 8-4
Platelet Serotonin Uptake: Schizophrenic Patients vs. Controls

Investigators	Number of Schizophrenic Subjects	Medicated	Platelet Serotonin Uptake
Modai et al., 1979	10	+ and –	Decreased in schizophrenic patients by 40%, V_{max} decreased
Rotman et al., 1979	22	+ and –	Decreased uptake and V_{max} in schizophrenic patients
Meltzer et al., 1981	17	–	NS*
Rotman et al., 1982a	22	+ and –	Decreased uptake and V_{max} in schizophrenic patients
Rotman et al., 1982b	12	+	Decreased in schizophrenic patients; positive correlation with ^{3}H-imipramine binding
Arora & Meltzer, 1982	43	–	NS*, with a trend toward decrease in schizophrenic patients
Kaplan & Mann, 1982	14	–	Decreased in schizophrenic patients, increased K_m
Arora & Meltzer, 1983	19	+ and –	NS* with increased K_m and V_{max}, and decreased uptake after medication
Lingjaerde, 1983	42	+ and –	Decreased in schizophrenic patients, decreased V_{max} while drug-free, and increased K_m with further decrease in uptake after medication
Wood et al., 1983	14	+	Decreased in schizophrenic patients; no correlation with ^{3}H-imipramine binding
Stahl et al., 1983	14	+ and –	NS*, 5-HT uptake decreased after medication
Jackman et al., 1983	41	+ and –	NS*, 5-HT uptake decreased after medication
Muck-Seler et al., 1988	55	+ and –	NS*

*No significant differences between groups.

5-HT Precursors

L-Tryptophan

The amino acid L-tryptophan is the normal dietary precursor of 5-HT, and its oral administration affects 5-HT synthesis in and release from 5-HT neurons. L-tryptophan can influence the synthesis of other neurotransmitters as it competes with other neutral amino acids to gain access from the blood into the brain. One of these amino acids is tyrosine, the precursor of DA and NA. Therefore, when high doses of tryptophan are administered, 5-HT levels in the brain increase, but it also should be noted that DA and NA levels decrease (Wurtman et al., 1981; van Praag et al., 1987b).

Bowers (1970) reported tranquilizing effects when he administered tryptophan (up to 4 g/day, for eight to 12 days), combined with pyridoxin (a decarboxylase cofactor), to six schizophrenic patients. In a placebo-controlled study, Gillin et al. (1976b) found tryptophan (up to 20 g/day, for 11–28 days), combined with pyridoxin, to be ineffective in the treatment of eight chronic schizophrenic patients. Chouinard et al. (1978) compared up to 6 g/day of tryptophan combined with benserazide (which inhibits tryptophan pyrrolase as well as 5-HT decarboxylase) with chlorpromazine in the treatment of 16 chronic schizophrenic patients. They found tryptophan to have a slight therapeutic effect, markedly inferior to that of chlorpromazine. Morand et al. (1983), focusing on aggressive behavior among chronic schizophrenics, reported that up to 5 g/day of tryptophan administration improved some aggressive variables, although the overall effect varied among individual patients.

5-Hydroxytryptophan (5-HTP)

5-HTP is the immediate precursor of 5-HT. As the enzyme 5-HTP–decarboxylase is found not only in 5-HT neurons, but in catecholamine (CA) neurons as well, the oral administration of 5-HTP leads to the formation of 5-HT not only in 5-HTergic neurons, but also in CA neurons, where it acts as a false transmitter, increasing CA metabolism as a compensatory mechanism. The net effect is probably an increase in CA function (van Praag et al., 1987a). Thus, by virtue of its CAergic effects, 5-HTP must be categorized as a nonselective 5-HT-active compound. The same is true for tryptophan in high doses.

In a placebo-controlled study, 10 g/day of 5-HTP in combination with carbidopa, a peripheral decarboxylase inhibitor, produced some clinical improvement in seven out of 11 chronic schizophrenics (Wyatt et al., 1972). In another placebo-controlled study, Bigelow et al. (1979) administered up to 6 g/day of 5-HTP with carbidopa to 15 patients who had been withdrawn from antipsychotic medication, seven patients who were maintained on haloperidol, and nine patients who were maintained on chlorpromazine. Individual responses were highly variable but the overall results suggested that 5-HTP treatment in chronic schizophrenics is not effective.

5-HT–Depleting Agents

Parachlorophenylalanine (pCPA)

pCPA is an inhibitor of tryptophan hydroxylase, the enzyme involved in the first and rate-limiting step of 5-HT synthesis. pCPA is known to cause a substantial decrease in brain 5-HT concentration in animals (Koe & Weissman, 1966) and to decrease CSF and urine 5-HIAA concentrations in humans (Cremata & Koe, 1966; Goodwin & Post, 1973). In a brief open trial of pCPA up to 1.25 g/day, Casacchia et al. (1975) found clinical improvement in three out of four acutely psychotic schizophrenic patients. In a placebo-controlled study, DeLisi et al. (1982) administered up to 3 g/day of pCPA to seven chronic schizophrenics, who demonstrated no overall improvement. The discrepancy between these two studies may be attributable to the difference in the patient populations examined (acutely psychotic versus chronic, treatment-resistant patients). Interestingly, both studies reported a decrease in withdrawal behavior (DeLisi et al., 1982) or an increase in socialization (Casacchia et al., 1975) among these patients after treatment.

Fenfluramine

Fenfluramine, an anorectic agent, promotes release of 5-HT and inhibits 5-HT uptake, and may have direct, weak 5-HT receptor agonist activity, as well (Murphy et al., 1986). Although these effects are 5-HT agonistic, fenfluramine's net effect is considered a 5-HT–depleting one: in animals, fenfluramine has been shown to induce a decrease in brain 5-HT (Clineschmidt et al., 1978), while in humans, CSF 5-HIAA was shown to be reduced following eight days of fenfluramine administration (Shoulson & Chase, 1975).

Two placebo-controlled studies using fenfluramine have been conducted. Shore et al. (1985) treated eight chronic schizophrenics with fenfluramine at doses of up to 120 mg/kg for eight weeks, and found no significant benefit, though a 50% decrease of blood 5-HT was demonstrated. Stahl et al. (1985) treated 12 chronic schizophrenics with fenfluramine at doses of up to 240 mg/day for 12 weeks, and found that negative symptoms improved in some individuals within the active treatment group but not within the placebo group. However, group comparisons of active treatment versus placebo were not significant, possibly because of the small sample size.

5-HT Receptor Antagonists

5-HT receptors differ according to their central or peripheral location, their occurrence on neurons or other cells (e.g., platelets or muscles), and their location on either presynaptic or postsynaptic 5-HT nerve terminals. In brain, 5-HT receptors have been classified into three main subtypes by radioligand binding: $5\text{-}HT_1$, $5\text{-}HT_2$, and $5\text{-}HT_3$ (Leysen et al., 1978; Peroutka et al., 1981). $5\text{-}HT_1$ receptors have been further subclassified into various subtypes ($5\text{-}HT_{1A}$, $5\text{-}HT_{1B}$, $5\text{-}HT_{1C}$, $5\text{-}HT_{1D}$, although our understanding of the functional importance of the various 5-HT receptors and subtypes is far from complete.

Methysergide

Methysergide is a 5-HT receptor antagonist with primarily $5\text{-}HT_1$ activity (Sills et al., 1984). Gallant et al. (1963) randomly administered methysergide (up to 16 mg/day), chlorpromazine (up to 800 mg/day), or placebo to a group of 40 chronic schizophrenics, and found that methysergide had no antipsychotic effects. Mendels (1967) used oral methysergide (15 mg/day) in 14 chronic schizophrenics, switching after 10 days to 5 mg/day intravenous methysergide in 12 patients, and changing again after eight more days to 2 mg/day intrathecal methysergide in six patients. No antipsychotic effect was found, and five patients (three of whom received the drug intravenously and two of whom received it intrathecally) showed temporary aggravation of psychosis.

Setoperone and Ritanserin

Setoperone is both a potent $5\text{-}HT_2$ and DA receptor antagonist (Ceulemans et al., 1985a), and ritanserin is a very selective $5\text{-}HT_2$ antagonist (Leysen et al., 1985). Ceulemans et al. (1985a) administered oral setoperone (15 mg/day) to 34 chronic schizophrenic patients with predominant negative symptomatology, who had been drug-free for one week, and compared its effect with that of previous antipsychotic treatment. After one month of treatment with setoperone, psychotic symptoms, as measured by the Brief Psychiatric Rating Scale (BPRS) (Overall & Gorham, 1962), improved by approximately 50%. Setoperone was specifically effective in diminishing negative symptoms, significantly decreasing emotional withdrawal, and improving blunted affect, and was also found to cause a marked euthymic effect, as shown by corresponding changes in BPRS ratings. It was also found to cause fewer extrapyramidal symptoms than antipsychotics combined with antiparkinsonian medication.

Studies with ritanserin (Ceulemans et al., 1985b; Gelders et al., 1985a, 1985b) show similar results. Ritanserin (20 mg/day) was administered to chronic, primarily type II schizophrenic patients, in three studies: (1) a comparison of ritanserin with placebo, both added to existing antipsychotic treatment, for six weeks in 35 patients (Gelders et al., 1985a); (2) a double-blind comparison of ritanserin and haloperidol, 10 mg/day, in 37 patients for a period of 60 days (Ceulemans et al., 1985b); and (3) a placebo-controlled design in which ritanserin, 20 mg/day, was compared with haloperidol, 10 mg/day, for six weeks in 57 patients (Gelders et al., 1985b). Overall results showed the efficacy of ritanserin in alleviating psychotic symptoms, as expressed by a significant decrease in total BPRS ratings and by ongoing clinical assessment. In the first study, when ritanserin was added to an antipsychotic, the total BPRS score decreased approximately 50%, while the BPRS negative symptom cluster decreased more than 60%. Placebo decreased BPRS (total and negative symptoms) by about 10% only.

In the second and third studies, where ritanserin was compared with haloperidol, both medications improved the total BPRS, while ritanserin alone improved the negative symptom cluster and haloperidol was superior in improving thought disorder. Moreover, ritanserin-treated patients showed significant improvement in extrapyramidal symptoms. The clearly superior efficacy of ritanserin in improving scores on the negative symptom cluster of the BPRS as compared with placebo suggests that the antipsychotic withdrawal effect was not significantly reflected in these results, since otherwise one would expect to see it demonstrated clearly in the placebo studies.

In conclusion, it appears that:

1. Treatment studies with 5-HT precursors give variable and inconsistent results, possibly because tryptophan and 5-HTP have pronounced effects on the DA and NA systems as well as on the 5-HT system.

2. 5-HT–depleting agents (pCPA and fenfluramine) do not appear to produce an overall clinical improvement in schizophrenics, although some may show some improvement in the cluster of negative symptoms.

3. Treatment studies with 5-HT2 antagonists suggest that these drugs may have antipsychotic activity, may significantly improve negative symptomatology, and may also be helpful to those patients who experience extrapyramidal side effects from antipsychotics.

DISCUSSION

At first glance, data on 5-HT in schizophrenia seem to be inconsistent, and even contradictory. Results of eight studies investigating approximately 200 chronic schizophrenic patients have demonstrated increased whole-blood or platelet 5-HT levels in this disorder. However, data on 5-HT uptake and ³H-imipramine binding in schizophrenia are inconsistent at this time. Direct evaluations of 5-HT, 5-HIAA, and tryptophan concentrations, as well as 5-HT receptor density in postmortem studies of brain specimens from schizophrenics, have produced contradictory and uninterpretable findings, probably owing to a number of technical problems and inconsistencies in experimental technique. Also, there appear to be no overall consistent differences in CSF 5-HIAA levels in schizophrenics as compared with controls, although decreased CSF 5-HIAA levels may well correlate significantly with specific characteristics, such as structural brain changes, within the schizophrenic population. Treatment studies with 5-HT precursors have not consistently demonstrated therapeutic effects. However, agents that are thought to decrease 5-HT function have shown antipsychotic effects, particularly when potent 5-HT$_2$ antagonists were employed. Such inconsistencies in clinical and biological research results may reflect the heterogeneity inherent in this disorder, as proposed by several authors (Bellak & Strauss, 1979; Buchsbaum & Rieder, 1979).

Integration of Data: The 5-HT Hypothesis

The two-syndrome paradigm proposed by Crow (1980a, 1980b) at the beginning of this decade seemed to offer the hope of substantial progress in the delineation of more homogenous subtypes of schizophrenia. Utilizing Crow's paradigm, a reexamination of clinical and biological 5-HT studies involving both CSF and blood measurements and treatment response to 5-HT–influencing agents reveals a fair consistency of findings within a subpopulation of schizophrenics. That is, chronic schizophrenic patients with a predominant type II syndrome seem to show 5-HT abnormalities or to have a positive response to 5-HT–influencing agents, thus suggesting the possible role of 5-HT dysfunction in type II schizophrenia.

A recent study by Lewine and Meltzer (1984) reporting elevated platelet MAO activity in male schizophrenics with predominant negative symptomatology may relate to multiple findings of increased whole-blood or platelet 5-HT levels in chronic schizophrenic patients (Todrick et al., 1960; Torre et al., 1970; Garelis et al., 1975; DeLisi et al., 1981; Freedman et al., 1981; Jackman et al., 1983; Stahl et al., 1983; King et al., 1985). The elevated platelet MAO activity in these patients might reflect a compensation for the elevation of the 5-HT concentration in the platelet.

The positive correlation between elevated blood 5-HT levels and degenerative brain changes (cortical atrophy or ventricular enlargement) found by DeLisi et al (1981) also suggests a possible link between elevated blood 5-HT and type II schizophrenia. It should be noted, however, that neither the clinical significance of elevated blood 5-HT nor its relationship to brain 5-HT is clear at this stage.

Several studies have also demonstrated that cortical atrophy, ventricular enlargement or increased VBR are significantly associated with decreased CSF 5-HIAA levels in schizophrenic patients (Nyback et al., 1983; Potkin et al., 1983; Losonczy et al., 1986a&b). These findings indicate a relationship between type II schizophrenia and decreased central 5-HT metabolism as reflected in lowered CSF 5-HIAA.

The apparent contradiction between increased blood 5-HT and decreased CSF 5-HIAA levels in the same subpopulation of schizophrenics (those with degenerative brain changes) might be explained, by the hypothesis of Freedman et al. (1981), as a consequence of increased uptake and utilization of tryptophan in the periphery, part of which may enter the 5-HT pathway. A possible net result would be decreased plasma tryptophan and diminished availability of tryptophan in the brain, and hence decreased central 5-HT and CSF 5-HIAA.

Another possible linkage between decreased central 5-HT metabolism and brain CT scan abnormalities in schizophrenia involves suicidality. Several studies (van Praag, 1983; Banki et al., 1984; Ninan et al., 1984) have found a correlation between decreased CSF 5-HIAA and suicide attempts among schizophrenics. Furthermore, Levy et al. (1984) demonstrated that a history of suicide attempts is also correlated with increased VBR among schizophrenics, suggesting a trivariate relationship among 5-HT function, suicidality, and type II schizophrenia that should be further studied.

Treatment studies using agents presumed to decrease 5-HT function further suggest the possible role of 5-HT dysfunction in type II schizophrenia. 5-HT–depleting agents such as pCPA (Casacchia et al., 1975; DeLisi et al., 1982) and fenfluramine (Stahl et al., 1985) appear to alleviate negative symptomatology in schizophrenic patients. Interestingly, fenfluramine has also been shown to improve certain symptoms of childhood autism (withdrawn behavior, inappropriate affect, and poor eye contact), which share some similarities with the negative symptoms of schizophrenia (Geller et al., 1982). Moreover, childhood autism has been reported to be associated with other features that may also occur in the type II syndrome, such as elevated blood 5-HT (Hanley et al., 1977) and ventricular enlargement (Hauser et al., 1975).

Finally, and most important, potent and/or selective 5-HT$_2$ antagonists, notably setoperone (Ceulemans et al., 1985a) and ritanserin (Ceulemans et al., 1985b; Gelders et al., 1985a, 1985b), have recently been reported to have a pronounced antipsychotic effect and to be especially effective in alleviating negative symptomatology and dysphoria in chronic schizophrenics with a predominant type II syndrome. These findings await corroboration.

These data all suggest a relationship between 5-HT dysfunction and type II schizophrenia. The reported effect of selective 5-HT$_2$ antagonists on the negative syndrome, as well as the decreased CSF 5-HIAA shown in type II schizophrenics, might suggest that the nature of this dysfunction involves 5-HT$_2$ postsynaptic receptor hypersensitivity. 5-HTergic postsynaptic receptor hypersensitivity would be expected to lead to a compensatory decrease of central 5-HT metabolism (lowered CSF 5-HIAA), as has indeed been shown in type II schizophrenia.

One possible mechanism for the mediation of receptor hypersensitivity may be a reduced level of available neurotransmitter (Charney et al., 1981). According to the hypothesis of Freedman et al. (1981), a subgroup of schizophrenics with elevated whole-blood 5-HT levels might have as a result a lowered level of 5-HT in the brain, through the mechanisms discussed above. This decreased brain 5-HT concentration might, in turn, mediate 5-HT receptor hypersensitivity.

The hypersensitivity hypothesis can be tested directly utilizing neuroendocrine challenge tests employing selective 5-HT agonists such as m-chlorophenylpiperazine (mCPP), which is a direct activator of the 5-HT (primarily 5-HT$_1$) receptor (Murphy et al., 1986), and antagonists such as ritanserin, a selective 5-HT$_2$ receptor blocker (Leysen et al., 1985), that have become available recently. The outcome of these tests should be correlated with (1) other central (CSF 5-HIAA) and peripheral (blood) 5-HT measures, (2) measures of (negative) symptomatology, and (3) CT scan results.

On the basis of the hypersensitivity hypothesis, one would expect 5-HT antagonists to be particularly effective in type II schizophrenia. Preliminary treatment studies are promising and should be replicated and expanded, and treatment response should be correlated with the aforementioned parameters.

5-HT/DA Modulation Effects

Chesire et al. (1982) have found that methysergide diminished akinesia induced by the section of nigrostriatal circuits in rats. Ceulemans et al. (1985a, 1985b) and Gelders et al. (1985a, 1985b) have reported that the administration of setoperone and ritanserin to schizophrenic patients caused fewer extrapyramidal symptoms than antipsychotics combined with antiparkinsonian medication. The fact that both drugs lack anticholinergic activity might support the hypothesis that 5-HT receptors have a modulating effect on the nigrostriatal DA system, which may provide the mechanism by which 5-HT–selective antagonists alleviate extrapyramidal symptoms.

The possibility of such a modulating effect is supported by the complex anatomical and functional interactions known to exist between DAergic and 5-HTergic neuronal systems in the forebrain. These interactions occur at axo-axonal synaptic connections between 5-HT–containing neurons originating from the medial and dorsal raphe nuclei and nigrostriatal as well as mesolimbic DA circuits (Waldmeier & Delina-Stula, 1979; Jenner et al., 1983).

Jenner et al. (1983) have reviewed literature on possible 5-HT/DA interactions involving 5-HT fibers that originate from the dorsal and medial raphe nuclei and that innervate DA-containing areas of the brain, such as the substantia nigra, corpus striatum, and nucleus accumbens. They indicate that manipulation of 5-HT system activity influences DA function, particularly as shown in data from electrophysiological recording studies and by certain behavioral models that are believed to express DA function (e.g., apomorphine- or amphetamine-induced circling behavior and stereotypy). From available data, it appears that 5-HT possesses an inhibitory modulating role on cerebral DA mechanisms and function, and that this effect is probably dependent on the relative state of activity of each system (Jenner et al., 1983). Recently, specific modes of 5-HTergic modulation of DA function have been identified. In the brains of rats, tyrosine hydroxylase, as well as DA release, has been found to be inhibited by 5-HT in a concentration-dependent manner in both striatal and nucleus acumbens synaptosomes (Ennis et al., 1981; Hetey et al., 1985; Hetey and Drescher 1986). These inhibitory effects of 5-HT are assumed to be mediated via 5-HT receptors at the DA terminals (5-HT heteroreceptors), because various 5-HT antagonists (methiothepine and methysergide) can attenuate these effects.

It should be noted that Geyer and Braff (1987) have also proposed an interactive 5-HT/DA theory of sensorimotor gating in schizophrenia. Based upon results of animal studies, they propose that DA overactivity in the nucleus accumbens may lead to a schizophrenia-like loss of sensory gating, consistent with hypotheses concerning mesolimbic DA overactivity in schizophrenia. They provide new evidence from animal models, extending earlier studies showing LSD-induced habituation deficits similar to those seen in schizophrenia, suggesting that 5-HT_2 receptors may play an important role in the modulation of startle habituation, and thus in primary schizophrenic deficits.

Assuming that 5-HT indeed modulates DAergic function, through the imposing of inhibitory tone, then excitation or disinhibition of the striatal DAergic system presumably produced by potent 5-HT antagonists might be effective for the amelioration of extrapyramidal symptoms, as has been suggested by the studies with ritanserin and setoperone cited above. Given the hypothesis proposed by Meltzer and Stahl (1976) and others that negative symptoms of schizophrenia may be the consequence of decreased DAergic activity, then the same disinhibition effects of 5-HT antagonists on the mesolimbic and mesocortical DAergic circuits might explain the improvement in negative symptomatology seen when they are administered. This hypothesis is further supported by controlled studies showing a decrease in negative symptoms in schizophrenics with the administration of DAergic agonists such as L-dopa or d-amphetamine (Buchanan et al., 1975; Gerlach

& Luhdorf, 1975; Inanaga et al., 1975; Alpert et al., 1978; Cesarec & Nyman, 1985).

CONCLUSION

We propose that while DA pathophysiology may be related more predominantly to type I schizophrenia, 5-HT dysfunction, and more specifically 5-HTergic postsynaptic receptor hypersensitivity, may be more directly associated with type II schizophrenia. Obviously, the presumed dysfunction of each neurotransmitter system should be considered in relation to the dynamic interactions among the systems, rather than as independent processes. Optimal pharmacotherapy of schizophrenia might include both a 5-HT antagonist and a DA blocking component, the former being more beneficial for negative symptomatology and the latter for overt psychotic symptoms.

We hope that this perspective will have promising implications for treating a disorder that, at the present time, has proved to be discouragingly resistant to treatment.

REFERENCES

Alpert, M., Friedhoff, A. J., Marcos, L. R., & Diamond, F. (1978). Paradoxical reaction to L-dopa in schizophrenic patients. *Am. J. Psychiatry*, *135*, 1327–1332.

Altar, C. A., Wasely, A. M., Neale, R. F., & Stone, G. A. (1986). Typical and atypical antipsychotic occupancy of D2 and S2 receptors: An autoradiographic analysis in rat brain. *Brain Res. Bull.*, *16*, 517–525.

Andreasen, N. C., Olsen, S. A., Dennert, J. W., & Smith, M. R. (1982). Ventricular enlargement in schizophrenia: Relationship to positive and negative symptoms. *Am. J. Psychiatry*, *139*, 297–301.

Angrist, B., Lee, H. K., & Gershon, S. (1974). The antagonism of amphetamine-induced symptomatology by a neuroleptic. *Am. J. Psychiatry*, *137*, 817–819.

Arora, R. C., & Meltzer, H. Y. (1982). Serotonin uptake by blood platelets of schizophrenic patients. *Psychiatry Res.*, *6*, 327–333.

Arora, R. C., & Meltzer, H. Y. (1983). Effects of chlorpromazine on serotonin uptake in blood platelets. *Psychiatry Res.*, *9*, 23–28.

Ashcroft, G. W., Crawford, T. B. B., Eccleston, D., Sharman, D. F., MacDougall, E. G., Stanton, J. B., & Binns, J. K. (1966). 5-hydroxyindole compounds in the cerebrospinal fluid of patients with psychiatric or neurologic disease. *Lancet*, *II*, 1049–1052.

Axelsson, S., & Nordgren, L. (1974). Indoleamines in blood plasma of schizophrenics: A critical study with sensitive and selective methods. *Life Sci.*, *14*, 1261–1270.

Banki, C. M., Arato, M., Papp, Z., & Kurcz, M. (1984). Cerebrospinal fluid amine metabolites and neuroendocrine changes in psychoses and suicide. In E. Usdin,

A. Carlsson, & A. Dahlstrom (Eds.), *Catecholamines: Neuropharmacology and central nervous system—Therapeutic aspects* (pp. 153–159). New York: Alan R Liss.

Bellak, L., & Strauss, J. S. (1979). Overview: The heuristic need for subgroups of the schizophrenic syndrome. *Schizophr. Bull.*, *5*, 441–442.

Bennett, J. P., Enna, S. J., Bylund, D., Gillin, J. C., Wyatt, R., & Snyder, S. H. (1979): Neurotransmitter receptors in frontal cortex of schizophrenics. *Arch. Gen. Psychiatry, 36*, 927–934.

Bigelow, L., Walls, P., Gillin, J. C., & Wyatt, R. J. (1979). Clinical effects of L-5-hydroxytryptophan administration in chronic schizophrenic patients. *Biol. Psychiatry, 14*, 53–67.

Bowers, M. B. (1970). Cerebrospinal fluid 5-hydroxyindoles and behavior after L-tryptophan and pyridoxine administration to psychiatric patients. *Neuropharmacology, 9*, 599–604.

Bowers, M. B. (1974). Central dopamine turnover in schizophrenic syndromes. *Arch. Gen. Psychiatry, 31*, 50–57.

Bowers, M. B., Heninger, G. R., & Gerbode, F. A. (1969). Cerebrospinal fluid, 5-hydroxyindoleacetic acid and homovanillic acid in psychiatric patients. *Int. J. Neuropharmacology, 8*, 255–262.

Bucci, L. (1987). The negative symptoms of schizophrenia and the monoamine oxidase inhibitors. *Psychopharmacology, 91*, 104–108.

Buchanan, F. H., Parton, R. V., & Warren, J. W. (1975). Double-blind trial of L-dopa in chronic schizophrenia. *Aust. N. Z. J. Psychiatry, 9*, 269–271.

Buchsbaum, M. S., & Rieder, R. O. (1979). Biologic heterogeneity and psychiatric research: Platelet MAO activity as a case study. *Arch. Gen. Psychiatry, 39*, 1163–1169.

Carpenter, W. T., Fink, E. B., Narasimhachari, N., & Himwich, H. (1975). A test of the transmethylation hypothesis in acute schizophrenic patients. *Am. J. Psychiatry, 132*, 1067–1071.

Carpenter, W. T., Heinrich, D. W., & Alphs, L. D. (1985). Treatment of negative symptoms. *Schizophr. Bull., 11*, 440–452.

Casacchia, M., Casati, C., & Fazio, C. (1975). P-chlorophenylalanine in schizophrenia. *Biol. Psychiatry, 10*, 109–110.

Cesarec, Z., & Nyman, A. K. (1985). Differential response to amphetamine in schizophrenia. *Acta Psychiatr. Scand., 71*, 523–528.

Ceulemans, D. L. S., Gelders, Y., Hoppenbrouwers, M. L., Reyntjens, A., & Janssen, P. (1985a). Effect of serotonin antagonism in schizophrenia: A pilot study with setoperone. *Psychopharmacology, 85*, 329–332.

Ceulemans, D. L. S., van Doren, J., Nuyts, J., & DeWit, P. (1985b). Therapeutic efficacy of serotonin and dopamine antagonism on positive and negative symptoms of chronic schizophrenic patients. Fourth World Congress of Biological Psychiatry. Philadelphia, Pa., p. 272.

Charney, D. S., Menkes, D. B., & Heninger, G. R. (1981). Receptor sensitivity and the mechanism of action of antidepressant treatment. *Arch. Gen. Psychiatry, 38*, 1160–1180.

Chesire, R. M., Cheng, J. T., & Teitelbaum, P. H. (1982). Antiserotonergic drugs reinstate galloping forward locomotion produced by pontine tegmentum damage in rats. In T. H. O. Beng, J. C. Schoolar, & E. Usdin (Eds.), *Serotonin in biological psychiatry* (pp. 315-317). New York: Raven Press.

Chouinard, G., Annabel, L., Young, S. N., & Sourke, T. L. (1978). A controlled study of tryptophan-benserazide in schizophrenia. *Commun. Psychopharmacology, 2,* 21-31.

Clineschmidt, B. V., Zacchei, A. G., Totaro, J. A., Pflueger, A. B., McGuffin, J. C., & Wishousky, T. I. (1978). Fenfluramine and brain serotonin. *Ann. N. Y. Acad. Sci., 305,* 222-241.

Corbett, L., Christina, S. T., Morin, R. D., Benington, F., & Smythies, J. R. (1978). Hallucinogenic N-methylated indolealkylamines in the cerebrospinal fluid of psychiatric and control populations. *Br. J. Psychiatry, 132,* 139-144.

Cowen, P. J., Gadhvi, H., Godsen, B., & Kolakowska, T. (1985). Responses of prolactin and growth hormone to L-tryptophan infusion: Effects in normal subjects and schizophrenic patients receiving neuroleptics. *Psychopharmacology, 86,* 164-169.

Cremata, V. Y., & Koe, K. B. (1966). Clinical-pharmacological evaluation of p-chlorophenylalanine: A new serotonin depleting agent. *Clin. Pharmacol. Ther., 7,* 768-776.

Crow, T. J. (1980a). Molecular pathology of schizophrenia: More than one disease process? *Br. Med. J., 280,* 66-68.

Crow, T. J. (1980b). Positive and negative schizophrenia symptoms and the role of dopamine. *Br. J. Psychiatry, 137,* 383-386.

Crow, T. J., Baker, H., Gross, A., Joseph, M., Lofthouse, R., Longden, A., Owen, F., Riley, G., Glover, V., & Killpack, W. (1979). Monoamine mechanisms in chronic schizophrenia: Post-mortem neurochemical findings. *Br. J. Psychiatry, 134,* 249-256.

Crow, T. J., Ferrier, I. N., & Johnstone, E. C. (1986). The two syndrome concept and neuroendocrinology of schizophrenia. *Psychiatr. Clin. N. Am., 9,* 99-113.

DeLisi, L. E., Freed, W. I., Gillin, J. C., Kleinman, J. E., Bigelow, L. B., & Wyatt, R. J. (1982). P-chlorophenylalanine trial in schizophrenic patients. *Biol. Psychiatry, 17,* 471-477.

DeLisi, L. E., Neckers, L. M., Weinberger, D. R., & Wyatt, R. J. (1981). Increased whole blood serotonin concentrations in chronic schizophrenic patients. *Arch. Gen. Psychiatry, 38,* 647-650.

Domino, E. F., & Krause, R. P. (1974). Free and bound serum tryptophan in drug-free normal controls and chronic schizophrenic patients. *Biol. Psychiatry, 8,* 265-279.

Ennis, E., Kemp, J. P., & Cox, B. (1981). Characterisation of inhibitory 5-hydroxytryptamine receptors that modulate dopamine release in the striatum. *J. Neurochem., 36,* 1515-1520.

Farely, I., Shannak, K., & Hornykiewicz, D. (1980). Brain monamine changes in chronic paranoid schizophrenia and their possible relation to increased dopamine receptor sensitivity. In G. Pepeu, M. Kuhar, & S. Enna (Eds.), *Receptors for neurotransmitters and peptide hormones* (pp. 427-433). New York: Raven Press.

Feldstein, A., Hoagland, H., & Freeman, H. (1959). Blood and urinary serotonin and 5-hydroxyindoleacetic acid levels in schizophrenic patients and normal subjects. *J. Nerv. Ment. Dis.*, *129*, 62–68.

Freedman, D. X., Belendiuk, K., Belendiuk, G. W., & Crayton, J. W. (1981). Blood tryptophan metabolism in chronic schizophrenics. *Arch. Gen. Psychiatry*, *38*, 655–659.

Gaddum, J. H. (1954). Drugs antagonistic to 5-hydroxytryptamine. In G. W. Wolstenholme (Ed.), *Ciba Foundation symposium on hypertension* (pp. 75–77). Boston: Little Brown.

Gallant, D. M., Bishop, M. P., Steele, C. A., & Noblin, C. D. (1963). The relationship between serotonin antagonism and tranquilizing activity. *Am. J. Psychiatry*, *119*, 882.

Garelis, E., Gillin, J., Wyatt, R. J., & Neff, N. (1975). Elevated blood serotonin concentration in unmedicated chronic schizophrenic patients: A preliminary study. *Am. J. Psychiatry*, *132*, 184–186.

Gattaz, W. F., Waldmeier, P., & Beckmann, H. (1982). CSF monoamine metabolism in schizophrenic patients. *Acta Psychiatr. Scand.*, *66*, 350–360.

Gelders, Y., Ceulemans, D.L.S., Hoppenbrouwers, M. L., Reyntjens, A., & Mesotten, F. (1985b). Ritanserin, a selective serotonin antagonist, in chronic schizophrenia. Fourth World Congress of Biological Psychiatry. Philadelphia, Pa., p. 338.

Gelders, Y., Ceulemans, D. L. S., Reyntjens, A., Hoppenbrouwers, M. L., & Ferange, M. (1985a). The influence of selective serotonin antagonism on conventional neuroleptic therapy. Fourth World Congress of Biological Psychiatry. Philadelphia, Pa., p. 417.

Geller, E., Ritvo, E. R., Freeman, B. J., & Yuwiler, A. (1982). Preliminary observations on the effect of fenfluramine on blood serotonin and symptoms in three autistic boys. *N. Engl. J. Med.*, *307*, 165–169.

Gentsch, C., Lichtsteiner, M., Gastpar, M., Gastpar, G., & Feer, H. (1985). (3H)Imipramine binding sites in platelets of hospitalized psychiatric patients. *Psychiatry Res.*, *14*, 177–187.

Gerlach, J., & Luhdorf, K. (1975). The effect of L-dopa on young patients with simple schizophrenia, treated with neuroleptic drugs. *Psychopharmacology*, *44*, 105–110.

Geyer, M. A., & Braff, D. L. (1987). Startle habituation and sensorimotor gating in schizophrenia and related animal models. *Schizophr. Bull.*, *13*, 643–668.

Gillin, J. C., Kaplan, J., Stillman, R., & Wyatt, R. J. (1976a). The psychedelic models of schizophrenia: The case of N,N-dimethyltryptamine. *Am. J. Psychiatry*, *133*, 203–208.

Gillin, J. C., Kaplan, J. A., & Wyatt, R. J. (1976b). Clinical effects of tryptophan in chronic schizophrenia. *Biol. Psychiatry*, *11*, 635–639.

Goodwin, F. K., & Post, R. M. (1973). The use of probenecid in high doses for the estimation of central serotonin turnover in affective illness and addicts on methadone. In J. Barchas, & E. Usdin (Eds.), *Serotonin and behavior* (pp. 476–480). New York: Academic Press.

Hanley, H. G., Stahl, S. M., & Freedman, D. X. (1977). Hyperserotonemia and amine metabolites in autistic and retarded children. *Arch. Gen. Psychiatry*, *34*, 521–523.

Hauser, S. L., Delong, G. R., & Rosman, N. P. (1975). Pneumographic findings in the infantile autism syndrome: A correlation with temporal lobe disease. *Brain*, *98*, 667–688.

Hetey, L., & Drescher, K. (1986). Influence of antipsychotics on presynaptic receptors modulating the release of dopamine in synaptosomes of the nucleus accumbens of rats. *Neuropharmacology*, *25*, 1103–1109.

Hetey, L., Kurdin, V. S., Shemanow, A. Y., Rayevsky, K. S., & Oelssner, W. (1985). Presynaptic dopamine and serotonin receptors modulating tyrosine hydroxylase activity in synaptosomes of the nucleus accumbens of rats. *Eur. J. Pharmacol.*, *113*, 1–10.

Hoshino, Y., Kaneko, M., Kumashiro, H., & Tachibana, R., (1985). Endocrinological function in schizophrenic patients under haloperidol treatment: Plasma PRL, HGH and 5HT levels after L-5HTP loading. *Folia Psychiatr. Neurol. Jpn.*, *39*, 25–31.

Inanaga, K., Nakasawa, T., Inoue, K., Tachibana, H., Oshima, M., Kotorii, T., Tanaka, M., & Ogawa, N. (1975). Double-blind controlled study of L-dopa therapy in schizophrenia. *Folia Psychiatr. Neurol. Jpn.*, *29*, 123–143.

Jackman, H., Luchins, D., & Meltzer, H. Y. (1983). Platelet serotonin levels in schizophrenia: Relationship to race and psychopathology. *Biol. Psychiatry*, *18*, 887–902.

Jenner, P., Sheehy, M., & Marsden, C. D. (1983). Noradrenaline and 5-hydroxytryptamine modulation of brain dopamine function: Implications for the treatment of Parkinson's disease. *Br. J. Clin. Pharmacol.*, *15*(suppl), 2779–2898.

Joseph, M., Owen, F., Baker, H., & Bourne, R. (1977). Platelet serotonin concentration and monoamine oxidase activity in unmedicated chronic schizophrenics and schizophrenic patients. *Psychol. Med.*, *7*, 159–162.

Joseph, M. H., Baker, H. F., Crow, T. J., Riley, G. J., & Rigsby, D. (1979). Brain tryptophan metabolism in schizophrenia: A postmortem study of metabolites on the serotonin and kynurenine pathways in schizophrenic and control subjects. *Psychopharmacology*, *62*, 279–285.

Kanof, P. D., Caccaro, E. F., Johns, C. A., Siever, L. J., & Davis, K. L. (1987). Platelet (3H)imipramine binding in psychiatric disorders. *Biol. Psychiatry*, *22*, 278–286.

Kaplan, J., Mandel, L. R., Stillman, R., Walker, R. W., Vanden-Heuvel, W. J. A., Gillin, J. C., & Wyatt, R. J. (1974). Blood and urine levels of N,N-dimethyltryptamine following administration of psychoactive dosage to human subjects. *Psychopharmacologia*, *38*, 239–266.

Kaplan, R. D., & Mann, J. J. (1982). Altered platelet serotonin uptake kinetics in schizophrenia and depression. *Life Sci.*, *31*, 583–588.

King, R., Faull, K. F., Stahl, S. M., Mefford, I. N., Thiemann, S., Barchas, J., & Berger, P. A. (1985). Serotonin and schizophrenia: Correlations between serotonergic activity and schizophrenic motor behavior. *Psychiatry Res.*, *14*, 235–240.

Koe, B. K., & Weissman, A. (1966). P-chlorophenylalanine: A specific depletor of brain serotonin. *J. Pharmacol. Exp. Ther.*, *154*, 499–516.

Kolakowska, T., & Molyneux, S. G. (1987). Platelet serotonin concentration in schizophrenic patients. *Am. J. Psychiatry*, *144*, 232–234.

Korpi, E. R., Kleinman, J. E., Goodman, S. I., Phillips, I., DeLisi, L. E., Linnoila, M., & Wyatt, R. J. (1986). Serotonin and 5-hydroxyindoleacetic acid in the brains of suicide victims. Comparison in chronic schizophrenic patients with suicide as cause of death. *Arch. Gen. Psychiatry, 43,* 594–600.

Langer, S. Z., Zarifian, E., Briley, M., Raisman, R., & Sechter, D. (1981). High affinity binding of (3H)imipramine in brain and platelets and its relevance to the biochemistry of affective disorders. *Life Sci., 29,* 211–220.

Levy, A. B., Kurtz, N., & Kling, A. S. (1984). Association between cerebral ventricular enlargement and suicide attempts in chronic schizophrenia. *Am. J. Psychiatry, 141,* 438–439.

Lewine, R. J., & Meltzer, H. Y. (1984). Negative symptoms and platelet monoamine oxidase activity in male schizophrenic patients. *Psychiatry Res., 12,* 99–109.

Leysen, J. E., Gommeren, W., Van Gompel, P., Wijnants, J., Janssen, P. F. M., & Laduron, P. M. (1985). Receptor binding properties in vitro and in vivo of ritanserin: A very potent and long-acting serotonin-S2 antagonist. *Mol. Pharmacol., 27,* 600–611.

Leysen, J. E., Niemegeers, C. J. E., Tollenaere, J. P., & Laduron, P. M. (1978). Serotonergic component of neuroleptic receptors. *Nature, 272,* 168–171.

Lingjaerde, O. (1983). Serotonin uptake and efflux in blood platelets from untreated and neuroleptic-treated schizophrenics. *Biol. Psychiatry, 18,* 1345–1356.

Lipinski, J. F., Mandel, L. R., Ahn, H. S., Vanden-Heuvel, W. J. A., & Walker, R. W. (1974). Blood dimethyltryptamine concentrations in psychotic disorders. *Biol. Psychiatry, 9,* 89–91.

Losonczy, M. F., Song, I. S., Mohs, R. C., Mathe, A. A., Davidson, M., Davis, B. M., & Davis, K. L. (1986a). Correlates of lateral ventricular size in chronic schizophrenia. I: Behavioral and treatment response measures. *Am. J. Psychiatry, 143,* 976–981.

Losonczy, M. F., Song, I. S., Mohs, R. C., Mathe, A. A., Davidson, M., Davis, B. M., & Davis, K. L. (1986b). Correlates of lateral ventricular size in chronic schizophrenia. II: Biological measures. *Am. J. Psychiatry, 143,* 1113–1118.

Manowitz, P., Gilmour, D. G., & Racevskis, J. (1973). Low plasma tryptophan levels in recently hospitalized schizophrenics. *Biol. Psychiatry, 6,* 109–118.

Meltzer, H. Y., & Stahl, S. M. (1976). The dopamine hypothesis of schizophrenia: A review. *Schizophr. Bull., 2,* 19–76.

Meltzer, H. Y., Arora, R. C., Baber, R., & Tricou, B. J. (1981). Serotonin uptake in blood platelets of psychiatric patients. *Arch. Gen. Psychiatry, 38,* 1322–1326.

Meltzer, H. Y., Duncavage, M., Arora, R. C., Tricou, B. J., Jackman, H., & Young, M. (1982). Effects of neuroleptic drugs on platelet monoamine oxidase in psychiatric patients. *Am. J. Psychiatry, 139,* 1242–1247.

Meltzer, H. Y., Sommer, A. A., & Luchins, D. J. (1986). The effect of neuroleptics and other psychotropic drugs on negative symptoms in schizophrenia. *J. Clin. Psychopharmacol., 6,* 329–338.

Mendels, J. (1967). The effect of methysergide (an antiserotonin agent) on schizophrenia: A preliminary report. *Br. J. Psychiatry, 124,* 157–160.

Miller, R. J., Horn, A. S., & Iverson, L. L. (1974). The action of neuroleptic drugs on dopamine-stimulated adenosine cyclic 3',5'-monophosphate production in rat neostriatum and limbic forebrain. *Mol. Pharmacol.*, *10*, 759–766.

Mita, T., Hanada, S., Nishino, N., Kuno, T., Nakai, H., Yamadori, T., Mizoi, Y., & Tanaka, C. (1986). Decreased serotonin-S2 and increased dopamine-D2 receptors in chronic schizophrenics. *Biol. Psychiatry*, *21*, 1407–1414.

Modai, I., Rotman, A., Munitz, H., Tjano, S., & Wijsenbeek, H. (1979). Serotonin uptake by blood platelets of acute schizophrenic patients. *Psychopharmacology*, *64*, 193–195.

Morand, C., Young, S. N., & Ervin, F. R. (1983). Clinical response of aggressive schizophrenics to oral tryptophan. *Biol. Psychiatry*, *18*, 575–578.

Muck-Seler, D., Jakovljevic, M., & Deanovic, Z. (1988). Time course of schizophrenia and platelet 5-HT level. *Biol. Psychiatry*, *23*, 243–251.

Murphy, D. L., Mueller, E. A., Garrick, N. A., & Aukakh, C. S. (1986). Use of serotonergic agents in the clinical assessment of central serotonin function. *J. Clin. Psychiatry*, *47*(suppl), 9–15.

Ninan, P. T., van Kammen, D. P., Scheinin, M., Linnoila, M., Bunney, W., & Goodwin, F. K. (1984). CSF 5-hydroxyindoleacetic acid levels in suicidal schizophrenic patients. *Am. J. Psychiatry*, *141*, 566–569.

Nyback, H., Berggren, B. M., Hindmarsh, T., Sedvall, G., & Wiesel, F. A. (1983). Cerebroventricular size and cerebrospinal fluid monoamine metabolites in schizophrenic patients and healthy volunteers. *Psychiatry Res.*, *9*, 301–308.

Overall, J. E., & Gorham, D. R. (1962). The brief psychiatric rating scale. *Psychol. Rep.*, *10*, 799–812.

Paul, S. M., Rehavi, M., Skolnick, P., & Goodwin, F. K. (1980). Demonstration of specific 'high affinity' binding sites for 3H-imipramine on human platelets. *Life Sci.*, *26*, 953–959.

Pearlson, G. D., Garbacz, D. J., Breaky, W. R., Ahn, H. S., & DePavlo, T. R. (1984). Lateral ventricular enlargement associated with persistent unemployment and negative symptoms in both schizophrenia and bipolar disorder. *Psychiatry Res.*, *12*, 1–9.

Peroutka, S. J., Lebovitz, R. M., & Snyder, S. H. (1981). Two distinct central serotonin receptors with different physiological functions. *Science*, *212*, 827–829.

Persson, T., & Roos, B. E. (1969). Acid metabolites from monoamines in cerebrospinal fluid of schizophrenics. *Br. J. Psychiatry*, *115*, 95–98.

Post, R. M., Fink, E., Carpenter, W. T., & Goodwin, F. K. (1975). Cerebrospinal fluid amine metabolites in acute schizophrenia. *Arch. Gen. Psychiatry*, *32*, 1063–1069.

Potkin, S. G., Cannon, H. E., Murphy, D. L., & Wyatt, R. J. (1978). Are paranoid schizophrenics biologically different from other schizophrenics? *N. Engl. J. Med.*, *298*, 61–66.

Potkin, S. G., Weinberger, D. R., Linnoila, M., & Wyatt, R. J. (1983). Low CSF 5-hydroxyindoleacetic acid in schizophrenic patients with enlarged cerebral ventricles. *Am. J. Psychiatry*, *140*, 21–25.

Reynolds, G. P., Rossor, M. N., & Iversen, L. L. (1983). Preliminary studies of human cortical 5HT2 receptors and their involvement in schizophrenia and neuroleptic drug action. *J. Neural Transm.*, *18*(Supp), 273–277.

Rimon, R., Roos, B. E., Rakkolainen, V., & Alonen, Y. (1971). The content of

5HIAA and HVA in the CSF of patients with acute schizophrenia. *J. Psychosom. Res.*, *15*, 375-378.

Rotman, A., Modai, I., Munitz, H., & Wijsenbeek, H. (1979). Active uptake of serotonin by blood platelets of schizophrenic patients. *FEBS Lett.*, *101*, 134-136.

Rotman, A., Munitz, H., Modai, I., Tjano, S., & Wijsenbeek, H. (1980). A comparative uptake study of serotonin, dopamine and norepinephrine by platelets of acute schizophrenic patients. *Psychiatry Res.*, *3*, 239-246.

Rotman, A., Zemishlany, Z., Munitz, H., & Wijsenbeek, H. (1982a). The active uptake of serotonin by platelets of schizophrenic patients and their families: Possibility of a genetic marker. *Psychopharmacology*, *77*, 171-174.

Rotman, A., Shatz, A., & Szekely, G. A. (1982b). Correlation between serotonin uptake and imipramine binding in schizophrenic patients. *Prog. Neuropsychopharmacol. Biol. Psychiatry*, *6*, 57-61.

Roy, A., Ninan, P., Mazonson, A., Pickar, D., van Kammen, D., Linnoila, M., & Paul, S. M. (1985). CSF metabolites in chronic schizophrenic patients who attempt suicide. *Psychol. Med.*, *15*, 335-340.

Sedvall, G., & Wode-Helgodt, B. (1980). Aberrant monoamine metabolite levels in CSF and family history of schizophrenia. *Arch. Gen. Psychiatry*, *37*, 1113-1116.

Shoulson, I., & Chase, T. N. (1975). Fenfluramine in man: Hypophagia associated with diminished serotonin turnover. *Clin. Pharmacol. Ther.*, *17*, 616-621.

Shore, D., Korpi, E. R., Bigelow, L. B., Zec, R. F., & Wyatt, R. J. (1985). Fenfluramine and chronic schizophrenia. *Biol. Psychiatry*, *20*, 329-352.

Sills, M. A., Wolf, B. B., & Frazer, A. (1984). Determination of selective and nonselective compounds for the 5HT 1A and 5HT 1B receptor subtypes in rat frontal cortex. *J. Pharmacol. Exp. Ther.*, *231*, 480-487.

Sneddon, J. M. (1969). Sodium-dependent accumulation of 5-hydroxytryptamine by rat blood platelets. *Br. J. Pharmacol.*, *37*, 680-688.

Sneddon, J. M. (1973). Blood platelets as a model for monoamine-containing neurons. *Prog. Neurobiol.*, *1*, 151-198.

Snyder, S. H. (1972). Catecholamines in the brain as mediators of amphetamine psychosis. *Arch. Gen. Psychiatry*, *27*, 169-179.

Snyder, S. H. (1973). Amphetamine psychosis: A model of schizophrenia mediated by catecholamines. *Am J. Psychiatry*, *120*, 61-67.

Snyder, S. H. (1976). The dopamine hypothesis of schizophrenia: Focus on the dopamine receptor. *Am. J. Psychiatry*, *133*, 197-202.

Stahl, S. M. (1977). The human platelet. *Arch. Gen. Psychiatry*, *34*, 509-516.

Stahl, S. M., Uhr, S. B., & Berger, P. A. (1985). Pilot study on the effects of fenfluramine on negative symptoms in twelve schizophrenic inpatients. *Biol. Psychiatry*, *20*, 1098-1102.

Stahl, S. M., Woo, D. J., Mefford, I. N., Berger, P. A., & Ciaranello, R. D. (1983). Hyperserotonemia and platelet serotonin uptake and release in schizophrenia and affective disorders. *Am J. Psychiatry*, *140*, 26-30.

Szara, S. (1967). Hallucinogenic amines and schizophrenia. In H. E. Himwich, S. S.

Kety & J. R. Smythies (Eds.), *Amines and schizophrenia* (pp. 181-197). New York: Pergamon Press.

Todrick, A., Tait, M. B., & Marshall, E. F. (1960). Blood platelet 5-HT levels in psychiatric patients. *J. Ment. Sci.*, *106*, 884-890.

Torre, M., Vergani, E., & Gaira, S. (1970). Livelli ematici di serotonina piastrinica in schizofrenic. *Acta Neurol. (Napoli)*, *25*, 740-746.

Van Kammen, D. P., Peters, J., & van Kammen, W. B. (1986). Cerebrospinal fluid studies of monoamine metabolism in schizophrenia. *Psychiatr. Clin. N. Am.*, *9*, 81-97.

van Praag, H. M. (1967). The possible significance of cerebral dopamine for neurology and psychiatry. *Psychiatr. Neurol. Neurochir.*, *70*, 361-379.

van Praag, H. M. (1983). CSF 5HIAA and suicide in non-depressed schizophrenics. *Lancet*, *3*, 977-978.

van Praag, H. M. (1986). Biological suicide research: Outcome and limitations. *Biol. Psychiatry*, *21*, 1305-1323.

van Praag, H. M., Kahn, R., Asnis, G. M., Lemus, C. Z., & Brown, S. L. (1987a). Therapeutic indications for serotonin-potentiating compounds: A hypothesis. *Biol. Psychiatry*, *22*, 205-212.

van Praag, H. M., Lemus, C., & Kahn, R. (1987b). Hormonal probes of central serotonergic activity: Do they really exist? *Biol. Psychiatry*, *22*, 86-98.

Waldmeier, P. C., & Delina-Stula, A. A. (1979). Serotonin-dopamine interactions in the nigrostriatal system. *Eur. J. Pharmacol.*, *55*, 363-373.

Weinberger, D. R. (1984). Computed tomography (CT) findings in schizophrenia: Speculation on the meaning of it all. *J. Psychiatr. Res.*, *18*, 477-490.

Weizman, A., Gonen, N., Tjano, S., Szekely, G. A., & Rehavi, M. (1987): Platelet (3H)imipramine binding in autism and schizophrenia. *Psychopharmacology*, *91*, 101-103.

Whitaker, P. M., Crow, T. J., & Ferrier, I. N. (1981). Tritiated LSD binding in frontal cortex in schizophrenia. *Arch. Gen. Psychiatry*, *38*, 278-280.

Winblad, B., Bucht, G., Gottfries, C. G., & Roos, B. E. (1979). Monoamines and monoamine metabolites in brains from demented schizophrenics. *Acta Psychiatr. Scand*, *60*, 17-28.

Wong, D. F., Wagner, H. N., Tune, L. E., Dannals, R. F., Pearlson, G. D., Links, J. M., Tamminga, C. A., Broussole, E. P., Ravert, H. T., Wilson, A. A., Toung, J. K. T., Malat, J., Williams, J. A., O'Tuama, L. A., Snyder, S. H., Kuhar, M. J., & Gjedde, A. (1986). Positron emission tomography reveals elevated D2 dopamine receptors in drug-naive schizophrenics. *Science*, *234*, 1558-1566.

Wood, P. L., Suranyi-Cadotte, B. E., Nair, N. P. V., LaFaille, F., & Schwartz, G. (1983). Lack of association between (3H)imipramine binding sites and uptake of serotonin in control, depressed and schizophrenic patients. *Neuropharmacology*, *22*, 1211-1214.

Woolley, D. W., & Shaw, E. (1954). A biochemical and pharmacological suggestion about certain mental disorders. *Proc. Natl. Acad. Sci. U.S.A.*, *40*, 228-231.

Wurtman, R. J., Heft, F., & Melamed, E. (1981). Precursor control of neurotransmitter synthesis. *Pharmacol. Rev.*, *32*, 315-335.

Wyatt, R. J., Vaughan, T., Galanter, M., Kaplan, J., & Green, R. (1972). Behavioral changes of chronic schizophrenic patients given L-5-hydroxytryptophan. *Science, 177,* 1124–1126.

Yuwiler, A., Brammer, G., Morley, J., Raleigh, M., Flannery, J., & Geller, E. (1981). Short-term and repetitive administration of oral tryptophan in normal men. *Arch. Gen. Psychiatry, 38,* 619–626.

9

Psychiatric Disorders of Childhood
The Role of Serotonin

ALAN APTER
SERENA-LYNN BROWN
MARTIN L. KORN
HERMAN M. van PRAAG

INFANTILE AUTISM

Recent research has extensively documented the fact that alterations in central nervous system (CNS) functioning underlie many of the symptoms of autism. Such dysfunctions have recently been well reviewed (Anderson & Hoshino, 1987; Golden, 1987; Ornitz, 1987).

Whole-Blood Serotonin Levels

The most robust and well-replicated neurochemical finding in this disease is the increase seen in whole-blood serotonin (WHBS) in autistic individuals (Schain & Freedman, 1961; Ritvo et al., 1970; Yuwiler et al., 1971; Goldstein et al., 1976; Hanley et al., 1976; Takahashi et al., 1976; Hoshino et al., 1984; Anderson et al., 1987). Golden (1987) has summarized research on disorders clinically seen to be associated with autism, such as Down's syndrome and infantile spasms, and has suggested that a possible unifying feature of this clinical triad might be an abnormality in the metabolism of serotonin (5-hydroxytryptamine, or 5-HT), as 5-HTergic abnormalities have been noted in all three of these illnesses separately. Much research effort has been expended both in trying to understand and elaborate on this finding, and in attempting to utilize such data to aid in devising new therapeutic strategies (Anderson & Hoshino, 1987).

A recent large-scale study by Anderson et al. (1987) examined whole-blood 5-HT and tryptophan in 40 autistic and 87 normal subjects. A 51%

215

elevation in WHBS in autistics as compared with normal controls was found. This was midway in the range of the 18% to 137% elevation found in other studies. Thirty-eight percent of the unmedicated autistics had WHBS levels above 220 ng/ml, which is in the upper 5% (mean + 1.65 SD) of the levels found in the normals studied. It should be noted that both the normal control group and the autistic subjects had WHBS levels that demonstrated a Gaussian distribution, suggesting that the elevation in group mean was not due to a subgroup of hyperserotonergic autistic individuals, but rather to an upward shift in WHBS in autism in general.

Cook et al. (1987) have presented evidence that this hyperserotonemia may have a familial basis. These investigators examined WHBS and plasma norepinephrine (NE) in 52 families of autistic probands. Siblings of affected probands were found to have decreased NE relative to their autistic siblings, and WHBS but not NE was significantly correlated between autistic children, mothers, fathers, and brothers, but not sisters. Four families were identified in which each family member studied had hyperserotonemia (5-HT > 270 ng/ml).

In normal individuals, 5-HT levels in general appear to decline with age. This may be especially marked in normal young males (Anderson et al., 1987). It appears that autistics do not show this normal maturational decline in 5-HT, however. Investigators in this area have not been able to explain this lack of maturational decline, but they have postulated that hyperserotonemia may reflect the failure of maturation seen in autism (Ritvo et al., 1970; Hoshino et al., 1984; Anderson et al., 1987).

Platelet Parameters

The factors influencing WHBS levels in normals include platelet structure and activity, 5-HT synthesis, and monoamine oxidase activity (Anderson et al., 1987). Differing hypotheses about the hyperserotonemia seen in autism therefore have been related to these three different areas.

It is not clear whether the increase in WHBS seen in autism might be due to abnormalities in the structure or number of blood platelets in autistic individuals, as was earlier postulated by Ritvo et al. (1970). 5-HT uptake by platelets of autistic children has been the subject of intensive but controversial research since 1962 (Guthrie & Wyatt, 1975). Rotman et al. (1980) and Boullin et al. (1982) initially described abnormal platelet 5-HT uptake in autistic children, and Katsui et al. (1986) subsequently reported that mean V_{max} (referring to the affinity of the uptake site for 5-HT) in both autistic and language-disabled children was significantly higher than in normal controls, and, furthermore, that in all autistic patients studied, the V_{max} of platelet 5-HT uptake was higher than the V_{max} of any of the normal controls. In contrast, Anderson (1984) found no difference in 5-HT uptake between autistic individuals and normal controls. There has also been one report of decreased platelet reactivity in autism (Safai-Kulti et al., 1985).

Urinary 5-HIAA

One method for examining the production rate of 5-HT involves the measurement of the primary 5-HT metabolite 5-hydroxyindoleacetic acid (5-HIAA). Since most 5-HT in the body is eventually metabolized to 5-HIAA and excreted in the urine (Udenfriend et al., 1959), it is thought that measurement of urinary 5-HIAA will accurately reflect the rate and amount of 5-HT metabolism in the body. Studies examining urinary 5-HIAA levels in autism, however, have produced contradictory results. While Hanley et al. (1977) have reported increased urinary 5-HIAA in autistic individuals, other investigators have not (Schain & Freedman, 1961; Partington et al., 1973; Jouve et al., 1986; Anderson et al., 1987b).

The evidence for a relationship between high WHBS and high levels of 5-HIAA in the urine is also ambiguous. Thus, Anderson and Hoshino (1987) concluded their comprehensive review of these studies by stating that, on balance, it seems that autistic individuals probably produce normal amounts of 5-HT. In addition, Anderson et al. (1987) point out that since they have observed normal or lowered levels of urinary 5-HT in autistic subjects, this would suggest that plasma-free 5-HT levels are not elevated and, therefore, that the platelets of autistic children are not exposed to higher levels of in vivo 5-HT.

CSF 5-HIAA

A limited number of studies of cerebrospinal fluid (CSF) 5-HIAA in autism have also been undertaken. Marked reductions of both dopamine (DA) and 5-HT acid metabolites have been found in the CSF of children with epilepsy (Shaywitz et al., 1975). Three studies used probenecid to block the egress of 5-HIAA from the CSF (Cohen et al., 1974, 1977; Winsberg et al., 1980). The former two studies compared autistic children with nonautistic psychotic controls and found no differences in CSF 5-HIAA. The last study, which used no controls, found that several autistic children did not show the expected increase in CSF 5-HIAA after probenecid. It should be noted that some investigators feel that measurements using probenecid may be problematic since CSF probenecid levels vary between subjects after oral probenecid administration (Anderson & Hoshino, 1987). Such problems may be purely dose dependent, however; when too much probenecid is administered, the transport mechanism is practically blocked.

One baseline, nonprobenecid study of 5-HIAA showed no differences between autistic children and controls (Gilberg et al., 1983), although nonprobenecid studies are also problematic. In reviewing literature in the field, Anderson and Hoshino (1987) have concluded that the data suggest there is some evidence for slightly decreased levels of 5-HIAA in the CSF of autistic individuals, but this still requires confirmation.

Tryptophan

The dietary precursor of 5-HT is tryptophan (TRP), and plasma-free TRP levels are thought to have a major effect on central TRP metabolism and 5-HT synthesis (Hoshino et al., 1984a). Decreased levels of plasma-free TRP have been found in Down's syndrome (Obuko, 1979), and this measurement is being explored in illnesses thought to be under 5-HTergic modulation. Coppen et al. (1973) have reported decreased plasma TRP in women with major depression, increasing after treatment but never reaching normal levels. Following on these findings, investigators have attempted to determine whether disturbances of TRP metabolism may be involved in autism.

Naruse et al. (1987) found a marked decrease in the intestinal transport of deuterated phenylalanine and TRP in several cases of infantile autism. They suggested that defective cellular transport of the aromatic amino acids may be of etiological significance in this disorder by causing decreased formation of brain 5-HT and catecholamines.

The measurement of levels of free TRP in the blood has yielded contradictory results. Hoshino et al. (1984a) found increased levels of plasma-free TRP and 5-HT in 37 autistic children as compared with normal children or adult controls. These autistic children showed a significant correlation between plasma TRP level, but not blood 5-HT level, and severity ratings on clinical assessment. Furthermore, Yamamoto (1982) found that the extent of clinical improvement on haloperidol correlated with the amount of reduction of WHBS in such individuals. On the other hand, three sets of investigators have reported that total plasma TRP is lower in autistic patients as compared with controls (Takatsu et al., 1965; Sylvester et al., 1970; Anderson et al., 1987).

Metabolism of 5-HT in autism has also been investigated using oral L-TRP challenge studies. Sutton et al. (1958) have reported that, after oral administration of 0.25 g/kg of L-TRP, an 18-month-old autistic girl excreted less urinary indoleacetic acid and 5-HIAA than did four nonpsychotic controls. These authors have postulated that autistic children may have a dysfunction in the metabolism of TRP to 5-HIAA. Hanley et al. (1977) reported that, after an oral dose of 1 g of L-TRP, children with both autism and mild mental retardation excreted increased urinary 5-HIAA, while urinary 5-HT excretion was decreased in the autistic children and increased in the mildly retarded children. However, Shaw et al. (1959) and Schain and Freedman (1961), using a lower dose of TRP, reported contradictory results.

5-HTP

5-hydroxytryptophan (5-HTP), the immediate metabolic precursor of 5-HT, crosses the blood–brain barrier and increases central 5-HT availability after oral administration. The administration of oral 5-HTP is a technique that has been employed in the investigation of the role of 5-HT in several neuropsychiatric disorders, including depression, myoclonic epilepsy, Lesch-Nyhan syndrome, schizophrenia, and Down's syndrome (Anderson & Hoshino, 1987).

Zarcone et al. (1973) gave two autistic boys 3.0 mg/kg of D-L-5-HTP for eight days. The only response noted was an increase in REM sleep. Sverd et al. (1978) gave a combination of L-5-HTP and carbidopa to three autistic children for six to 10 weeks, also without any improvement noted.

Using the neuroendocrine challenge paradigm, Hoshino et al. (1984a) have challenged autistic children with 3 mg/kg of L-5-HTP, and have shown a suppressed increase of WHBS in the autistic children as compared with normal controls, even though baseline levels of 5-HT were higher in patients than in controls. However, lower baseline levels of prolactin and a blunted prolactin response to 5-HTP were present in the autistic group. These results may be due to diminished 5-HTergic tone in the CNS or to enhanced activity of tuberoinfundibular DA neurons, which have powerful inhibitory control over prolactin release. Watanabe et al. (1980) also challenged autistic children and normal adult controls with 3 mg/kg of L-5-HTP, and reported that the normal adults, but not the autistic children, had a significant rise in WHBS, thus suggesting defective absorption or metabolism of 5-HTP to 5-HT in these children.

Normal prolactin response to DA blockers in autistics (Anderson & Hoshino, 1987) suggests that the former explanation, that of lowered 5-HTergic tone in the CNS, may be more correct. In addition, pre- and post-stimulation levels of growth hormone were found to be no different for autistic subjects and normal controls. Many investigators have noted the fact that 5-HTergic neurons appear to be involved in the control of prolactin, growth hormone, and cortisol release. This suggests that further research using 5-HTP and TRP loading to stimulate hormone release may prove to be a fruitful way to examine central 5-HTergic function in autistic children.

MAO

The enzyme responsible for the catabolism of 5-HT is monoamine oxidase (MAO). This enzyme is also of interest to workers in the field of autism, as it has been reported to be decreased in schizophrenia (Wyatt et al., 1980). Given findings of increased 5-HT and TRP in autism, some researchers in this field have suggested that, since the metabolic system appears to be under the control of plasma-free TRP, 5-HT metabolism may be abnormally increased in autism, possibly by an increase in degradation of 5-HT by MAO (Hoshino et al., 1984b). In fact, however, several studies have shown no difference in MAO-B activity between autistics and controls (Boullin et al., 1976; Roth et al., 1976; Cohen et al., 1977; Lake et al., 1977). The significance of this finding is uncertain for two reasons: (1) the relationship of platelet MAO to brain MAO is controversial, and (2) most peripheral 5-HT is catabolized by MAO-A in the lung and liver. Thus, only studies of MAO in these tissues will finally elucidate what role, if any, MAO plays in the hyperserotonemia of autism. Interestingly, children with childhood schizophrenia have been reported to have higher platelet MAO levels than both patients and normal controls (Rogeness et al., 1985), a finding opposite to that found in chronic adult schizophrenics (Gattaz et al., 1981).

Drug Treatment Studies

Interest in 5-HT and autism has also spurred therapeutic endeavors, and a number of treatment studies have been performed. 6R-L-erythro-5, 6, 7, 8-tetrohydrobiopterin (R-THBP) is the natural cofactor of tryptophan and tyrosine hydroxylase. These are the rate-limiting enzymes involved, respectively, in the synthesis of 5-HT and the catecholamines (CAs). Both intraventricular (Miwa et al., 1985) and peripheral (Watanabe et al., 1984) administrations of this substance increase the biosynthesis of these amines in rat brain. The effect of R-THBP in autistics has been extensively studied by Naruse and his colleagues. In a preliminary open study, two typical cases of infantile autism were treated and significant improvement was noted. Subsequently, 17 other autistic patients were given this compound and seven showed marked improvement in clinical symptoms. Finally, a large double-blind study was conducted with 84 patients (Naruse et al., 1987), and marked improvement was noted in the R-THBP group, especially in the under-five-year-old group. These findings await confirmation by other workers.

Based on the finding that autistic children have high WHBS, Ritvo et al. (1971) gave L-dopa to four autistic patients for six months in an attempt to lower their plasma 5-HT levels and thus attempt to relieve their symptoms. They chose L-dopa because it has been reported to decrease 5-HT levels in animals (Weigand & Perry, 1961; Everett & Borcherding, 1970). Ritvo et al. (1971) have hypothesized that such an effect may be due to competition between DA and 5-HT for available platelet binding sites, or for reactive sites on aromatic amino acid decarboxylase, or reaction between DA and pyridoxal phosphate to form isotetraquinolines, thus decreasing 5-HT formation by removing pyridoxal phosphate from aromatic amino-acid decarboxylase. In this open study, although blood 5-HT levels fell significantly in the three younger children, clinical improvement did not occur. Campbell et al. (1976) also administered L-dopa to 12 children diagnosed as schizophrenic with autistic features, five of whom showed some improvement, primarily in the areas of a decrease in negativism and a stimulation of play, energy, motor initiation, language production, and affective responsiveness. However, these changes did not correlate with changes in 5-HT levels.

Segawa et al. (1987) treated 32 autistic children with 20–32 mg of 5-HTP daily for two months. Seventeen children showed a favorable response, 11 showed no response, and four worsened. In the same study, L-dopa produced a favorable effect in eight cases, no effect in eight cases, and an unfavorable effect in four patients. 5-HTP was especially efficacious for such symptoms as hyperkinesia, self-stimulation, aggressiveness, and self-mutilation. On the basis of their results, the authors have hypothesized that 5-HTergic neurons may be involved in the early symptoms of autism, while DAergic neurons may be involved in the later stages of the disease.

5-HT antagonists have also been used to treat autism. Bender et al. (1963) administered lysergic acid diethylamide (LSD) and its methylated derivative methysergide (both 5-HT antagonists) to 54 autistic and schizophrenic children six to 12 years of age. Increased activity and alertness and decreased stereotypic behavior were reported. However, Fish et al. (1969) treated 11 autistic children with methysergide and obtained mixed results.

In contrast to the findings with 5-HTP, Campbell et al. (1971) gave the tricyclic antidepressant imipramine (6–125 mg/day) to 10 autistic and schizophrenic children for seven to 18 weeks, and found a mixture of stimulating, tranquilizing, and disorganizing effects, with half the children showing improvement and half developing worsening of symptoms. It was felt that if increased 5-HT is pathogenic in some autistic and schizophrenic children, the increase in 5-HT caused by imipramine may have caused the worsening of symptoms in this subset of children.

Geller et al. (1982) treated three hyperserotonemic autistic boys with fenfluramine, an anorexic agent that markedly decreases brain 5-HT (Clineschmidt et al., 1978). Doses were given that reduced blood 5-HT levels to normal. Behavioral improvements were noted in all the patients, and IQ improved in two of them. These gains lasted at least six weeks after the drug was discontinued. In a double-blind, crossover study, Ritvo et al. (1983) treated 14 autistic outpatients aged two-and-a-half to 18 years with 1.5 mg/kg fenfluramine, with one month of placebo, four months of drug, then two months of placebo. Seven of these patients had hyperserotenemia (WHBS levels above 300 ug/ml). Blood levels of 5-HT fell an average of 51% in both normal and hyperserotonemic patients after one month of fenfluramine, and returned to baseline within a month after return to placebo; 10 of 14 patients showed a rebound effect and blood 5-HT levels were higher than baseline two months later. Platelet count, however, remained constant, suggesting that hyperserotonemia in autism may be related to higher 5-HT concentration in each platelet, rather than to higher platelet number (Ritvo et al., 1983). During the four-month treatment period, all the patients showed improvement. Changes noted were decreased restlessness, decreased motility disturbances, improved sleep patterns, increased eye contact, increased socialization, increased spontaneous use of language, decreased echolalia, more appropriate affect, and increased social awareness. There were no differences in response for the hyperserotonemic and normoserotonemic subjects. The therapeutic effect disappeared two to four weeks after discontinuing the drug. Side effects included weight loss, lethargy, irritability, restlessness, and sleep disruption.

More recently, Campbell et al. (1987) reported a double-blind, placebo-controlled, 12-week study on the effects of fenfluramine in autism. Behavioral assessments were done at specified times by multiple independent raters on a number of different rating scales. Laboratory assessment of the effects of drug on discrimination learning were also obtained. Twenty-four subjects completed the protocol. Doses of fenfluramine ranged from 1.25 mg/kg/day to 2.068 mg/kg/day. The only symptom to improve was withdrawal ($p < .03$). Rebound deterioration was noted in fidgetiness, hyperactivity, and stereotypies. Discriminant learning was adversely affected by the fenfluramine. It has been suggested that the sedative side effects of this drug are due to early release of 5-HT from presynaptic terminals, while the agitation, irritability, crying, and sleep pattern disturbances are due to its later 5-HT–depleting effect (Realmuto et al., 1986). One of the cases described by Realmuto et al. (1986) developed unmanageably aggressive behavior, stimulating animal reactions to 5-HT depletion.

Finally, it should be pointed out that 5-HT is elevated in other diseases, some of which have behavioral characteristics similar to those in autism. These include mental retardation, schizophrenia, motor neuron disease (Belendiuk et al., 1981), Lesch-Nyhan syndrome (Castells et al., 1979), and a subgroup of children with attention deficit disorder (ADD) (Anderson et al., 1987). Inverse correlations between 5-HT levels and IQ have been reported (Campbell et al., 1974; Hanley et al., 1977), as have positive correlations with activity (Campbell et al., 1974; Takahashi et al., 1976). In mentally retarded patients, hyperactivity has been shown to be accompanied by low platelet 5-HT levels (Greenberg & Coleman, 1976). Anderson et al. (1987) did not find correlations between platelet 5-HT levels and IQ but did find negative correlations between 5-HT and stereotypies, echolalia, and self-injurious behavior.

A final provocative line of evidence supporting the indoleamine hypothesis of autism is the finding of 5-HT receptor antibodies in some autistic children (Todd & Ciaranello, 1985). Investigators are currently searching for such antibodies in other illnesses possibly related to autism, as above.

These findings, taken as a group, imply that a functional or dimensional, as compared with a strictly nosological, approach to classifying psychopathology, as first proposed by van Praag (1986) in relation to 5-HT and depression, might also be important to consider in autism. Another hypothesis is that elevated 5-HT levels may reflect nonspecific neuronal damage. The latter hypothesis is supported by the fact that in motor neuron disease, WHBS levels rise with increasing neuronal damage (Belendiuk et al., 1981).

In conclusion, it appears that:

1. There is hyperserotonemia in autism. Many studies have demonstrated an increase in WHBS in autistic individuals. Autistics also do not show the maturational decline in 5-HT seen in normals.
2. As yet, there are no data suggesting that this hyperserotonemia is due to an abnormality of structure or number of platelets.
3. As yet, data on the possible role of MAO activity in the hyperserotonemia of autism mainly concern MAO-B, and are inconclusive.
4. Studies examining the possibility of increased 5-HT synthesis in autism have also produced inconclusive or mixed findings. Investigations of urinary 5-HIAA, plasma-free TRP, and CSF 5-HIAA have given contradictory results.
5. Treatment studies using 5-HTergic agents that both increase and decrease 5-HT synthesis or availability have given mixed results, as well.

Thus, while the hyperserotonemia of autism continues to be investigated, there are still no answers concerning its etiology or function. We suggest that an examination of this illness functionally, by symptom complex (e.g., aggression-dysregulation), rather than nosologically, as a separate disease entity, may help in the determination of the etiology of this dysfunction.

ANOREXIA NERVOSA

Anorexia nervosa (AN) is a syndrome of self-starvation occurring primarily in adolescent girls. Several lines of evidence suggest involvement of 5-HTergic mechanisms in the pathogenesis of this disorder. An extensive animal literature has established the importance of brain indoleamine systems in the normal regulation of appetite (Zemishlany et al., 1987). It is believed that 5-HT is involved in the regulation of feeding behavior via an inhibitory effect on food intake. 5-HT agonists generally act as anorexic agents and cyproheptadine, a 5-HT antagonist, is an appetite stimulant (Goldberg et al., 1979).

In addition, there appears to be a close link between mood disorders and AN. Depressive symptoms are common in these patients, and many anorectics meet the revised third edition of the *Diagnostic and Statistical Manual of Mental Disorders* (DSM III-R) criteria for major mood disorders (Zemishlany et al., 1987). On follow-up, as many as 25% of anorectics have been noted to have developed a mood disorder, and anorectic probands have an excess of mood disorders in their relatives as compared with normal controls (Cantwell et al., 1977). Given the large body of data on 5-HT dysfunction in depression, then (see Chapter 5 of this volume for a review of this area), it is not surprising that a number of investigators have been tempted to search for the link between these two conditions via the 5-HT system.

Gilberg (1983) reported that two anorectic girls had the lowest CSF 5-HIAA and homovanillic acid (HVA, the primary metabolite of DA) values ever seen in his laboratory, where 116 children aged two to 16 years with a wide variety of different diseases had previously been tested. He proposed the raising of 5-HT and/or NE levels as a therapeutic strategy for this disorder. It should be noted that part of the decrease in the levels of these neurotransmitters might also be attributable to the decrease in food intake seen in this disorder. There is some disagreement as to whether this may be contributory, however, since some studies have shown that underweight anorectics have normal monoamine precursor amino-acid concentrations (Kaye et al., 1984), whereas other studies have reported low plasma TRP levels in these individuals (Coppen et al., 1976).

Riederer et al. (1982) showed that anorectics excreted lower levels of both 5-HT and CA metabolites in their urine, suggesting an overall reduction of CA and indoleamine metabolism in this disorder. Kaye et al. (1984) studied 10 older underweight anorectic patients and found a 30% decrease in CSF HVA and a 20% decrease in CSF 5-HIAA. These values returned to normal shortly after weight recovery. On the basis of animal studies linking monoamine metabolism to control of appetite and weight, these investigators have suggested that some disturbance in monoamine function in AN may drive weight loss, and might be responsible for the hormonal and mood changes seen in this disorder, since brain monoamine metabolism, appetitive behavior, and weight loss are likely to be linked in AN. However, in contrast, it should be noted that Gerner et al. (1984) were not able to demonstrate differences in CSF 5-HIAA between anorectics and controls.

There are conflicting data about TRP levels in AN. While Russell (1967) and Kaye et al. (1984) have not found lowered plasma TRP levels in anorectic patients, Coppen et al. (1976) and Gerner et al. (1984) have reported decreased plasma TRP levels in anorectics as compared with normals. With such findings, it is difficult to decide between cause and consequence.

Another avenue of investigation has involved the study of peripheral 5-HT parameters, including platelet 5-HT uptake and ^{3}H-imipramine binding. Weizmann et al. (1986) compared 17 anorectic adolescents with matched controls. B_{max}, the number of platelet binding sites, was decreased in the anorectic subjects. K_d, the affinity of imipramine for the binding sites, did not differentiate between the two groups. Both 5-HT parameters V_{max}, the affinity of the binding sites for 5-HT, and K_m, the dissociation constant, were similar in patients and controls. Neither the presence or absence of mood-related symptoms, nor a family history of depression, influenced either parameter. A similar study, using different methodology for the measurement of platelet 5-HT uptake, yielded similar results (Zemishlany et al., 1987).

As in autism, there has been a great deal of interest in the therapeutic use of 5-HT antagonists for AN. Cyproheptadine has a structure resembling that of the phenothiazine H_1 (histamine) receptor antagonists and is an effective H_1 blocker. It also has prominent 5-HT blocking activity on various smooth-muscle tissues. Strober (1981) has found that cyproheptadine has appetite-stimulating properties in asthmatic children. Goldberg et al. (1979) established the safety and efficacy of cyproheptadine used in high doses of 32 mg/day to treat anorectic inpatients. They randomly allocated 81 female anorectics to one of four treatment conditions involving cyproheptadine and placebo with or without behavior therapy. Cyproheptadine induced weight gain in a subgroup of more severely affected patients, with a greater weight loss, a history of prior treatment failures, and a history of birth complications. Halmi et al. (1986) compared cyproheptadine with amitriptyline and placebo in 72 anorectic patients. Cyproheptadine was significantly efficacious in treatment of the nonbulimic patients, but made the bulimic anorectics worse. Those patients who improved also showed an elevation in mood. In addition, the 5-HT reuptake inhibitor fluonetine has also been reported to be effective in AN (Ferguson, 1987). Taken as a whole, such data suggest that 5-HT antagonists may have a role in the management and treatment of some types of AN.

Finally, there is some evidence that "true" anorexia (i.e., appetite loss) is related to altered 5-HT metabolism. Hyman et al. (1986) reported a case of a metabolically stable seven-and-a-half-year-old girl with arginosuccinic aciduria who had severe anorexia for four and a half years. CSF HIAA was markedly elevated (79 ng/ml versus a normal of $33 +/- 11$ ng/ml). Altered 5-HT metabolism was also reflected in her sleep recordings, which showed decreased REM periods. Reduction of her TRP intake led to a CSF 5-HIAA level of 20 ng/ml, increased REM sleep, and the onset of spontaneous eating for the first time in four and a half years. Reintroduction of TRP up to 25 mg/kg/day led to recrudescence of the anorectic and sleep disturbance symptoms.

In conclusion, it appears that:

1. 5-HT is certainly involved in the regulation of feeding behavior. Drugs with 5-HTergic actions affect AN, and thus 5-HT would seem to have a major role in AN. In light of work linking AN and the mood disorders, with the recent surge of interest in 5-HT and depression, such a link appears even more likely.

2. Studies of 5-HT precursors and metabolites in AN are inconclusive because of their contradictory results.

3 There are some very preliminary data suggesting the possibility that platelet 5-HT uptake and ^{3}H-imipramine binding may be decreased in this disorder.

4 Treatment studies suggest that 5-HT antagonists may have efficacy in a subgroup of patients with AN.

Clearly, a great deal of work remains to be done in this area.

ENURESIS

Functional nocturnal enuresis is usually defined as repeated involuntary voiding of urine during sleep and after the age at which continence is expected, with no concomitant physical disorder that might explain the symptoms. Enuresis has been classified into primary and secondary types. In primary enuresis, the individual has never achieved continence; in secondary enuresis, the person is currently incontinent, but in the past has had a period of continence for at least one year. Primary enuresis is considered to be more rooted in developmental and psychobiological issues than secondary enuresis. It is common in children and there is often a positive family history. The exact etiology of the condition is unclear.

Tricyclic antidepressants such as imipramine are widely used in the treatment of enuresis, but while clinical efficacy is well documented, their mode of action is unclear. The antienuretic action of tricyclics is immediate, within a few hours or days, whereas their antidepressant action generally takes at least two to four weeks. Thus, it seems that the antienuretic action of these medications is independent of their antidepressant actions.

The first suggestion of a 5-HTergic influence on enuresis was made by Traskman-Bendz (1983) as a chance observation, during one of a series of classic studies on suicide. Thirty-two depressed patients, 12 with low CSF 5-HIAA, were evaluated for suicidality and were subsequently followed up. The low CSF HIAA values appeared to be a trait rather than a state-related phenomenon, since these values remained constant over time rather than showing responsivity to state-related variables. Subjects with low CSF 5-HIAA had a greater incidence of enuresis (four out of 12) after age five than subjects with high CSF 5-HIAA (2 out of 20). The author postulated a developmental imbalance of central cholinergic and 5-HTergic systems as being the pathogenetic basis of enuresis.

Based upon this report, and to examine possible 5-HTergic changes in this disorder, Weizmann et al. (1985) assayed platelet ^{3}H-imipramine binding in 16 enuretic children between the ages of two and 16, and in 22 matched controls. No significant change in the dissociation constant (K_d) was noted. However, the number of binding sites (B_{max}) was 22% lower in enuretics than in controls. Neither major mood disorders in the children themselves nor a family history of mood disorders appeared to be related to the reduction in the number of binding sites, since neither was reported for any of the subjects. To eliminate the possibility that this finding might be secondary to treatment with tricyclics, the study was repeated with a group of untreated adolescent enuretics (Weizmann et al., 1986), and platelet 5-HT uptake was also assayed. Once again, there was a significant decrease in the number of binding sites for imipramine in subjects relative to controls. However, all the other parameters (i.e., K_d for imipramine binding, V_{max} and K_m for 5-HT uptake) did not distinguish between the two groups. Interestingly, the reduction in binding sites was more marked in adolescents (29%) than in children (22%), possibly a reflection of the fact that enuresis in adolescents is considered a more serious disorder than childhood enuresis.

In conclusion, it would seem that 5-HT systems might be involved in the pathogenesis of enuresis, but until controlled studies of central 5-HT function, such as central neuroendocrine challenge studies using more specific 5-HTergic agents, are undertaken, preferably in older adolescents (for ethical reasons), this involvement cannot be defined more accurately.

TOURETTE'S SYNDROME

Tourette's syndrome (TS) is characterized by recurrent, involuntary, repetitive, rapid, purposeless motor movements and various vocal tics. Such movements can be voluntarily suppressed for minutes to hours, and the intensity of symptoms may vary over weeks to months. TS occurs more frequently in males than in females.

Three studies have shown that CSF 5-HIAA concentration is reduced in

TS, thus suggesting involvement of the 5-HT system in this condition (Cohen et al., 1978, 1979; Butler et al., 1979). In addition, there has been one report of decreased excretion of 5-HT in the urine of a TS patient (Yergani et al., 1983).

Singer et al. (1978) studied 14 patients with TS and have found no similarity to the Lesch-Nyhan syndrome, as has been suggested by other authors. Based upon the finding that haloperidol (a butyrophenone DA receptor blocker) is helpful in the treatment of TS, while symptoms of this illness increase with central stimulators, and based upon 5-HTergic findings, such as the induction of aggression by inhibition of 5-HT, they postulate that TS may be due to an imbalance between central DA and 5-HT, analogous to other movement disorders such as Parkinson's disease and Huntington's chorea.

More recently, interest in 5-HTergic systems in TS has reemerged with the finding that clonidine may be beneficial in the treatment of certain patients with TS, and with new research on the complex biological effects of clonidine in this condition. Bunney and DeRiemer (1982) and Leckman et al. (1984) have suggested that clonidine, primarily a specific alpha$_2$ agonist, has indirect effects on the 5-HT system as well, by decreasing NE influence on 5-HT neurons. They have also hypothesized that clonidine acts on the DAergic system by activating NE systems, with 5-HT pathways acting as a link between the two. To test the effects of clonidine on TS, Leckman et al. (1984) challenged TS patients and controls with 2.5–5.1 ng/kg of oral clonidine, and found no difference in WHBS. Subsequently, these investigators treated nine boys with TS with 0.15–0.3 mg/day of clonidine for 12 weeks. No significant changes in WHBS or platelet 5-HT levels were shown, although nonsignificant mean increases in WHBS and platelet 5-HT levels reached a peak 52 hours after the last clonidine dose (Leckman et al., 1986). These authors suggest that new techniques are needed to study in vivo central DAergic and 5-HTergic function (Riddle et al., 1986), in order to establish the role of these systems in mediating the beneficial effect of clonidine on TS.

KLEIN-LEVINE SYNDROME

Klein-Levine syndrome is a sleep disorder of adolescents, involving hypersomnia, hyperphagia, and hypersexuality. High levels of CSF 5-HIAA have been reported in both a patient with Klein-Levine syndrome and a patient with "subwakefulness" (Livrea et al., 1977). An autopsy report on another adolescent with Klein-Levine syndrome showed mild depigmentation of the locus coeruleus and the substantia nigra. Postmortem CSF levels of 5-HTP and 5-HIAA were elevated (Koerber, 1984).

These findings may indicate that some of the symptoms of Klein-Levine syndrome are a result of a neurotransmitter imbalance involving brain-stem 5-HTergic pathways. Clearly, a great deal of research remains to be done in this largely unexplored field.

DEPRESSION

The past decade has seen a revolution in the attitudes of child psychiatrists toward the subject of major depressive disorder in prepubertal children and adolescents. Formerly considered extremely rare, or even a theoretical impossibility (Rie, 1966), childhood depression is now thought to be a commonly encountered condition in child psychiatry (Kashani & Cantwell, 1983). In addition, it is now widely accepted that adult DSM-III criteria for depression apply for children as well and that there is no further need for ambiguous concepts such as "masked depression" (Cytrin et al., 1980).

Given this new descriptive resemblance to adult depression, it is natural that attempts have been made to explore the role of 5-HT in childhood depression (Kashani & Cantwell, 1983).

Rehavi et al. (1984) examined platelet ^{3}H-imipramine binding in children with major depressive disorder, comparing them with a group of normal controls and with children with conduct disorders. No differences were found, nor did the presence of a family history of major depression effect the ^{3}H-imipramine binding. Similarly, Ambrozini et al. (1987) found no differences in the V_{max} and K_m of platelet 5-HT uptake among actively depressed, recovered, or nondepressed child psychiatric patients, although V_{max} and K_d were significantly correlated in the actively depressed sample only. On the other hand, Rogeness et al. (1985) reported significantly lower platelet MAO and WHBS for children with major depression compared with schizophrenics and with schizotypal children, while Plizka et al. (1987) found that WHBS was significantly lower in depressed and anxious adolescents, compared with a group of adolescents with conduct disorder. Finally, reports that children with major depression respond to antidepressants that affect 5-HT also provide evidence that 5-HT dysfunction may be involved in childhood depression.

In conclusion, little work has been done to date on the role of 5-HT in childhood depression. However, given the huge body of data on the significance of the role of 5-HT in adult major depression, and with the proved efficacy of 5-HT–potentiating compounds in the treatment of both adult and childhood major depression, considerably more study in this area is warranted.

OBSESSIVE COMPULSIVE DISORDER

Obsessive compulsive disorder (OCD) often has its onset during or before puberty (Rapoport, 1986). In childhood, OCD is commonly associated with anorexia nervosa and Tourette's syndrome, as well as with encephalitis (Rapoport, 1986). As with OCD in adulthood, symptoms of childhood OCD include recurrent, persistent, ego-dystonic obsessions and repetitive stereotyped behaviors designed to affect future events or situations, which are carried out in a compulsive, excessive manner and are not connected to such future events in any realistic way.

As has been reported with adults, the tricyclic antidepressant clorimipramine hydrochloride, which is a potent 5-HT reuptake inhibitor, has beneficial effects for children with OCD (Flament et al., 1985). This has suggested that 5-HT mechanisms may be involved in childhood OCD. It should also be noted, however, that desmethylclorimipramine (clorimipramine's primary metabolite) and its 8-hydroxylated metabolites are powerful reuptake inhibitors of both 5-HT and NE (Linnoila et al., 1982), although more selective 5-HT blockers have not been shown to be as efficacious in this disorder as clomipramine (Flament et al., 1985).

Weizman et al. (1986) found that maximal platelet ^{3}H-imipramine binding in adult and adolescent OCD patients was lower than that of controls. 5-HT uptake parameters and affinity of binding of imipramine for platelets did not differ between patients and controls. These findings were no different in adults than in adolescents, suggesting that the duration of the disorder is not the explanation for this finding.

The most comprehensive study of 5-HT function in childhood OCD done to date was undertaken by Flament et al. (1987). These investigators found no significant difference in platelet 5-HT levels between drug-free OCD children and controls. Both platelet 5-HT concentration and platelet MAO activity were significantly and negatively correlated with pretreatment severity scores. In contrast, plasma epinephrine and NE levels showed no relationship to any measure of psychopathology. During five weeks of treatment with clorimipramine, platelet 5-HT concentration fell markedly in all patients, as did platelet MAO, although not significantly. Plasma NE levels increased significantly, while plasma epinephrine was left unchanged by treatment. Pretreatment platelet 5-HT levels correlated with response to treatment, as did the decrement in concentration during treatment.

It seems, therefore, that the 5-HT uptake inhibition effect of clorimipramine may be related to its antiobsessional properties in children.

LESCH-NYHAN SYNDROME

Another severe developmental disorder of childhood, the Lesch-Nyhan syndrome, is a sex-linked enzyme-deficiency disorder of purine metabolism characterized by self-mutilation, spasticity, mental and growth retardation, choreoathetosis, and hyperuricemia (Lesch & Nyhan, 1964). Since it has been hypothesized that abnormalities of 5-HT metabolism are also involved in this disorder, 5-HTP has been used in an attempt to treat it. Castells et al. (1979) have reported on a patient with Lesch-Nyhan syndrome who showed a decrease in CSF 5-HIAA and CSF HVA. 5-HTP administration did not affect retardation and neurological deficits in this patient, but did lead, at least temporarily, to a reduction in self-mutilation. Of course, considerably more work remains to be done in this area.

CONCLUSION

It is apparent from the foregoing that, as has been shown in adult psychopathology, there appears to be significant involvement of 5-HT mechanisms in a wide variety of childhood psychopathological entities. The ubiquitous nature of this involvement does not necessarily mean that these 5-HT mechanisms lack specificity. Rather, as van Praag has suggested for the range of adult psychiatric disorders, such dysfunctions may be more directly related to basic psychopathological dimensions, such as anxiety, aggressivity, impulsivity, and mood dysregulation, which cut across nosological boundaries (van Praag et al., 1987a, 1987b).

The most consistent abnormality found across the childhood psychiatric disorders discussed above involves the high blood levels of 5-HT in autism and other pervasive developmental disorders. Thus, 5-HT mechanisms may be disrupted by abnormalities in development (or vice versa), which are concomitantly found in these different diagnostic entities in child psychiatry.

Although ethical and technical problems remain, there is now an increased interest in using neuroendocrine challenges in children. These methods, in addition to recent advances in brain-imaging techniques, should allow us to obtain greater insight into the role of 5-HT in normal and disturbed development. It is to be hoped that these insights will enable us to develop specific pharmacological tools for what appear to be 5-HT–based disturbances of developmental psychopathology.

REFERENCES

Ambrozini, P., Metz, C., Kregel, L., Aurora, R., & Meltzer, H. (1987). Platelet serotonin in child and adolescent major depression. Presented at the American Academy of Child and Adolescent Psychiatry, Washington, D. C.

Anderson, G. M., Freedman, D. X., Cohen, D. J., Volkmar, F. R., Hoder, E. L., McPhedran, P., Minderaa, R. B., Hansen, C. R., & Young, J. G. (1987).

Whole blood serotonin in autistic and normal subjects. *J. Child Psychol. Psychiatry, 28*, 885–900.

Anderson, G. M., & Hoshino, Y. (1987). Neurochemical studies of autism. In D. J. Cohen & A. M. Donnellan (Eds.), *Handbook of autism and pervasive developmental disorders* (pp. 166–191). New York: Wiley.

Anderson, G. M., Minderaa, R. B., van Bentem, P. G., Volkmar, F. R., & Cohen, D. J. (1984). Platelet imipramine binding in autistic subjects. *Psychiatry Res., 11*, 133–141.

Belendiuk, K., Belendiuk, G. W., Freedman, D. X., & Antel, J. P. (1981). Neurotransmitter abnormalities in motor neurone disease. *Arch. Neurol., 38*, 15–417.

Bender, L., Faretra, G., & Combrinik, L. (1963). LDS and UML treatment of hospitalized disturbed children. In J. Wortis (Ed.), *Recent advances in biological psychiatry*, Vol. 6 (pp. 84–92). New York: Plenum Press.

Boullin, D. J., Bhagavan, H. N., O'Brien, R. A., & Youdin, M. B. H. (1976). Platelet monoamine oxidase in children with infantile autism. In M. Coleman (Ed.), *The autistic syndromes* (pp. 51–56). Amsterdam: North-Holland.

Boullin, D. J., Freeman, B. J., Geller, E., Ritvo, E., Rutter, M., & Yuwiler, A. (1982). Toward the resolution of conflicting findings. *J. Autism Dev. Disord., 12*, 97–98.

Bunney, B. S., & DeRiemer, S. A. (1982). Effect of clonidine on dopaminergic neuron activity in the substantia nigra: Possible indirect mediation by noradrenergic regulation of the serotonergic raphe system. *Adv. Neurol., 35*, 99–104.

Butler, I. J., Koslow, S. H., Seifert, W. E., Caprioli, R. M., & Singer, H. S. (1979). Biogenic amine metabolism in Tourette syndrome. *Ann. Neurol., 6*, 37–39.

Campbell, M., Fish, B., Shapiro, T., & Floyd, A. (1971). Imipramine in preschool autistic and schizophrenic children. *J. Autism Child. Schiz., 1*, 267–282.

Campbell, M., Friedman, E., DeVito, E., Greenspan, L., & Collins, P. J. (1974). Blood serotonin in psychotic and brain damaged children. *J. Autism Child. Schiz., 4*, 33–41.

Campbell, M., Small, A. M., Collins, P. J., Friedman, E., Daid, R., & Genieser, N. B. (1976). Levodopa and levoamphetamine: A crossover study in schizophrenic children. *Curr. Ther. Res., 19*, 70–86.

Campbell, M., Small, A., Adams, P., Curren, E., Spencer, E., Perry, R., & Lynch, N. (1987). Fenfluramine in infantile autism: A double blind controlled study. Presented at the American Academy of Child and Adolescent Psychiatry, Washington, D.C.

Cantwell, D. P., Sturzenberger, S., Burroughs, J., Salkin, B., & Green, J. (1977). Anorexia nervosa—an affective disorder? *Arch. Gen Psychiatry, 34*, 1087–1093.

Castells, C., Chakrabati, C., Winsberg, B. G., Hurwic, M., Perel, J. M., & Nyhan, W. L. (1979). Effects of L-5-hydroxytryptophan on monoamine and amino acid turnover in the Lesch-Nyhan syndrome. *J. Autism Dev. Disord., 9*, 95–103.

Clineschmidt, B. V., Zacchei, A. G., Totaro, J. A., Pflueger, A. D., McGuffin, J. C. & Wishonsky, T. I. (1978). Fenfluramine and brain serotonin. *Ann. N. Y. Acad. Sci., 305*, 222–241.

Cohen, D. J., Caparulo, B. K., Shaywitz, B. A., & Bowers, M. B. (1977). Dopamine and serotonin metabolism in neuropsychiatrically disturbed children. *Arch. Gen. Psychiatry, 34*, 545–550.

Cohen, D. J., Shaywitz, B. A., Caparulo, B., Young, J. G., & Bowers, M. B. (1978). Chronic multiple tics of Gilles de la Tourette's disease. CSF acid monoamine metabolites after probenecid administration. *Arch. Gen. Psychiatry, 35*, 245–250.

Cohen, D. J., Shaywitz, B. A., Johnson, W. T., & Bowers, M. (1974). Biogenic amines in autistic and atypical children. *Arch. Gen. Psychiatry, 31*, 845–853.

Cohen, D. J., Shaywitz, B. A., Young, J. G., Carbonari, C. M., Nathanson, J. A., Lieverman, D., Bowers, M. B., & Maas, J. W. (1979). Central biogenic amine metabolism in children with the syndrome of chronic multiple tics of Gilles de la Tourette: Norepinephrine, serotonin, and dopamine. *J. Am. Acad. Child Psychiatry, 18*, 320–341.

Cohen, D. J., Young, J. G., & Roth, J. A. (1977). Platelet monoamine oxidase in early childhood autism. *Arch. Gen. Psychiatry, 34*, 534–537.

Cook, E. H., Leventhal, B. L., Freedman, D. X., & Ravitz, A. (1987). Relationships of whole blood serotonin and plasma norepinephrine within families. Presented at the American Academy of Child and Adolescent Psychiatry, Washington, D. C.

Coppen, A. J., Eccleston, E. G., & Peet, M. (1973). Total and free tryptophan concentration in the plasma of depressive patients. *Lancet, 2*, 60–63.

Coppen, A. J., Gupta, K., & Eccleston, E. G. (1976). Plasma tryptophan in anorexia nervosa. *Lancet, 1*, 961.

Cytrin, L., McKnew, D. H., & Bunney, W. (1980). Diagnosis of depression in children: A reassessment. *Am. J. Psychiatry, 137*, 22–25.

Dugas, M., Mouren, M. C., Halfon, O., & Moron, P. (1985). Treatment of childhood and adolescent depression with mianserin. *Acta Psychiatr. Scand., 72*, (S320), 48–53.

Everett, G. M., & Borcherding, J. W. (1970). L-dopa: Effect on concentrations of dopamine, norepinephrine and serotonin in brains of mice. *Science, 168*, 849–850.

Ferguson, J. M. (1987). Treatment of an anorexia nervosa patient with fluoxetine. *Am. J. Psychiatry, 144*, 1239.

Fish, B., Campbell, M., Shapiro, T., & Floyd, A. (1969). Schizophrenic children treated with methysergide (Sansert). *Dis. Nerv. Sys., 30*, 534–540.

Flament, M. F., Rapoport, J. L., Berg, C. B., Sceery, W., Kilts, C., Mellstrom, B., & Linnoila, M. (1985). Clomipramine treatment of childhood obsessive-compulsive disorder: A double-blind controlled study. *Arch. Gen. Psychiatry, 42*, 977–983.

Flament, M. F., Rapoport, J. L., Murphy, D. L., Berg, C. J., & Lake, C. R. (1987). Biochemical changes during clomipramine treatment of childhood obsessive-compulsive disorder. *Arch. Gen. Psychiatry, 44*, 219–225.

Gattaz, W. F., Kaspar, S., & Propping, P. (1981). Low platelet MAO activity and schizophrenia. Sex differences. *Acta Psychiatr. Scand., 64*, 167–174.

Geller, E., Ritvo, E., Freeman, E., & Yuwiler, A. (1982). Preliminary observations on the effect of fenfluramine on blood serotonin and symptoms in three autistic boys. *N. Engl. J. Med.*, *307*, 165–169.

Gerner, R. H., Cohen, D. J., Fairbanks, L., Anderson, G. M., Young, J. G., Scheinin, M., Linnoila, M., Shaywitz, B. A., & Hare, T. A. (1984). CSF neurochemistry of women with anorexia nervosa and normal women. *Am. J. Psychiatry*, *141*, 1441–1444.

Gilberg, C. (1983). Low dopamine and serotonin levels in anorexia nervosa. *Am. J. Psychiatry*, *140*, 948–949.

Gilberg, C., Svennerholm, L., & Hamilton-Hellberg, C. (1983). Childhood psychosis and monoamine metabolites in spinal fluid. *J. Autism Dev. Disord.*, *13*, 383–396.

Goldberg, A. C., Halmi, K. A., Eckert, E. D., Casper, R., & Davis, J. M. (1979). Cyproheptadine in anorexia nervosa. *Br. J. Psychiatry*, *134*, 67–70.

Golden, G. S. (1987). Neurological functioning. In D. J. Cohen & A. M. Donnellan (Eds.), *Handbook of autism and pervasive developmental disorders* (pp. 133–147). New York: Wiley.

Goldstein, M., Mahanand, P., Lee, J., & Coleman, M. (1976). Dopamine-beta-hydroxylase and endogenous total 5-hydroxylindole levels in autistic patients and controls. In M. Coleman (Ed.), *The autistic syndrome* (pp. 57–63). Amsterdam: North-Holland.

Greenberg, A. S., & Coleman, M. (1976). Depressed 5-hydroxyindole levels associated with hyperactive and aggressive behavior. Relationship to drug response. *Arch. Gen. Psychiatry*, *33*, 331–336.

Guthrie, R. D., & Wyatt, R. J. (1975). Biochemistry and schizophrenia. III. A review of childhood psychosis. *Schizophr. Bull.*, *1*, 18–32.

Halmi, K. A., Eckert, E., LaDu, T. J., & Cohen, J. (1986). Anorexia nervosa. *Arch. Gen. Psychiatry*, *43*, 177–181.

Hanley, G., Stahl, S. M., & Freedman, D. X. (1977). Hyperserotonemia and amine metabolites in autistic and retarded children. *Arch. Gen. Psychiatry*, *34*, 521–531.

Hoshino, Y., Tachibana, R., Watanabe, M., Murata, S., Yokoyama, F., Kaneko, M., Yashima, &., & Kumashiro, H. (1984a). Serotonin metabolism and hypothalamic-pituitary function in children with infantile autism and minimal brain dysfunction. *Jpn. J. Psychiatry*, *26*, 937–945.

Hoshino, Y., Yamamoto, T., Kaneko, M., Tachibana, R., Watanabe, M., Ohno, Y., & Kumashiro, H. (1984b). Blood serotonin and free-tryptophan concentration in autistic children. *Neuropsychobiology*, *11*, 22–27.

Hyman, S. L., Coyle, J. T., Parke, J. C., Porter, C., Thomas, G. H., Jankel, W., & Batshaw, M. L. (1986). Anorexia and altered serotonin metabolism in a patient with argininosuccinic aciduria. *J. Pediatr.*, *108*, 705–709.

Jouve, J., Martineau, J., Mariotee, N., Barthelemy, C., Muh, J. P., & LeLord, G. (1986). Determination of urinary serotonin using liquid chromatography with electrochemical detection. *J. Chromatogr.*, *378*, 437–443.

Kashani, J. H., & Cantwell, D. P. (1983). Etiology and treatment of childhood depression: A biopsychological perspective. *Compr. Psychiatry*, *24*, 476–486.

Katsui, T., Okuda, M., Usuda, S., & Koizumi, T. (1986). Kinetics of 3H-serotonin uptake by platelets in infantile autism and developmental language disorder (including five pairs of twins). *J. Autism Dev. Disord.*, *6*, 69-76.

Kaye, W. H., Ebert, M. H., Raleigh, M., & Lake, R. (1984). Abnormalities in CNS monoamine metabolism in anorexia nervosa. *Arch. Gen. Psychiatry*, *41*, 350-355.

Koerber, R. K., Torkelson, R., Haven, G., Donaldson, J., Cohen, S. M., & Case, M. (1984). Increased cerebrospinal fluid 5-hydroxytryptamine and 5-hydroxyindoleacetic acid in Klein-Levine syndrome. *Neurol.*, *34*, 1597-1600.

Lake, R., Zeigler, M. G., & Murphy, D. L. (1977). Increased norepinephrine levels and decreased DBH activity in primary autism. *Arch. Gen. Psychiatry*, *35*, 553-556.

Leckman, J. F., Anderson, G. M., Cohen, D. J., Ort, S., Harcherik, D. F., Hoder, E. L., & Shaywitz, B. A. (1984). Whole blood serotonin and tryptophan levels in Tourette's disorder: Effects of acute and chronic clonidine treatment. *Life Sci.*, *35*, 2497-2503.

Leckman, J. F., Ort, S., Caruso, K. A., Anderson, G. M., Riddle, M. A., & Cohen, D. J. (1986). Rebound phenomena in Tourette's syndrome after abrupt withdrawal of clonidine. *Arch. Gen. Psychiatry*, *43*, 1168-1176.

Lesch, M., & Nyhan, W. L. (1964). A familial disorder of uric acid metabolism and central nervous system function. *Am. J. Med.*, *36*, 561-570.

Linnoila, M., Insel, T., Kilts, C., Potter, W. Z., & Murphy, D. L. (1982). Plasma steady-state concentrations of hydroxylated metabolites of clomipramine. *Clin. Pharmacol. Ther.*, *32*, 208-211.

Livrea, P., Puca, F. M., Barnaba, A., & Di Reda, L. (1977). Abnormal central monamine metabolism in humans with "true hypersomnia" and "subwakefulness." *Eur. J. Neurol.*, *15*, 71-76.

Miwa, S., Watanabe, Y., & Hayaishi, O. (1985). 6R-L-Erythro-5,6,7,8-tetrahydrobiopterin as a regulator of dopamine and serotonin biosynthesis in the rat brain. *Arch. Biochem. Biophys.*, *239*, 234-241.

Naruse, H., Hayashi, T., Takesada, M., Nakane, A., Yamazaki, K., Noguchi, T., Watanabe, Y., & Hayaishi, O. (1987). Therapeutic effect of tetrahydrobiopterin in infantile autism. *Proc. Jpn. Acad.*, *63*, 231-233.

Obuko, S., Hoshino, Y., & Kumashiro, H. (1979). Serum total and free tryptophan concentration in patients with Down's Syndrome. *Jpn. J. Brain Res.*, *5*, 78-79.

Ornitz, E. M. (1987). Neurophysiologic studies of infantile autism. In D. J. Cohen & A. M. Donnellan (Eds.), *Handbook of autism and pervasive developmental disorders* (pp. 148-165). New York: Wiley.

Partington, M. W., Tu, J. B., & Wong, C. Y. (1973). Blood serotonin levels in severe mental retardation. *Dev. Med. Child Neurol.*, *15*, 616-627.

Plizka, S. R., Rogeness, G. A., & Renner, P. (1987). Higher whole blood serotonin in aggressive juvenile delinquents. Presented at the American Academy of Child and Adolescent Psychiatry, Washington, D.C.

Rapoport, J. L. (1986). Childhood obsessive compulsive disorder. *J. Child Psychol. Psychiatry*, *27*, 289-295.

Realmuto, G. M., Jensen, J., Klykylo, W., Piggot, L., Stubbs, G., Yuwiler, A., Geller, E., Freeman, B. J., & Ritvo, E. (1986). Untoward effects of fenfluramine in autistic children. *J. Clin. Psychopharmacol.*, *6*, 350-355.

Rehavi, M., Weizman, R., Carel, C., Apter, A., & Tyano, S. (1984). High affinity 3H-imipramine binding in platelets of children and adolescents with major affective disorders. *Psychiatry Res.*, *13*, 31–39.

Riddle, M. A., Shaywitz, B. A., Leckman, J. F., Anderson, G. M., Shaywitz, S. E., Hardin, M. I., Ort, S., & Cohen, D. J. (1986). Brief debrisoquin loading to assess central dopaminergic function in children and adults. *Life Sci.*, *38*, 1041–1048.

Rie, H. E. (1966). Depression in childhood: A survey of some pertinent contributors. *J. Am. Acad. Child Psychiatry*, *5*, 653–685.

Riederer, P., Toifl, K., & Kruizik, P. (1982). Excretion of biogenic amine metabolites in anorexia nervosa. *Clin. Chim. Acta*, *123*, 27–32.

Ritvo, E., Freeman, B., Geller, E., & Yuwiler, A. (1983). Effects of fenfluramine on 14 outpatients with the syndrome of autism. *J. Am. Acad. Child Psychiatry*, *22*, 549–558.

Ritvo, E. R., Yuwiler, A., Geller, E., Kales, A., Rashkis, S., Schicor, A., Plotkin, S., Axelrod, R., & Howard, C. (1971). Effects of L-dopa in autism. *J. Autism Child Schiz.*, *1*, 190–205.

Ritvo, E. R., Yuwiler, A., Geller, E., Ornitz, E. M., Saeger, K., & Plotkin, S. (1970). Increased blood serotonin and platelets in early infantile autism. *Arch. Gen. Psychiatry*, *23*, 566–572.

Rogeness, G. A., Mitchell, E. L., Custer, G. J., & Harris, W. R. (1985). Comparison of whole blood serotonin and platelet MAO in children with schizophrenia and major depressive disorder. *Biol. Psychiatry*, *20*, 270–275.

Roth, J. A., Young, J. G., & Cohen, D. J. (1976). Platelet monoamine oxidase activity in children and adolescents. *Life Sci.*, *18*, 919–924.

Rotman, A., Caplan, R., & Szekely, G. A. (1980). Platelet uptake of serotonin in psychotic children. *Psychopharmacology*, *67*, 245–248.

Russell, G. F. M. (1967). The nutritional disorder in anorexia nervosa. *J. Psychosom Res.*, *11*, 141–149.

Safai-Kulti, S., Kulti, J., & Villberg, C. (1985). Impaired in vivo platelet reactivity in infantile autism. *Acta Paediatr. Scand.*, *74*, 799–800.

Schain, R. J., & Freedman, D. X. (1961). Studies on 5-hydroxyindole metabolism in autistic and other mentally retarded children. *J. Pediatr.*, *58*, 315–320.

Segawa, M., Noda, Y., Nezu, A., Uchiyama, A., Soda, M., & Nomura, Y. (1987). Trials of 5-hydroxytryptophan and low dose l-dopa on early infantile autism. Presented at the American Academy of Child and Adolescent Psychiatry, Washington, D. C.

Shaw, C. R., Lucas, J., & Rabinovitch, R. D. (1959). Metabolic studies in childhood schizophrenia. *Arch. Gen. Psychiatry*, *1*, 366–371.

Shaywitz, B. A., Cohen, D. J., & Bowers, M. B. (1975). Reduced cerebrospinal fluid 5-hydroxyindoleacetic acid and homovanillic acid in children with epilepsy. *Neurol.*, *25*, 74–79.

Singer, H. S., Pepple, J. M., Ramage, A. L., & Butler, I. J. (1978). Gilles de la Tourette syndrome: Further studies and thoughts. *Ann. Neurol.*, *4*, 21–25.

Strober, M. (1981). The significance of bulimia in juvenile anorexia nervosa. An exploration of possible etiologic factors. *Int. J. Eating Disord.*, *1*, 28–43.

Sutton, H. E., Read, J. H., & Arbor, A. (1958). Abnormal amino acid metabolism in a case suggesting autism. *Am. J. Dis. Child.*, *96*, 23–28.

Sverd, J., Kuptetz, S. S., Winsberg, B. G., Hurwic, M. J., & Becker, L. (1978). Effects of L-5-hydroxytryptophan in autistic children. *J. Autism Child. Schiz.*, *8*, 171–180.

Sylvester, O., Jorgensen, E., Mellerup, T., & Rafaelsen, O. J. (1970). Amino acid excretion in urine of children with various psychiatric diseases. *Dan. Med. Bull.*, *17*, 166–170.

Takahashi, S., Kanai, H., & Miyamoto, Y. (1976). Reassessment of elevated serotonin levels in blood platelets in early infantile autism. *J. Autism Child. Schiz.*, *6*, 317–326.

Takatsu, T., Onizawa, J., & Nakahato, M. (1965). Tryptophan metabolism disorder and therapeutic diet in children with infantile autism. *Amino Acids*, *5*, 13–14.

Todd, R. D., & Ciaranello, R. D. (1985). Demonstration of inter- and intraspecies differences in serotonin binding sites by antibodies from an autistic child. *Proc. Natl. Acad. Sci. U.S.A.*, *82*, 612–616.

Traskman-Bendz, L. (1983). CSF 5HIAA and a family history of psychiatric disorder. *Am. J. Psychiatry*, *140*, 1257.

Udenfriend, S., Titus, E., Weissbach, H., & Peterson, R. E. (1959). Biogenesis and metabolism of 5-hydroxyindole compounds. *J. Biol. Chem.*, *219*, 335–344.

van Praag, H. M. (1983). CSF 5HIAA in non-depressed schizophrenics. *Lancet*, *2*, 977-978.

van Praag, H. M. (1986). Biological suicide research: Outcome and limitations. *Biol. Psychiatry*, *21*, 1305–1323.

van Praag, H. M., Kahn, R., Asnis, G. M., Lemus, C. Z., & Brown, S. L. (1987a). Therapeutic indications for serotonin potentiating compounds: A hypothesis. *Biol. Psychiatry*, *22*, 205–212.

van Praag, H. M., Lemus, C., & Kahn, R. (1987b). Hormonal probes of central serotonergic activity: Do they really exist? *Biol. Psychiatry*, *22*, 86–98.

Watanabe, M., Hoshino, Y., & Kumashiro, H. (1980). The change of blood HGH, serotonin and cyclic AMP levels after L-5HTP loading in children with infantile autism. *Brain Res.*, *6*, 124–125.

Watanabe, Y., Miwa, S., Inoue, M., Fugiwara, M., & Hayaishi, O. (1984). Increase in monoamine biosynthesis in rat brain by peripheral administration of biopterin analogues. *Jpn. J. Pharmacol.*, *36*(suppl), 148P.

Weigand, R., & Perry, J. (1961). Effects of L-dopa, N-methyl N-benzyl-2 propanolamine HCl on DOPA, dopamine, norepinephrine, and serotonin levels in mouse brain. *Biochem. Pharmacol.*, *1*, 181–186.

Weizman, A., Carel, C., Tyano, S., & Rehavi, M. (1985). Decreased high affinity 3H-imipramine binding in platelets of enuretic children and adolescents. *Psychiatry Res.*, *14*, 39–46.

Weizman, R., Carmi, M., Tyano, S., Apter, A., & Rehavi, M. (1986). High affinity imipramine binding and serotonin uptake in platelets of adolescent females suffering from anorexia nervosa. *Life Sci.*, *38*, 1235–1242.

Weizman, R., Carmi, M., Tyano, S., & Rehavi, M. (1986). Reduced 3H-imipramine binding but unaltered 3H-serotonin uptake in platelets of adolescent enuretics. *Psychiatry Res.*, *19*, 37–42.

Winsberg, B. G., Sverd, J., Castells, S., Hurvic, M., & Perel, J. M. (1980). Estimation of monoamine and cyclic-AMP turnover and amino acid concentrations of spinal fluid in autistic children. *Neuropediatrics, 11*, 250–255.

Wyatt, R. J., Potkin, S. G., Bridge, T. P., Phelps, B. H., & Wise, C. D. (1980). Monoamine oxidase in schizophrenia: An overview. *Schizophr. Bull., 6*, 199–207.

Yamamoto, T., Hoshino, Y., Ono, Y., Okubo, S., Tachibana, R., Watanabe, M., Kaneko, M., & Kumashiro, H. (1982). Plasma-free tryptophan concentration before and after haloperidol treatment in autistic children. *Jpn. J. Brain Res., 8*, 102–103.

Yergani, V. K., Blackman, M., & Baker, G. B. (1983). Biological and psychological aspects of a case of Gilles de la Tourette's syndrome. *J. Clin. Psychiatry, 44*, 27–29.

Yuwiler, A., Ritvo, E. R., Bald, D., Kuyper, D., & Kopen, A. (1971). Examination of circadian rhythmicity of blood serotonin and platelets in autistic and nonautistic children. *J. Autism Child. Schiz., 1*, 421–435.

Zarcone, V., Kales, A., Scharf, M., Tan, T. L., Simmons, J. O., & Dement, W. C. (1973). Repeated oral ingestion of 5-hydroxytryptophan. *Arch. Gen. Psychiatry, 28*, 843–846.

Zemishlany, Z., Modai, I., Apter, A., Jerushalmy, Z., Samuel, E., & Tyano, S. (1987). Serotonin (5HT) uptake by platelets in anorexia nervosa. *Acta Psychiatr. Scand., 75*, 127–130.

10

Serotonin Dysregulation in Bulimia Nervosa
Neuroendocrine and Headache Responses

TIMOTHY D. BREWERTON
DENNIS L. MURPHY
HARRY A. BRANDT
MICHAEL D. LESEM
DAVID C. JIMERSON

A HISTORICAL PERSPECTIVE

Bulimia nervosa was originally described in the context of anorexia nervosa, first by Morton and later by others (Casper, 1983). It was only much later that bulimic symptoms were reported to occur in the context of obesity (Stunkard, 1959) and normal weight (Boskind-Lodahl, 1976; Crisp, 1981; Palmer, 1979; Russell, 1979). While the term "bulimia" often refers simply to the presence of binge eating and its associated counteractive measures, the current term "bulimia nervosa" was coined in 1979 by Gerald Russell to describe "an ominous variant of anorexia nervosa." Russell noted that bulimia nervosa occurs in the context of both low and normal weight and is characterized by intractable urges to eat, counteractive behaviors against resultant weight gain, and a morbid dread of fatness (Russell, 1979). The third edition of the *Diagnostic and Statistical Manual of Mental Disorders* (DSM-III) (American Psychiatric Association, 1980) defined the "bulimia" syndrome as fundamentally distinct from anorexia nervosa. Meanwhile, Russell (1985) clarified his original criteria for bulimia nervosa and required a past history of anorexia nervosa. Such a stipulation is complicated by differences in criteria for anorexia nervosa as well as by Rus-

TABLE 10-1
DSM-III-R Criteria for Bulimia Nervosa

A. Recurrent episodes of binge eating (rapid consumption of a large amount of food in a discrete period of time).
B. A feeling of lack of control over eating behavior during the eating binges.
C. The person regularly engages in either self-induced vomiting, use of laxatives or diuretics, strict dieting or fasting, or vigorous exercise in order to prevent weight gain.
D. A minimum average of two binge eating episodes a week for at least three months.
E. Persistent overconcern with body shape and weight.

sell's use of the term "cryptic anorexia" (Russell, 1985). Currently, the revised DSM-III (DSM-III-R) (American Psychiatric Association, 1987) uses Russell's term "bulimia nervosa" to describe the syndrome (see Table 10-1), but absent are the previous exclusion criteria for anorexia nervosa, as well as Russell's inclusion criteria requiring a past history of anorexia nervosa. For the purposes of this chapter, bulimia nervosa will refer to DSM-III-R criteria.

Suffice it to say that the relationship between bulimia nervosa and anorexia nervosa remains controversial. However, recent data document that bulimia nervosa patients, regardless of weight, have similar degrees and types of psychopathology (Garner et al., 1985a, 1985b; Mickalide & Andersen, 1985). This psychopathology tends to be qualitatively distinct from, and more severe than, that of nonbulimic anorexics (Beumont et al., 1976; Casper et al., 1980; Garfinkel et al., 1980; Strober, 1981). Comparative studies of biological variables in bulimic and nonbulimic patients with and without anorexia nervosa may contribute to the improved understanding and treatment of these enigmatic and perplexing conditions. One important biological system that is likely to be involved in the pathophysiology of bulimia nervosa is serotonin (5-HT).

RELATIONSHIP TO SEROTONIN DYSREGULATION

There are a number of reasons to suspect that the pathophysiology of bulimia nervosa involves 5-HT dysregulation (Brewerton et al., 1990). One of the strongest suggestions comes from links between bulimia nervosa and mood illnesses, particularly major depression. Bulimic patients have been noted by several authors to have high frequencies of depressed mood (Abraham & Beumont, 1982; Weiss & Ebert, 1983; Hatsukami et al., 1984; Johnson & Larson, 1982; Weiss & Ebert, 1983; Hatsukami et al., 1984; Walsh et al., 1985) and family histories of major depression (Hudson et al., 1984a, 1987; Walsh et al., 1985; Kassett et al., 1989). The hypothesis that major depression involves a reduction in serotonin function is a longstanding one, and is supported by several lines of evidence that have been reviewed elsewhere (Murphy et al., 1978; Coppen & Wood, 1982; Meltzer & Lowy, 1987; see Chapter 5 of this volume). Of particular relevance to this chapter are reports of blunted prolactin responses to intravenous L-tryptophan (L-TRP) in depressed patients (Charney et al., 1984; Cowen & Charig, 1987). Depressed mood has been reported to be induced in subjects blindly receiving diets low in L-TRP (Young et al., 1985; Smith et al., 1987), presumably as a result of lowering brain 5-HT.

Serotonergic manipulations are also known to result in marked changes in feeding behaviors, particularly satiety responses (Blundell, 1977, 1984, 1986; Samanin et al., 1982; Silverstone & Goodall, 1986), which are dysfunctional in bulimic patients (Chiodo & Latimer, 1986; Kissileff et al., 1986; Owen et al., 1985). Pharmacological enhancement of 5-HT neurotransmission in animals and humans generally leads to increased satiety (Blundell, 1984, 1986), with the exception of 5-HT_{1A} receptor activation, which induces feeding in animals in specific paradigms (Dourish et al., 1985, 1986, 1988). Conversely, attenuation of 5-HT neurotransmission by various methods leads to decreased satiety and increased food consumption and weight gain (Blundell 1984, 1986). The effects of 5-HT on feeding are thought to be mediated centrally via the medial hypothalamus (Leibowitz & Shor-Posner, 1986), although there is some evidence that peripheral mechanisms may play a part (Davies et al., 1983; Pollock & Rowland, 1981).

Disinhibited behavior may be modulated by 5-HT neurotransmission (Asberg et al., 1976a, 1976b, 1987; Brown et al., 1982; Brown & Goodwin, 1986; Linnoila et al., 1983), and may include more loosely defined forms of self-destructive, impulsive behaviors such as binge eating and self-induced vomiting, or purging. Bulimic anorexics share clinical features with normal-weight bulimics, in addition to binge eating, that are indicative of impulsivity, such as increased frequency of suicide attempts, alcohol/drug abuse, stealing, and capricious sexual behavior (Crisp et al., 1980; Garfinkel & Garner, 1982; Russell, 1979). Interestingly, several authors have noted the association between disturbed eating behaviors and self-mutilation (French & Nelson, 1972; Goldney & Simpson, 1975; Rosenthal et al., 1972; Simpson, 1975).

THE CHALLENGE PARADIGM

For these reasons and others, we studied in double-blind, randomized fashion a number of response measures following challenge with the postsynaptic 5-HT agonist, m-chlorophenylpiperazine (mCPP) (0.5 mg/kg p.o.), and separately, the dietary precursor of 5-HT, L-TRP (100 mg/kg in-

TABLE 10-2
A Summary of Prolactin Responses Following mCPP and L-TRP
in Normal-Weight Bulimia and Anorexia Nervosa
Relative to Healthy Controls

	mCPP	*L-TRP*
Normal-weight bulimia		
All subjects	↓	0
Depressed	↓	↓
Nondepressed	↓	0
Anorexia Nervosa		
Low weight	↓	↓
Goal weight	↓	↓

travenously). Subjects were age-matched females with bulimia nervosa ($n = 36$) and healthy female controls ($n = 15$). Methods have been described in detail elsewhere (Brewerton et al., 1988, in press).

This chapter will review neuroendocrine data and present new data on headache responses in anorexic and normal-weight patients with bulimia nervosa and healthy controls. The responses of patients with and without concurrent anorexia nervosa, as well as those with and without concurrent major depression, will be compared in an attempt to assess the potential effects of starvation and mood disorders on several measures of 5-HT function in bulimic patients using two similar but unique challenge agents. Data from nonbulimic anorexics have been excluded and are not reported at this time because of the very small sample sizes.

NEUROENDOCRINE RESPONSES

Previous Studies

Neuroendocrine results following challenge with each agent in normal-weight patients with bulimia nervosa and in patients with anorexia nervosa (with and without bulimia nervosa) have been reported in detail elsewhere and are summarized in Table 10-2. Prolactin, but not cortisol, responses to mCPP were blunted in patients with normal-weight bulimia (Brewerton et al., 1986b, 1987b; submitted) and in patients with anorexia nervosa at low weight and after refeeding to a predetermined goal weight (Brewerton et al., 1987a). Blunted prolactin, but not cortisol, responses to L-TRP were also observed in low-weight and goal-weight anorexic patients (Brewerton et al., 1987a), but not in the normal-weight patients with bulimia nervosa (Brewerton et al., 1987b, submitted). However, prolactin responses to L-TRP were significantly blunted in the subgroup of normal-weight bulimics with concurrent major depression (Brewerton et al., 1987b).

A Comparison of Prolactin Responses in Bulimia Nervosa

Peak delta prolactin levels following mCPP were comparable for all patient groups; however, each patient group was significantly lower than the group of controls. There were no significant differences between the normal-weight bulimics (6.5 ± 5.9 ng/ml) and the bulimic anorexics, either at low weight (3.7 ± 3.2 ng/ml) or at goal weight (6.8 ± 6.8 ng/ml). Peak delta prolactin did not significantly increase in the paired group of bulimic anorexics after refeeding. When the low-weight bulimic anorexics were combined with the normal-weight bulimics into one bulimia nervosa group, their mean peak delta prolactin ($n = 36$, 5.7 ± 5.4 ng/ml) was significantly lower than that of the controls ($n = 15$, 27.3 ± 28.7 ng/ml, $p < 0.0002$, Mann-Whitney test). There was no significant difference in peak delta prolactin in patients with DSM-III major depression ($n = 13$, 4.4 ± 4.0 ng/ml) compared with patients without this diagnosis ($n = 23$, 6.5 ± 6.0 ng/ml, unpaired t test).

Normal-weight bulimics had higher peak delta prolactin following L-TRP (17.6 ± 10.1 ng/ml) than the bulimic anorexics, both at low weight (7.2 ± 6.8 ng/ml, $p \leq 0.006$, unpaired t test) and at goal weight (10.4 ± 6.6 ng/ml, $p \leq 0.06$). Peak delta prolactin did not significantly increase in the paired group of bulimic anorexics after refeeding ($n = 9$, $p = 0.12$, paired t test). If the low-weight bulimic anorexics are combined with the normal-weight bulimics, prolactin responses following L-TRP are not significantly different from controls. However, bulimia nervosa patients with major depression have blunted peak delta prolactin responses ($n = 11$, 8.1 ± 7.3 ng/ml) in comparison with nondepressed patients ($n = 22$, 17.0 ± 10.4 ng/ml, $p \leq 0.02$, unpaired t test) and controls (25.4 ± 21.0 ng/ml, $p < 0.02$, Mann-Whitney test).

Comparison of Cortisol Responses in Bulimia Nervosa

Peak delta cortisol levels following both mCPP and L-TRP were comparable for all groups regardless of the presence of anorexia nervosa or mood disorder. There were no significant differences between the normal-weight bulimics and the bulimic anorexics, either at low weight or at goal weight. There was a trend for peak delta cortisol following mCPP (but not L-TRP) to increase in the paired group of bulimic anorexics after refeeding ($n = 7$, $p \leq 0.09$, paired t test), although this appears to be due to higher mCPP plasma levels in the goal-weight patients. When the low-weight bulimic anorexics were combined with the normal-weight bulimics into one bulimia nervosa group, the mean peak delta cortisol remained similar to that of the controls. There was no significant difference in peak delta cortisol responses in patients with DSM-III major depression compared with patients without this diagnosis.

HEADACHE AS A MEASURE OF 5-HT RECEPTOR SENSITIVITY

In the course of the challenge studies described above, severe headaches with features of common migraine were noted in 54% of subjects eight to 12 hours after receiving mCPP (Brewerton et al., 1988). None of the same subjects developed similar late-occurring headaches following placebo or L-TRP. Headache incidence was significantly greater in subjects with a personal and/or family history of migraine. Headache ratings were also significantly correlated with peak concentration of mCPP in plasma occurring several hours earlier, whether or not there was a predisposition to migraine (Figure 10-1.) Although the frequency of the migrainelike headaches was not significantly different among normal-weight bulimics, anorexics, and controls, the data presented below suggest that patients with bulimia nervosa, regardless of weight, mood, or migraine history, demonstrate a greater susceptibility to the development of severe migrainelike headaches than controls. The mechanism by which mCPP induces migrainelike headache responses is discussed in detail elsewhere (Brewerton et al., 1988c), but may involve a "rebound" vasodilatory response to stimulation of 5-HT receptors in vascular tissues. Although the specific 5-HT receptor type involved is uncertain, contraction of vascular smooth muscle is thought to be mediated primarily via $5\text{-}HT_2$ receptors (Van Nueten et al., 1985a, 1985b).

Headache Ratings

Headache ratings were not significantly different at any time between bulimic patients with and without concurrent anorexia nervosa; hence these data have been combined for further analysis. The mean maximum headache ratings for the different groups are shown in Figure 10-2; the total group of bulimic patients have significantly higher ratings than controls ($p \leq 0.003$, Mann-Whitney test). In the seven bulimic anorexic patients rechallenged at goal weight, headache ratings were almost identical to their paired low-weight ratings, so they are not reported. As seen in Figure 10-3, patients with bulimia nervosa reported greater head pain than controls eight ($p \leq 0.1$) and 12 hours ($p < 0.01$) after receiving mCPP. The overall frequency of late-onset "severe" headaches (defined by a self-rating of "3 = severe" at the eight- or 12-hour point) following mCPP was significantly higher in the patients (23 of 36, 64%) than in the controls 5 of 15, 33%) ($p < 0.05$, Fisher's exact test). In addition, more patients (31 of 36, 86%) than controls (nine of 15, 60%; $p < 0.05$, Fisher's exact test) reported some degree of head pain.

MAXIMUM HEADACHE RATINGS FOLLOWING
m-CPP vs PEAK m-CPP CONCENTRATIONS

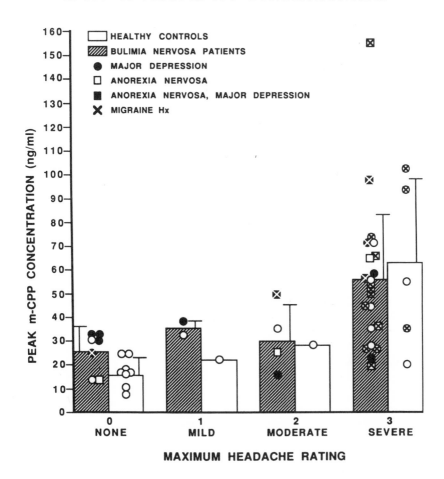

Figure 10-1. Mean maximum headache ratings following mCPP are correlated with the peak plasma level of mCPP occurring several hours earlier as well as the presence of a personal or family history of migraine.

Migrainous Symptoms

Symptoms typical of common migraine—nausea, involuntary vomiting, photophobia, unilaterality, and throbbing (Ad Hoc Committee on Classification of Headache, 1962)—were higher in the patient group than in the controls (Figure 10-4). There were significantly more patients (23 of 36,

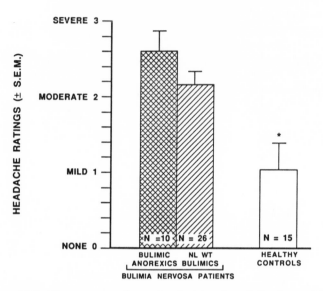

Figure 10-2. The mean maximum headache ratings following mCPP are not significantly different between bulimic anorexics and normal weight (NL WT) bulimics. The combined group of bulimia nervosa patients have significantly higher ratings than controls (*, $p \leq 0.003$, Mann-Whitney test)

64%) than controls (three of 15, 20%; $p < 0.005$, Fisher's exact test) reporting two or more of these symptoms in conjunction with headaches. Headaches associated with two or more of the migrainous symptoms were operationally defined as "migrainelike." No subject reported sensory or motor symptoms indicative of classical migraine.

Migraine History

To clarify further the relationship of mCPP-induced headaches to migraine, subjects were categorized based on personal and family history of migraine (Tables 10-3 and 10-4). Since most subjects with a personal or family history of migraine experienced a severe migrainelike headache following mCPP (Brewerton et al., 1988), increased vulnerability to the drug effect in bulimia nervosa patients could be assessed only by comparing personal and family history negative subjects. More patients with a negative personal and family history (eight of 19) than matched controls (one of 12) developed a severe migrainelike headache ($p < 0.05$, Fisher's exact test) (Table 10-3). Mean maximum headache ratings after mCPP were significantly

MEAN HEADACHE RATINGS FOR m-CPP STUDY DAY

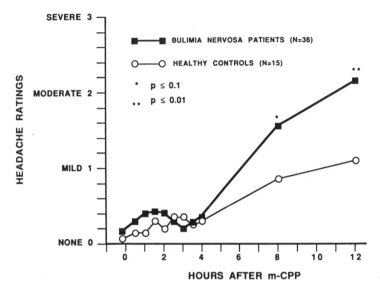

Figure 10-3. Mean headache ratings are higher in patients with bulimia nervosa than in controls at 8 (*, $p \leq 0.1$, Mann-Whitney test) and 12 hours (**, $p \leq 0.01$) after receiving mCPP.

higher in patients with negative histories (1.8 ± 1.3) than their control counterparts (0.6 ± 1.2, $p < 0.02$, Mann-Whitney test). These patients also had a significantly greater number of migrainous symptoms ($p \leq 0.001$, Mann-Whitney test) (Table 10-4).

mCPP Levels

Maximum headache ratings were correlated to peak mCPP levels in the controls (rho = 0.77, $p \leq 0.0007$), in the patients (rho = 0.58, $p \leq 0.0002$), and in the total group (rho = 0.70, $p \leq 0.0001$). When predisposed subjects were excluded, peak mCPP levels were significantly higher in the patients (35.5 ± 16.5 ng/ml) than in the controls (21.8 ± 12.5 ng/ml, $p < 0.02$), and there remained a significant correlation between maximum headache ratings and peak mCPP levels in the controls (rho = 0.63, $p \leq 0.03$), the patients (rho = 0.54, $p \leq 0.02$), and the total group (rho = 0.61, $p \leq 0.003$).

Relationship to Other Measures

Maximum headache ratings were correlated to peak delta prolactin following mCPP in the patients (rho = 0.51, $p \leq 0.0015$), but not in the con-

FREQUENCY OF MIGRAINOUS SYMPTOMS ASSOCIATED WITH m-CPP HEADACHES

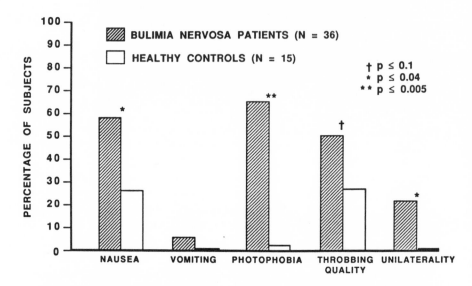

Figure 10-4. The frequency of migrainous symptoms associated with mCPP headaches is higher in patients than controls: nausea (*, $p \leq 0.04$); vomiting (NS); photophobia (**, $p \leq 0.005$); throbbing quality (+, $p \leq 0.1$), and unilaterality (*, $p \leq 0.04$). Significantly more patients (23 of 36, 64%) than controls (three of 15, 20%; $p < 0.005$, Fisher's exact test) reported two or more of these symptoms in conjunction with headaches.

trols or in the total group. Maximum headache ratings were also correlated to peak delta temperature following mCPP in the patients (rho = 0.45, $p \leq 0.006$) and the total group (rho = 0.25, $p \leq 0.05$), but not in the controls. Maximum headache ratings were also correlated to Hamilton Depression ratings in the total group ($n = 50$, rho = 0.26, $p \leq 0.07$), but not in the

TABLE 10-3
Frequency of Severe Migrainelike Headaches Following mCPP Sorted by Personal and Family History (Hx) of Migraine

Personal Hx	Family Hx	Patients	Controls
−	−	8/19*	1/12
+	−	3/4	−
−	+	8/9	2/3
+	+	4/4	−

*$p < 0.05$, Fisher's exact test.

TABLE 10-4
Mean Number of Migrainous Symptoms Following mCPP
Sorted by Personal and Family History (Hx) of Migraine

Personal Hx	Family Hx	Patients	Controls
−	−	1.4*	0.2
+	−	2.5	—
−	+	3.1	2.0
+	+	3.0	—

*$p < 0.001$, Mann-Whitney test.

patients ($n = 30$) or the controls ($n = 15$) alone. There were no significant correlations between maximum headache ratings and weight, other neuroendocrine responses, temperature responses, or Beck Depression Inventory scores. However, the one patient with a past history of migraine who did not develop a severe migrainelike headache was depressed, whereas none of the other seven predisposed patients with headaches were depressed. In the group of 23 patients with severe migrainelike headaches, there was a trend toward an inverse relationship between the presence of a personal history of migraine and the presence of concurrent major depression ($p < 0.06$, Fisher's exact test). No relationship between maximum headache ratings and menstrual phase was evident. In subjects who had had lumbar punctures three to 10 days prior to challenge with mCPP, maximum headache ratings were not significantly correlated with cerebrospinal fluid (CSF) 5-hydroxyindoleacetic acid (5HIAA), the primary metabolite of 5HT, or with CSF homovanillic acid (HVA), the primary metabolite of dopamine, in the patients, the controls, or the total group. However, there were notable negative correlations between maximum headache ratings and CSF MHPG (3-methoxy-4-hydroxyphenethyleneglycol, the principal metabolite of norepinephrine) in the total ($n = 35$, rho $= -0.43$, $p = 0.01$) and bulimic groups ($n = 30$, rho $= -0.35$, $p = 0.057$), but not in the controls, although this was a small sample size ($n = 5$).

Comment

These results suggest that patients with bulimia nervosa, irrespective of a personal or family history of migraine, are more sensitive than controls to the induction of severe migrainelike headaches by mCPP. Although the patients without a predisposition to migraine had higher peak mCPP concentrations than comparable controls, it is unlikely that this factor alone accounts for the severity of headaches experienced by the bulimic patients. From a purely clinical perspective, these headaches were extremely incapacitating. Such severe migrainelike headaches have not been reported or noted by other investigators in either normal controls (Mueller et al., 1985; Zohar et al., 1987) or other nonbulimic patients (Zohar et al., 1987) who achieved similar or higher peak mCPP concentrations (the original samples having been assayed in the same laboratory). This is also true for studies of subjects without migraine histories using intravenous mCPP, which results in much higher concentrations than those produced by oral administration (Lawlor et al., 1989; Murphy, personal communication).

It should also be noted that the method used to classify a family history of migraine relied solely on patient report and was not based on direct interviews with relatives, thereby probably favoring type I errors. Since migraine affects approximately 3 to 15% of the general population (Adams & Victor, 1981; France & Keefe, 1987), the fact that 16 (44%) of 36 patients reported a family history of migraine does indeed suggest overinclusion of bulimics in the positive family history group. A true difference in headache response between bulimics and controls would then have been diluted. On the other hand, a genetic link between bulimia nervosa and migraine is viable, particularly in light of the abundant evidence for 5-HT dysfunction in migraine (Eadie & Tyrer, 1985). A study of the families of 56 anorexia nervosa patients revealed that 30% of the mothers had a history of migraine (Kalucy et al., 1977), although it was not stated whether the anorexic patients were bulimic or not. Given the role of 5-HT in the mediation of pain (Roberts, 1984), another possible interpretation of these data is that bulimics are more sensitive to pain induction than controls, but further studies are needed to clarify this.

Even though bulimia nervosa and migraine appear unrelated, they actually share many common features. Both are often characterized by vomiting (often associated with an experience of relief), alterations in appetite, relief or termination of the episode with sleep, and depressive and autonomic symptomatology (Sicuteri, 1982; France & Keefe, 1987). Bulimia and migraine occur predominantly in females, and both can involve perceptual distortions of body image (Klee, 1975). Furthermore, the psychological attributes described in migraine patients, such as increased emotionality, anxiety, hostility, somatization (Henryk-Gutt & Rees, 1973), and depression (Crisp et al., 1977), are similar to those described in bulimic patients. Pharmacological treatments, such as antidepressant medications, are effective in both migraine (Raskin, 1981; Ziegler et al., 1987) and bulimia nervosa (Gwirtsman et al., 1984), and are thought to work largely via their effects on 5-HT function, particularly downregulation of 5-HT receptors (Fozard, 1982; Fuxe et al., 1983; Wilner, 1985).

These data imply a complicated relationship between migraine and depression. On the one hand, Hamilton depression ratings are positively correlated with headache responses; on the other hand, the presence of a major depression appears to be associated with a dampened headache response. The literature on this subject is unclear. While depression appears to be a common symptom associated with migraine (Harrigan et al., 1984), Crisp (1981) describes an inverse relationship between migraine and levels of depression. Philips and Hunter (1982) did not find an association between the diagnosis of depression and headache, although headache patients had higher depressive ratings. Garvey and colleagues (1984) reported that the prevalence of migraine is higher in depressed males, but not females, with RDC-defined major depressive disorder compared with the general population (Garvey et al., 1984). Other, more recent investigations have also supported a positive familial association between migraine and depression (Merikangas & Angst, 1988; Sandler et al., 1989).

Although circumstantial, these links between bulimia and migraine, bulimia and depression, and migraine and depression are consistent with the possibility of a common underlying dysregulation of 5-HT function in these disorders. Further studies of the relationships among bulimia nervosa, migraine, and mood disorder are warranted.

Since maximum headache ratings were negatively correlated to CSF MHPG, it appears that the overall "adrenergic tone" of the CNS influences vascular responses to 5-HT agonists. This is not surprising given the extensive data indicating an elaborate anatomical and functional network involving the adrenergic and serotonergic systems (Ortmann et al., 1981; Stockmeier et al., 1985; Rappaport et al., 1985; Houston & Vanhoutte, 1986; Limberger et al., 1986; Sulser & Sanders-Bush, 1987). In particular, beta-adrenergic blockade has been reported to enhance 5-HT$_2$ receptor sensitivity in animals (Cowen et al., 1982) and to lower CSF 5-HIAA in humans (Scheinin et al., 1984). The adrenergic system is also thought to play a role in the pathogenesis of migraine (Eadie & Tyrer, 1985).

SUMMARY AND CONCLUSIONS

Evidence has been reviewed and presented in support of 5-HT dysregulation in bulimia nervosa. Prolactin responses following mCPP are markedly blunted in patients with bulimia nervosa, regardless of the presence of anorexia nervosa or major depression, whereas prolactin responses following L-TRP are blunted only in the presence of anorexia nervosa or major depression. Cortisol responses following both serotonergic agents are similar in all diagnostic groups. However, headache responses following mCPP were greater in bulimic patients, regardless of the presence of anorexia nervosa or major depression. These findings suggest that postsynaptic 5-HT receptor sensitivity is altered in hypothalamic-pituitary serotonergic pathways and the vascular tissues of bulimia nervosa patients. Additional disturbances in 5-HT function, perhaps presynaptic ones, may be associated with anorexia nervosa and major depression. Similar alterations in other 5-HT pathways at or above the level of the hypothalamus may contribute to binge eating and other behavioral symptoms of bulimia nervosa. Whether 5-HT receptor sensitivity is decreased or increased probably depends on anatomical location and differential involvement of 5-HT receptor subtypes, as well as on the influence of other neurochemical systems. Further studies exploring the functional integrity of 5-HT receptors and their subtypes are warranted in bulimia nervosa patients, as well as in patients with nonbulimic anorexia nervosa, minor and major depression without an eating disorder, and migraine and other headache patients. The present results also emphasize the relevance of testing serotonergic drugs in the treatment of bulimia nervosa and related disorders.

REFERENCES

Abraham, S. F., & Beumont, P. J. V. (1982). How patients describe bulimia or binge eating. *Psychol. Med.*, *12*, 625-635.

Adams, R. D., & Victor, M. (1981). Headache and other craniofacial pains. In R. D. Adams & M. Victor (Eds.), *Principles of neurology* (2nd ed.) (pp. 117-135). New York: McGraw-Hill.

Ad Hoc Committee on Classification of Headache (1962). Classification of headache. *Arch. Neurology, 6*, 173-176.

American Psychiatric Association (1980). *Diagnostic and Statistical Manual of Mental Disorders* (2nd ed.). Washington, D.C.: American Psychiatric Association.

American Psychiatric Association (1987). *Diagnostic and Statistical Manual of Mental Disorders* (3rd ed. rev.). Washington, D.C.: American Psychiatric Association.

Asberg, M., Thoren, P., & Traskman, L. (1976a). "Serotonin depression"—A biochemical subgroup within the affective disorders? *Science, 191*, 478.

Asberg, M., Traskman, L., & Thoren, P. (1976b). 5-HIAA in the cerebrospinal fluid a biochemical suicide predictor? *Arch. Gen. Psychiatry, 33*, 1193.

Asberg, M., Schalling, D., Traskman-Bendz, L., & Wagner, A. (1987). Psychobiology of suicide, impulsivity, and related phenomena. In H. Meltzer (Ed.), *Psychopharmacology: The third generation of progress* (pp. 655-668). New York: Raven Press.

Beumont, P. J. V., George, G. C. W., & Smart, D. E. (1976). 'Dieters' and 'vomiters and purgers' in anorexia nervosa. *Psychol. Med.*, *6*, 617-622.

Blier, P., de Montigny, C., & Chaput, Y. (1987). Modifications of the serotonin system by antidepressant treatments: Implications for the therapeutic response in major depression. *J. Clin. Psychopharmacol., 7*, 24S-35S.

Blundell, J. E. (1977). Is there a role for serotonin (5-hydroxy-tryptamine) in feeding? *Int. J. Obes.*, *1*, 15-42.

Blundell, J. E. (1984). Serotonin and appetite. *Neuropharmacology, 23*, 1537-1551.

Blundell, J. E. (1986). Serotonin manipulations and the structure of feeding behaviour. *Appetite, 7,* 39–56.

Boskind-Lodahl, M. (1976). Cinderella's stepsisters: A feminist perspective on anorexia nervosa and bulimia. *J. Wom. Cult. Soc., 2,* 342–356.

Brewerton, T. D., Brandt, H. A., Lesem, D. T., Murphy, D. L., & Jimerson, D. C. (1990). Serotonin in eating disorders. In E. Coccaro & D. Murphy (Eds.), *Serotonin in major psychiatric disorders.* Washington, D.C.: American Psychiatric Press.

Brewerton, T. D., Murphy, D. L., Mueller, E. A., & Jimerson, D. C. (1988). The induction of migraine-like headaches by the serotonin agonist, m-chlorophenylpiperazine. *Clin. Pharmacol. Ther., 43,* 605–609.

Brewerton, T. D., Heffernan, M. M., & Rosenthal, N. E. (1986a). Psychiatric aspects of the relationship between eating and mood. *Nutr. Rev., 44*(Suppl), 78–88.

Brewerton, T. D., Mueller, E. A., George, D. T., Brandt, H. A., Lesem, M. D., Narang, P. K., Jimerson, D. C., & Murphy, D. L. (1986b). Blunted prolactin response to the serotonin agonist m-chlorophenylpiperazine (m-CPP) in bulimia. *Book of abstracts and poster sessions.* 15th Collegium Internationale Neuro-Psychopharmacologium Congress. San Juan, Puerto Rico, p. 186.

Brewerton, T. D., & McLaughlin, D. (1985). Circannual cyclicity of affective illness in Hawaii. IVth World Congress of Biological Psychiatry. Philadelphia, Pa., Abstract #528.3, p. 404.

Brewerton, T. D., Mueller, E. A., Brandt, H. A., Lesem, M. D., Murphy, D. L., & Jimerson, D. C. (1987a). Evidence for serotonin dysregulation in anorexia. *New research abstracts,* 140th Annual Meeting of the American Psychiatric Association (p. 123). Washington, D.C.: American Psychiatric Association.

Brewerton, T. D., Mueller, E. A., Murphy, D. L., & Jimerson, D. C. (1987b). Neuroendocrine effects of 5-HT agents in bulimia. *CME syllabus and scientific proceedings summary,* 140th Annual Meeting of the American Psychiatric Association, p. 85. Washington, D.C.: American Psychiatric Association.

Brewerton, T. D., Mueller, E. A., Lesem, D. T., Brandt, H. A., Quearry, B., George, D. T., Murphy, D. L. & Jimerson, D. C. (submitted). Neuroendocrine responses to m-chlorophenylpiperazine and L-tryptophan in bulimia.

Brown, G. L., & Goodwin, F. K. (1986). Human aggression and suicide. *Suicide Life Threat. Behav., 16,* 223–243.

Brown, G. L., Ebert, M. H., Boyer, P. F., et al. (1982). Aggression, suicide, and serotonin: relationships to c.s.f. amine metabolites. *Am. J. Psychiatry, 139,* 741–746.

Casper, R. C. (1983). On the emergence of bulimia nervosa as a syndrome: A historical view. *Int. J. Eating Dis., 2,* 3–16.

Casper, R. C., Eckert, E. D., Halmi, D. A., Goldberg, S. C., & Davis, J. M. (1980). Bulimia. Its incidence and clinical importance in patients with anorexia nervosa. *Arch. Gen. Psychiatry, 37,* 1030–1035.

Charig, E. M., Anderson, I. M., Robinson, J. M., Nutt, D. J., & Cowen, P. J. (1986). L-tryptophan and prolactin release: Evidence for interaction between 5-HT$_1$ and 5-HT$_2$ receptors. *Hum. Psychopharmacol., 1,* 93–97.

Charney, D. S., Heninger, G. R., Reinhard, J. F., Sternberg, D. E., & Hafstead, K.

M. (1982). The effect of intravenous l-tryptophan on prolactin and growth hormone and mood in healthy subjects. *Psychopharmacology, 7*, 217–222.

Charney, D. S., Heninger, G. R., & Sternberg, D. E. (1984). Serotonin function and mechanism of action of antidepressant treatment. Effects of amitriptyline and desipramine. *Arch. Gen. Psychiatry, 41*, 359–365.

Charney, D. C., Menkes, D. B., & Heninger, G. R. (1981). Receptor sensitivity and the mechanism of action of antidepressant treatment: Implications for the etiology and therapy of depression. *Arch. Gen. Psychiatry, 38*, 1160–1180.

Chiodo, J., & Latimer, P. R. (1986). Hunger perceptions and satiety responses among normal-weight bulimics and normals to a high-calorie, carbohydrate-rich food. *Psychol. Med., 16*, 343–349.

Coppen, A., & Wood, K. (1982). 5-Hydroxytryptamine in the pathogenesis of affective disorders. In B. T. Ho, J. C. Schoolar, & E. Usdin (Eds.), *Serotonin in biological psychiatry* (pp. 249–258). New York: Raven Press.

Cowen, P. J., & Charig, E. M. (1987). Neuroendocrine responses to intravenous tryptophan in major depression. *Arch. Gen. Psychiatry, 44*, 958–966.

Cowen, P. J., Grahame-Smith, D. G., Green, A. R., & Heal, D. J. (1982). B-Adrenoceptor agonists enhance 5-hydroxytryptamine-mediated behavioural responses. *Br. J. Pharmac., 76*, 265–270.

Crisp, A. H., Shu, L. K. G., & Harding, B. (1980). The string hoarder and verocious spender: Stealing in anorexia nervosa. *J. Psychosomatic Res., 24*, 225–231.

Crisp, A. H. (1981a). Laterality of migraine and reported affect. *J. Affect. Dis., 3*, 71–75.

Crisp, A. H. (1981b). Anorexia nervosa at normal body weight! The abnormal weight control syndrome. *Int. J. Psychiatry Med., 11*, 203–234.

Crisp, A. H., Kalucy, R. S., McGuinness, B., Ralph, P. C., & Harris, G. (1983). Some clinical, social, and psychological characteristics of migraine subjects in the general population. *Postgraduate Medical Journal, 53*, 691–697.

Davies, R. F., Rossi, J., Panksepp, J., Bean, N. J., & Zolovick, A. J. (1983). Fenfluramine anorexia: A peripheral locus of action. *Physiol. Behav., 30*, 723–730.

Dourish, C. T., Cooper, S. J., Gilbert, F., Coughlan, J., & Iversen, S. D. (1988). The 5-HT$_{1A}$ agonist 8-OH-DPAT increases consumption of palatable wet mash and liquid diets in the rat. *Psychopharmacol., 94*, 58–63.

Dourish, C. T., Hutson, P. H., & Curzon, G. (1985). Low doses of the putative serotonin agonist 8-hydroxy-2-(di-n-propylamino) tetralin (8-OH-DPAT) elicit feeding in the rat. *Psychopharmacol., 86*, 197–204.

Dourish, C. T., Hutson, P. H., Kennett, G. A., & Curzon, G. (1986). 8-OH-DPAT-induced hyperphagia: Its neural basis and possible therapeutic relevance. *Appetite, 7*(Suppl), 127–140.

Eadie, M. J., & Tyrer, J. H. (1985). *The biochemistry of migraine* (pp. 45–97). Lancaster, England: MTP Press.

Fairburn, C. G. (1984). Bulimia: Its epidemiology and management. In A. J. Stunkard & E. Stellar (Eds.), *Eating and its disorders* (p. 235). New York: Raven Press.

Fairburn, C. G., & Cooper, P. J. (1982). Self-induced vomiting and bulimia nervosa: An undetected problem. *Br. Med. J.*, *284*, 1153–1155.

Fairburn, C. G., & Cooper, P. J. (1984). The clinical features of bulimia nervosa. *Br. J. Psychiatry*, *144*, 238–246.

Fozard, J. R. (1982). Basic mechanisms of antimigraine drugs. *Adv. Neurol.*, *33*, 295–307.

France, R. D., & Keefe, F. J. (1987). Chronic pain. In R. Michels, J. O. Cavenar, A. M. Cooper, S. B. Guze, L. L. Judd, G. L. Klerman, & A. J. Solnit (Eds.), *Psychiatry*. Vol. 2, Ch. 104 (pp. 1–12). New York: Basic Books.

French, A. P., & Nelson, H. L. (1972). Genital self-mutilation in women. *Arch. Gen. Psychiatry*, *27*, 618–620.

Fuxe, K., Ogren, S. O., Agnati, L. F., Benfenati, F., Fredholm, B., Andersson, K., Zini, I., & Eneroth, P. (1983). Chronic antidepressant treatment and central 5-HT synapses. *Neuropharmacology*, *22*, 389–400.

Garfinkel, P. E., & Garner, D. M. (1982). Subtypes of anorexia nervosa. In P. E. Garfinkel & D. M. Garner (Eds.), *Anorexia nervosa: A multidimensional perspective* (pp. 40–57). New York: Brunner/Mazel.

Garfinkel, P. E., Moldofsky, H., & Garner, D. M. (1980). The heterogeneity of anorexia nervosas. Bulimia as a distinct subgroup. *Arch. Gen. Psychiatry*, *37*, 1036–1040.

Garner, D. M., Garfinkel, P. E., & O'Shaughnessy, M. (1985a). The validity of the distinction between bulimia with and without anorexia nervosa. *Am. J. Psychiatry*, *142*, 581–587.

Garner, D. M., Olmsted, M. P., & Garfinkel, P. E. (1985b). Similarities among bulimic groups selected by different weights and weight histories. *J. Psychiatr. Res.*, *19*, 129–134.

Garvey, M. J., Tollefson, G. D., & Schaffer, C. B. (1984). Migraine headaches and depression. *Am. J. Psychiatry*, *141*, 986–988.

Goldney, R. D., & Simpson, I. G. (1975). Female genital self-mutilation, dysorexia and the hysterical personality: The Caenis syndrome. *Can. Psychiatr. Assoc. J.*, *20*, 435–441.

Gwirtsman, H. E., Kaye, W., Weintraub, M., & Jimerson, D. C. (1984). Pharmacologic treatment of eating disorders. *Psychiatr. Clin. N. Am.*, *7*, 863–877.

Harrigan, J. A., Kues, J. R., Ricks, D. F., & Smith, R. (1984). Moods that predict coming migraine headaches. *Pain*, *20*, 385–396.

Hatsukami, D. K., Mitchell, J. E., & Eckert, E. D. (1984). Eating disorders: A variant of mood disorders? *Psychiatr. Clin. N. Am.*, *7*, 349–365.

Heal, D. J., Philpot, J., O'Shaughnessy, K. M., & Davies, C. L. (1986). The influence of central noradrenergic function on 5-HT₂-mediated head-twitch responses in mice: Possible implications for the actions of antidepressant drugs. *Psychopharmacology*, *89*, 414–420.

Henryk-Gutt, R., & Rees, W. L. (1973). Psychological aspects of migraine. *J. Psychosom. Res.*, *17*, 141–153.

Herzog, D. (1982). Bulimia: The secretive syndrome. *Psychosomatics*, *23*, 481–487.

Houston, D. S., & Vanhoutte, P. M. (1986). Serotonin and the vascular system. Role in health and disease, and implications for therapy. *Drugs, 31*, 149–163.

Hudson, J. I., Pope, H. G., Jonas, J. M., & Yurgelun-Todd, D. (1984a). Phenomenologic relationship of eating disorders to major affective disorder. *Psychiatry Res., 9*, 345–354.

Hudson, J. I., Pope, H. G., & Jonas, J. M. (1984b). Treatment of bulimia with antidepressants: Theoretical considerations and clinical findings. In A. J. Stunkard & E. Stellar (Eds.), *Eating and its disorders* (pp. 259–273). New York: Raven Press.

Hudson, J. I., Pope, H. G., Yurgelun-Todd, D., Jonas, J. M., & Frandenburg, F. R. (1987). A controlled study of lifetime prevalence of affective and other psychiatric disorders in bulimic outpatients. *Am. J. Psychiatry, 144*, 1283–1287.

Hughes, P. L., Wells, L. A., Cunningham, C. J., & Ilstrup, D. M. (1986). Treating bulimia with desipramine: A double-blind, placebo-controlled study. *Arch. Gen. Psychiatry, 43*, 182–186.

Johnson, C., & Larson, R. (1982). Bulimia: An analysis of moods and behavior. *Psychosom. Med., 44*, 341–351.

Kalucy, R. S., Crisp, A. H., & Harding, B. (1977). A study of 56 families with anorexia nervosa. *Br. J. Med. Psychol., 50*, 381.

Kassett, J., Brandt, H., & Jimerson, D. (1989). A family history study of bulimia nervosa. *Proceedings of the 142nd Annual Meeting of the American Psychiatric Association*. San Francisco: American Psychiatric Association.

Kissileff, H. R., Walsh, B. T., Kral, J. G., & Cassidy, S. M. (1986). Laboratory studies of eating behavior in women with bulimia. *Physiol. Behav., 38*, 563–570.

Klee, A. (1975). Perceptual disorders in migraine. In J. Pearce (Ed.), *Modern topics in migraine* (pp. 45–51). London: Heinemann Medical Books.

Lawlor, B. A., Sunderland, T., Mellow, A. M., Hill, J. L., Molchan, S. E., & Murphy, D. L. (1989). Hyperresponsivity to the serotonin agonist m-chlorophenylpiperazine in Alzheimer's disease. *Arch. Gen. Psychiatry, 46*, 542–549.

Leibowitz, S. F., & Shor-Posner, G. (1986). Brain serotonin and eating behavior. *Appetite, 7*(Suppl), 1–14.

Limberger, N., Bonanno, G., Spath, L., & Starke, K. (1986). Autoreceptors and alpha$_2$-adrenoceptors at the serotonergic axons of rabbit brain cortex. *Naunyn-Schmiedeberg's Arch. Pharmacol., 332*, 324–331.

Linnoila, M., Virkhunen, M., Scheinin, M., Nuutila, A., Rimon, R., & Goodwin, F. K. (1983). Low cerebrospinal fluid 5-hydroxyindoleacetic acid concentration differentiates impulsive from nonimpulsive violent behavior. *Life Sci., 33*, 2609–2614.

Meltzer, H. Y., & Lowy, M. T. (1987). The serotonin hypothesis of depression. In H. Y. Meltzer (Ed.), *Psychopharmacology: The third generation of progress* (pp. 513–526). New York: Raven Press.

Merikangas, K. R., & Angst, J. (1988). Psychopathology and migraine. *Abstracts of Panels and Posters*, Annual Meeting of the American College of Neuropsychopharmacology, p. 181.

Mickalide, A. D., & Andersen, A. E. (1985). Subgroups of anorexia nervosa and bulimia: Validity and utility. *J. Psychiatr. Res., 19*, 121–128.

Mitchell, J. E., Hatsukami, D., Eckert, E. D., & Pyle, R. L. (1985). Characteristics of 275 patients with bulimia. *Am. J. Psychiatry*, *142*, 482–485.

Mitchell, J. E., Hatsukami, K., Pyle, R. L., & Eckert, E. D. (1986). The bulimia syndrome: Course of the illness and associated problems. *Compr. Psychiatry*, *27*, 165–170.

Mueller, E. A., Murphy, D. L., & Sunderland, T. (1985). Neuroendocrine effects of m-chlorophenylpiperazine, a serotonin agonist, in humans. *J. Clin. Endocrinol. Metab.*, *61*, 1179–1184.

Murphy, D. L., Campell, I., & Costa, J. L. (1978). Current status of the indoleamine hypothesis of affective disorders. In M. A. Lipton, A. DiMascio, & K. F. Killam (Eds.). *Psychopharmacology: A generation of progress* (pp. 1234–1248). New York: Raven Press.

Ortmann, R., Martin, S., Radeke, E., & Delini-Stula, A. D. (1981). Interaction of B-adrenergic agonists with the serotonergic system in rat brain. A behavioral study using the L-5-HTP syndrome. *Naunyn-Schmiedeberg's Arch. Pharmacol.*, *316*, 225–230.

Owen, W. P., Halmi, K. A., Biggs, J., & Smith, G. P. (1985). Satiety responses in eating disorders. *J. Psychiatry Res.*, *19*, 279–284.

Palmer, R. L. (1979). The dietary chaos syndrome: A useful new term? *Br. J. Med. Psychol.*, *52*, 43–52.

Philips, C., & Hunter, M. (1982). Headache in a psychiatric population. *J. Nerv. Ment. Dis.*, *170*, 34–40.

Pollock, J. D., & Rowland, N. (1981). Peripherally administered serotonin decreases food intake in rats. *Pharmacol. Biochem. Behav.*, *15*, 179–183.

Pyle, R. L. (1985). The epidemiology of eating disorders. *Pediatrician*, *12*, 102–109.

Rappaport, A., Sturtz, F., & Guicheney, P. (1985). Regulation of central alpha-adrenoceptors by serotoninergic denervation. *Brain Res.*, *344*, 158–161.

Raskin, N. H., (1981). Pharmacology of migraine. *Ann. Rev. Pharmacol. Toxicol.*, *21*, 463–478.

Roberts, M. H. T. (1984). 5-HT and antinociception. *Neuropharmacology*, *23*, 1529–1536.

Rosenthal, R. J., Rinzler, C., Walsh, R., & Klausner, E. (1972). Wrist-cutting syndrome: The meaning of a gesture. *Am. J. Psychiatry*, *11*, 1363–1368.

Russell, G. F. M. (1979). Bulimia nervosa: An ominous variant of anorexia nervosa. *Psychol. Med.*, *9*, 429–448.

Russell, G. F. M. (1985). Bulimia revisited. *Int. J. Eating Dis.*, *4*, 681–692.

Sandler, M., Jarman, J., & Glover, V. (1989). Endogenous depression in a migraine clinic population—identification by use of the oral tyramine test. *Program and Abstracts*, World Federation of Societies of Biological Psychiatry, Biological Aspects of Non-psychotic Disorders Regional Congress, Jerusalem, p. 21.

Samanin, R., Mennini, T., & Ferraris, A. (1982). M–chlorophenylpiperazine: A central serotonin agonist causing powerful anorexia in rats. *Naunyn-Schmiedebergs Arch. Pharmacol.*, *308*, 605.

Scheinin, M., van Kammen, D. P., Ninan, P. T., et al. (1984). Effect of propranolol on monoamine metabolites in cerebrospinal fluid of patients with chronic schizophrenia. *Clin. Pharmacol. Ther.*, *36*, 33–39.

Scott, J. A., & Crews, F. T. (1985). Increase in serotonin$_2$ receptor density in rat cerebral cortex slices by stimulation of beta-adrenergic receptors. *Biochem. Pharmacol.*, *34*, 1585–1588.

Sicuteri, F. (1982). *Advances in neurology, volume 33*. M. Critchley, A. P. Friedman, S. Gorini, & F. Sicuteri (Eds.), (pp. 65–74). New York: Raven Press.

Silverstone, T., & Goodall, E. (1986). Serotonergic mechanisms in human feeding: The pharmacological evidence. *Appetite*, *7*(Suppl), 85–97.

Simpson, M. A. (1975). The phenomenology of self-mutilation in a general hospital setting. *Can. Psychiatr. Asso. J.*, *20*, 429–434.

Smith, S. E., Pihl, R. O., Young, S. N., et al. (1987). A test of possible cognitive and environmental influences on the mood lowering effect of tryptophan depletion in normal males. *Psychopharmacology*, *91*, 451–457.

Stockmeier, C. A., Martino, A. M., & Kellar, K. J. (1985). A strong influence of serotonin axons on B-adrenergic receptors in rat brain. *Science*, *230*, 323–325.

Strober, M. (1981). The significance of bulimia in juvenile anorexia nervosa: An exploration of possible etiologic factors. *Int. J. Eating Dis.*, *1*, 28–43.

Stunkard, A. J. (1959). Eating patterns and obesity. *Psychiatric Quarterly*, *33*, 284–292.

Sulser, F., & Sanders-Bush, E. (1987). The serotonin-norepinephrine link hypothesis of affective disorders: Receptor-receptor interactions in brain. In Y. H. Ehrlich, R. H. Lenox, E. Kornecki, & W. O. Berry (Eds.), *Molecular mechanisms of neuronal responsiveness* (pp. 489–502). New York: Plenum Press.

Van Nueten, J. M., Janssens, W. J., & Vanhoutte, P. M. (1985a). Serotonin and vascular reactivity. *Pharmacol. Res. Comm.*, *17*, 585–608.

Van Nueten, J. M., Janssens, W. J., & Vanhoutte, P. M. (1985b). Serotonin and vascular smooth muscle. In P. M. Vanhoutte (Ed.), *Serotonin and the cardiovascular system* (pp. 95–103). New York: Raven Press.

Walsh, B. T., Roose, S. P., Glassman, A. H., Gladis, M., & Sadik, G. (1985). Bulimia and depression. *Psychosom. Med.*, *47*, 123–131.

Walsh, B. T., Stewart, J. W., Roose, S. P., Gladis, M., & Glassman, A. H. (1984). Treatment of bulimia with phenelzine: A double-blind, placebo-controlled study. *Arch. Gen. Psychiatry*, *41*, 1105–1109.

Weiss, S. R., & Ebert, M. H. (1983). Psychological and behavioral characteristics of normal-weight bulimia and normal-weight controls. *Psychosomatic Medicine*, *45*, 293–303.

Wilner, P. (1985). Antidepressants and serotonergic neurotransmission: An integrative review. *Psychopharmacol.*, *85*, 387–404.

Young, S. N., Smith, R. O., Pihl, F. R., et al. (1985). Tryptophan depletion causes a rapid lowering of mood in normal males. *Psychopharmacology*, *87*, 173–177.

Ziegler, D. K., Hurwitz, A., Hassanein, R. S., Kodanaz, H. A., Preskorn, S. H., &

Mason, J. (1987). Migraine prophylaxis: A comparison of propranolol and amitriptyline. *Arch. Neurol.*, *44*, 486–489.

Zohar, J., Mueller, E. A., Insel, T. R., Zohar-Kadouch, R. C., & Murphy, D. L. (1987). Serotonergic responsivity in obsessive-compulsive disorder. *Arch. Gen. Psychiatry*, *44*, 946–951.

11

Serotonin, Seasonality, and Mood Disorders

DEMITRI F. PAPOLOS

> Many features of internal temporal organization—the mutual timing of constituent events—are historical exploitations of earlier organization that was evolved initially purely as adaptation to the temporal order of the external world.
> —COLIN S. PITTENDRIGH
> *The Handiwork of Darwin's Demon*
> Princeton University, January 19, 1961

Since ancient times, remarkably regular seasonal recurrences of depression and mania have been an intriguing but unexplained phenomenon. According to Eastwood and Stiasny (1979), Hippocrates (460–370 B.C.) considered mania and depression to be disorders of spring, while Pinel (1806) wrote that "maniacal paroxysms generally begin immediately after the summer solstice, . . . are continued during the heat of the summer, and commonly terminate towards the decline of autumn." Kraepelin (1921) documented seasonal episodes of illness in some manic-depressive patients with a preponderance of manic episodes in the spring and depressions in winter.

While there are differences in their specific findings, most contemporary studies have shown that spring and fall are peak times for depression (Eastwood & Peacocke, 1976; Frangos et al., 1980). Hospital admissions for mania undergo seasonal variations as well, with a peak in the summer months (Walter, 1977). Milstein (1976) reported that manic-depressive episodes increase with the difference between maximum and minimum daily temperatures. A high correlation has also been reported between monthly admission rates for mania in Great Britain and seasonal changes in mean monthly day length, daily hours of sunshine, and daily temperature (Myers & Davies, 1978) that correspond to the vernal and autumnal equinox.

The seasonal nature of suicides has been recognized since the late 19th century, when Durkheim (1897) reported a higher incidence of suicide in spring and summer than in fall and winter. Subsequent studies have noted a bimodal distribution of suicides, with peaks in April and May and an additional, smaller peak in the fall (Eastwood & Peacocke, 1976; Lester, 1979; Souetre et al., 1987). A study by Egeland and Sussex (1985) reporting on suicide and family loading for mood disorders over a 100-year period (1880–1980) among the Old Order Amish found that the majority (92%) of the suicides were among four primary family pedigrees with heavy loading for mood disorders. Eighteen of the 26 suicides showed a clear seasonal pattern with peaks in the spring and fall.

Despite the compelling evidence documenting the influence of seasonal phenomena in the natural course of major mood disorders, relatively few studies have investigated psychobiological variables with seasonal variations. While serotonergic mechanisms have been heavily implicated in the etiology of mood disorders, there is little work to date examining the role that serotonin (5-HT) may play in the apparent seasonal vulnerability of patients with general mood disturbances. In fact, seasonal changes have been found in humans for a variety of parameters related to 5-HT metabolism. Discrete seasonal patterns have been observed in both platelet 5-HT content and platelet 5-HT uptake. Carlson et al. (1980) reported that hypothalamic 5-HT content from the postmortem brains of individuals who died from nonneurological, nonpsychiatric conditions showed a marked seasonal variation, with the lowest levels in the fall and winter months.

Within the pineal gland, the concentration of 5-HT is higher than in any other part of the central nervous system (CNS), and varies inversely with the concentration of melatonin. Pineal 5-HT levels are at their peak during the day and fall abruptly after dusk, at which time 5-HT is converted to melatonin (Klein, 1985). In addition to circadian and menstrual-cycle fluctuations, serum melatonin in humans has been observed to vary seasonally with peak levels in both summer and winter (Arendt, 1979). An inverse relationship has been noted between the circannual rhythm of plasma melatonin and that of suicide (Souetre et al., 1987), and the incidence of depression has been reported to be higher in spring and autumn when melatonin values are naturally reduced as a result of seasonal changes in total secretion (Arendt, 1979).

Recently, research interest in these phenomena has been spurred by (1) reports that patients with mood disorders have disturbed circadian rhythms (Teicher et al., 1988; Souetre et al., 1988; Sack et al., 1988; Avery et al., 1986; Kripke et al., 1978; Mendlewicz et al., 1980); (2) the accumulation of more detailed knowledge about the neural mechanisms that regulate circadian and circannual rhythms (Moore-Ede et al., 1982; Weitzman et al., 1979; Hastings et al., 1985); and (3) the establishment of diagnostic criteria for a form of mood disorder characterized by regularly occurring summer depressions and winter depressions that frequently alternate with summer hypomania (Wehr et al., 1989), both of which have been shown to be responsive to phototherapy.

CIRCADIAN RHYTHM DYSFUNCTIONS

Circadian rhythms are an evolved adjustment of the time course of metabolism to the temporal pattern of the environmental day and are major components of animals' adaptation to their environments, determining such events as the timing of activity and feeding and, for many species, the patterns of reproduction (Moore & Card, 1985). Circadian rhythms are generated by endogenous pacemakers, or "clocks," that establish rhythms with a period that approximates 24 hours. These rhythms are not learned or "impressed" on the organism by an immediate experience of a periodic environment; rather, they are innate, inherited features of the physiological system (Pittendrigh, 1961).

There has long been thought to be an association between circadian rhythm disruption and mental illness, and a number of formulations link these disturbances exclusively to the mood disorders. A variety of hypotheses concerning circadian rhythm dysfunctions have been proposed in depression, including (1) desynchronization in rhythms (Halberg, 1968), (2) critical interval (Kripke, 1984), (3) loss of amplitude (Schultz & Lund, 1985), (4) phase advance (Papousek, 1975), (5) deficiency of a sleep substance (Borbely et al., 1984), (6) inappropriate entrainment (von Zerssen et al., 1985), and (7) dysregulation of a central circadian pacemaker (Siever & Davis, 1985).

Most of these hypotheses are complementary, having in common the assumption of loss of strength of central pacing functions, and are unified by the notion that the cyclic nature of the mood disorders can be linked to a condition in which biological rhythms regulated by multiple pacemakers or oscillators in the central nervous system fail to be entrained effectively to external time cues or to each other. Recent studies have lent support to a model of the circadian system (Moore-Ede & Sulzman, 1981; Moore, 1983; Czeislar et al., 1981) in which the external light–dark cycle synchronizes the endogenous circadian oscillator (Carpenter & Grossberg, 1985), which, in turn, governs the internal organization and spontaneous duration of sleep. According to one hypothesis, periodic changes in day length trigger winter depressions by alternating the pattern of nocturnal melatonin secretion, which acts as a hormonal signal of darkness. In those susceptible to developing a mood disorder, a predisposition of endogenous pacemakers to drift may be reflected in the greater ease with which melatonin is suppressed by light in bipolar patients (Lewy et al., 1981), or in the persistence of electroencephalographic sleep abnormalities even after recovery from illness (Kupfer & Reynolds, 1983). Kripke et al. (1978) has suggested that continuously advancing free-running rhythms in rapidly cycling manic-depressives, and advanced but synchronized rhythms in more stable depressive syndromes, might be quantitative variants of a similar circadian oscillator disorder.

For many species, phase maps have been compiled that demonstrate the multiplicity of circadian rhythms within an animal and the specific phase relationship of each rhythm (Moore-Ede & Sulzman, 1982). If one examines several different circadian rhythms within an individual subject, the highly specific order of the circadian system becomes apparent (Rasmussen, 1986). The various rhythms play in intricate counterpoint, reaching their peaks (acrophases) and troughs (nadirs) at different phases of the circadian day (Moore-Ede & Sulzman, 1982). If the organization of rhythmicity falters (i.e., if two oscillators lose their coupling strength), some rhythms will desynchronize from others, some may phase advance, amplitude will be lost, and rhythms released from mutual entrainment may entrain inappropriately to some other competing signal. This alteration in the relative coordination of mutually timed events could cause a breakdown in internal temporal order, and, as a result, physiological systems that normally prime each other would fail to do so, leading to many physiological functions not being switched on or off at the appropriate times during the circadian day.

Moore-Ede and Sulzman (1976), in their review of the literature on periodic internal temporal order, underscore the elaborate counterpoint of rhythms in a host of physiological functions, and point to some of the potential consequences of failures in the circadian system. Seasonal affective disorder (SAD) is the first psychiatric disorder defined in the revised third edition of the *Diagnostic and Statistical Manual of Mental Disorders* (DSM-III-R) that could be characterized as a temporal disorder, in which the timing of circannual or circadian biological rhythms is pathologically altered.

SEASONAL AFFECTIVE DISORDER

Criteria for this syndrome were first published by the National Institute of Mental Health Intramural Research Program group (Rosenthal et al., 1984). More recently, DSM-III-R, under the category of mood disorders, made provision for designation of a seasonal pattern in the course of recurrent major depression and bipolar disorder. DSM-III-R further stipulates that these recurrent episodes must occur within a particular 60-day period of the year, and that there must be a history of at least three episodes in three separate years that demonstrate a clear seasonal pattern. While there is general agreement concerning the diagnostic and clinical criteria for winter depression or SAD (Rosenthal et al., 1985), limited epidemiological data are available that would help to determine the true incidence and prevalence of the condition. Moreover, the difference between this syndrome and a milder form of bipolar disorder remains to be delineated. These recurrent, mostly bipolar depressions occur in winter, and show atypical signs of increased appetite, carbohydrate craving, weight gain, and hypersomnia (Rosenthal, 1984; Thompson & Issacs, 1988). The fact that a preponderance of patients with SAD experience hypomanic episodes in spring and summer, and that a high percentage of patients with bipolar disorder (approximately 80%) manifest atypical features during the depressed phase of the illness (Akiskal, 1983), suggests that this syndrome may be a variant of bipolar disorder. With regard to SAD, the serotonin system appears likely to be dysregulated, as evidenced by abnormal psychological and hormonal responses to m-chlorophenylpiperazine (mCPP) (Jacobsen et al., 1987), abnormal responses to carbohydrate-rich meals (Rosenthal, 1987), and the beneficial therapeutic effects of d-fenfluramine, a 5-HT releasing agent (O'Rourke et al., 1987). 5-HT dysregulation, while not unique to SAD, may provide an integrative frame of reference in the investigation of underlying mechanisms involved in the response to phototherapy effects.

THE PHOTOPERIODIC RESPONSE AND LIGHT THERAPY OF SAD

The circadian–photoperiod rationale for phototherapy in SAD implies that the timing of light treatments is critical for its therapeutic efficacy. The pattern of seasonal occurrence and the relief of winter depression by bright-light treatment in SAD suggest that there may be perturbation of the normal circannual or circadian rhythmicity that has been shown in sleep and a broad range of other physiological processes (Aschoff, 1981), and that some aspect of a photoperiodic mechanism may be involved in its pathogenesis. Since mechanisms that regulate photoperiodic control of seasonal behaviors in animals are related to circadian rhythm phase (Pengelley, 1974), disrupted photoperiodic mechanisms in humans could be a source of the depressive symptoms in SAD.

In mammals, the photoperiodic response has an important biological function in sleep, activity, and reproductive behavior, particularly through its influence on seasonal breeding patterns. Animal studies have shown that light exerts a dual action on sleep and motor activity. The 24-hour light-dark (LD) cycle acts as a synchronizer for the circadian rest–activity (RA) and sleep–wake (SW) rhythms, determining their period and phase relationship. The length of the photoperiod influences the RA and SW patterns, and short light periods may have a potent direct action on the vigilance and arousal states and on motor activity (Borbely et al., 1978).

The photoperiod determines the light fraction of the total LD cycle. Under natural conditions, the photoperiod exhibits seasonal variations whose magnitude is a function of the northern and southern latitudes (Borbely, 1978). The circadian "clock" is used as part of the timing device that can measure the duration of either darkness or light. The resolution of a clock is a measure of its ability to detect the temporal order of two events closely spaced in time. If the events are closer together than a clock can resolve, the clock will not be able to distinguish reliably which events precede the other events (Moore-Ede et al., 1982). Exposure to a brief pulse of light causes a change in phase that depends on when the light pulse occurs. If the pulse of light occurs during the subjective day (in constant conditions), there is relatively little change in phase. If the pulse of light occurs during the first half of subjective night, there is a phase advance (shift to an earlier time) (Lewy, 1987a, 1987b). Therefore, in the middle of the night there is an inflection point that separates phase-delay from phase-advance responses. The closer they are to the middle of the night, the greater is the magnitude of these phase shifts (Moore-Ede & Sulzman, 1982). Phase-advance and phase-delay responses of different magnitudes vary according to when the light pulse occurs and can be plotted as a phase-response curve (DeCoursey, 1960).

In most mammals, light is a potent physical *zeitgeber* (time giver or cue), and the absence of changes in light will cause many rhythms to "free run" or desynchronize, losing their circadian time periods (Wever, 1974). The resetting of biological clocks by light has been characterized in nearly all species studied. Until recently, human circadian rhythms were thought to be insensitive to light. However, Czeisler et al. (1986) have reported that, in humans, light exposure is indeed capable of shifting circadian rhythms in the direction predicted on the basis of the phase-response curve generated from animal experiments (DeCoursey, 1960). They demonstrated an intensity-dependent neuroendocrine response to light in an elderly woman who experienced a six-hour phase shift of her circadian pacemaker, as indicated by recordings of body temperature and cortisol secretion, suggesting that exposure to bright light can reset the human circadian pacemaker.

It has been suggested that phase advances and delays—essential for entrainment—occur when bright light strikes the eye at particular states of visual sensitivity (Terman & Terman, 1985). Findings from various studies of photoperiodic time measurement in animals all support the hypothesis of a rhythm of photosensitivity underlying the photoperiodic response (Elliot, 1976). The principle is that the duration of either darkness or light entrains a circadian rhythm of sensitivity to light such that, if a second light pulse (or a continuation of the first) falls into a light-sensitive phase (or window) occurring later in the day, then the appropriate neuroendocrine response will follow (Hastings et al., 1985). It is likely that this neuroendocrine response—which acts to translate the photoperiodic stimulus into an endocrine signal—involves various neuronal and endocrine functions, including the modulation of the hypothalamic pulsing of luteinizing hormone releasing hormone (LHRH) (Rasmussen, 1986); the firing rate of cells in the suprachiasmatic nucleus (SCN), the neuronal pathways leading from retina to the SCN, terminating at the level of the pineal; and, possibly, those 5-HT terminals coursing from the raphe nucleus to the SCN (Ajika & Ochi, 1978).

In addition to the reported therapeutic effects of phototherapy in SAD, the hypothesis that depression can result from abnormalities of photoperiodic regulation is supported by evidence of abnormal melatonin concentrations and abnormal melatonin suppressibility by bright light in patients with a mood disorder (Lewy, 1981; Mendlewicz et al., 1980; Brown et al., 1985). The efficacy of phototherapy for SAD has been debated, yet a number of well-controlled studies support its effectiveness (Rosenthal, 1985; Lewy et al., 1983, 1985, 1987b). Indeed, most studies have found that phototherapy can induce complete remission in recurrent seasonal depression within a few days. By contrast, antidepressant medications require weeks to months to exert their therapeutic effects. Interestingly, the only other treatment that has been found to reverse the symptoms of depression so rapidly is sleep deprivation—another method of circadian intervention. While its mechanism of action remains unknown, several hypotheses have been proposed to explain the therapeutic effects of light, including extension of the winter photoperiod (Lengthening duration of exposure to light) (Rosenthal et al., 1985) and increased light intensity (Wehr et al., 1985). Lewy et al. (1987a) proposed that light may exert its antidepressant action through its phase-shifting effects on circadian rhythms. This proposition relies on a key property of entrainable circadian systems—the periodically changing sensitivity to light—and the known properties of light to act as a *zeitgeber* and entrain the circadian timing system.

According to these investigators, patients with SAD have endogenous circadian rhythms that are either phase advanced or phase delayed with respect to sleep; thus, light would have two potential antidepressant effects—a phase-shifting effect that corrects an abnormal phase position and an energizing effect (Lewy et al., 1986). The former effect is thought to depend on the timing, intensity, and duration of light treatment. In a series of experiments in normal volunteers, Lewy et al. (1985) found that advancing the time of bright-light exposure in the evening advanced the circadian phase position in the timing of melatonin production, as well as core body temperature rhythm, and that delaying bright-light exposure in the morning delayed circadian phase position. In a subsequent study (Lewy et al., 1987b), eight patients who regularly became depressed in the winter (as day length shortens) significantly improved after one week of exposure to bright light in the morning, but not after one week of bright light in the evening. This antidepressant response to morning light was accompanied by an advance (shift to an earlier time) in the onset of melatonin production at night. Lewy et al. (1987b) have used the response of circadian rhythms to light as a means of subtyping SAD patients, and suggest that such subtyping may have predictive value in determining the optimal timing of treatment.

The causal relationship between phase shifting and the therapeutic effect of light treatment has been called into question, however, by several studies with conflicting results, indicating that the timing of treatment may not necessarily be related to its therapeutic effects (Rosenthal et al., 1987; Thompson et al., 1988).

A strategy developed by Czeisler et al. (1986) provides an objective protocol for quantifying changes in phase position of the circadian pacemaker before and after a therapeutic intervention, and, therefore, makes it possible to devise studies that would correlate changes in internal phase relationships of circadian rhythms with clinical response to treatment. This protocol, and the availability of more sensitive assays for melatonin, will now make it more feasible for researchers to resolve questions about the hypothesized role of a circadian dysfunction in mood disorders.

THE PINEAL

Many studies support the view that, in mammals, the pineal gland participates in photoperiod-related seasonal changes of endocrine activity, particularly in reproduction (Reiter, 1983). In seasonal breeders, its role is to synchronize breeding activities through the translation of photic cues into hormonal agents that regulate reproductive competence (Hastings et al., 1985). Changes in day length are principally responsible for synchronizing breeding with time of year in mammals (Yates & Herbert, 1976). The seasonal changes in day length are the principal cues that regulate the pulsatile release of hypothalamic releasing factors (Clarke & Cummins, 1982), which, in turn, activate the pituitary–gonadal axis, and the pineal is an essential mediator of this photoperiodic response (Vaughn, 1981).

If the melatonin signal is to be interpreted accurately by its target system, there must be periods free of the compound to generate a clear pattern. Once initiated, periods of elevated melatonin must be sustained without interruption to generate a clear signal. These periods must be of critical duration for the signal to be effective, and such periods must be separated by periods of low or absent melatonin (Hastings, 1985). Therefore, some disturbance in the secretion of melatonin could potentially alter behavioral functions that are keyed to the pattern of its circadian release.

On the basis of studies in rodents (Klein & Weller, 1972) and nonhuman primates (Reppert et al., 1981), the melatonin rhythm in mammals is thought to be generated by a circadian pacemaker in the suprachiasmatic nucleus of the anterior hypothalamus. The melatonin rhythm is entrained to the 24-hour period by the daily LD cycle, with peak levels occurring at night (Klein, 1985). In humans, the melatonin rhythm appears to be regulated in a similar manner, and is expressed in blood and cerebrospinal fluid (Reppert et al., 1988).

The principal perturbation causing the daily rhythm in melatonin synthesis is the increase in the rate of N-acetylation of 5-HT. In the rat, the enzyme responsible for this step, 5-HT N-acetyltransferase (NAT) (Voisin et al., 1984), increases in activity at night 70–100-fold (Klein & Weller, 1972). The rhythm of this enzymatic activity is circadian, with its highest levels taking place during the dark phase. Light falling during this phase blocks melatonin production, truncates the pineal signal, and produces LD response by the CNS (Klein, 1985). The rise of NAT activity at night is initiated by norepinephrine release from sympathetic nerve terminals in the pineal gland. Beta-adrenergic receptors are stimulated, which, in turn, cause a stimulation of pineal adenylate cyclase. As a consequence, the concentration of intracellular cyclic adenosine monophosphate (cAMP) rises and induces protein synthesis (Klein, 1985). This increase in cAMP is orchestrated by a photoneural mechanism located in the SCN (Moore & Card, 1985).

Illernova and Vanecek (1982) have provided convincing evidence that this SCN clock is actually composed of two dependent clocks, and the degree to which their pineal stimulatory periods overlap is determined by the photoperiod. Long nights appear to allow the clocks to drift apart, so that the pineal gland will be stimulated for a longer time than seen in animals kept in short nights. Light rapidly terminates the autonomic stimulation of the pineal (Klein & Weller, 1972), resulting in a rapid decrease in N-acetyltransferase activity and in melatonin production (Namboodiri et al., 1985). In this two-oscillator model, an evening oscillator in the SCN controls the rise of NAT, and a morning one controls the NAT decline. According to their proposition, the evening oscillator (coupled to dusk) controls the evening rise of NAT and the morning oscillator (coupled to dawn) controls the morning component.

MELATONIN SECRETION IN PATIENTS
WITH MOOD DISORDERS

A number of studies in patients with mood disorders have found that those with major depression have a reduced nocturnal rise of melatonin. Mendlewicz et al. (1980) described an absence of the usual nocturnal increase of melatonin in three of four depressed patients, compared with that measured in five normal subjects. Brown et al. (1985) also found lower nocturnal concentrations of serum melatonin in patients with major depressive disorder, melancholic subtype, compared with that in either healthy control subjects or patients with major depressive disorder without melancholia.

While several studies of nonseasonal depressives have shown abnormally low nocturnal melatonin secretion, Skwerer et al. (1988) have reported a similar profile of low plasma melatonin in 15 SAD patients compared with 11 normal controls studied under conditions of ordinary room light. In this study, bright-light treatment, however, had no effect on mean nocturnal melatonin secretion or on the timing of its onset or offset.

Lewy et al. (1988) have phase-shifted patients' melatonin cycles relative to sleep by selective morning and evening light exposures, with greater therapeutic benefit for early morning light accompanied by a melatonin phase advance. Furthermore, these investigators found that, in comparison with normals, several patients with SAD have a pattern of nocturnal melatonin secretion that is phase-delayed in winter.

Effects of Antidepressant Agents on Melatonin Secretion

Several studies have reported an enhancement of nocturnal melatonin secretion in depressed patients, but not in normal subjects, following three weeks of desipramine treatment (Thompson et al., 1985), and an increased melatonin concentration at night and during the day after chronic clorgyline administration (Murphy et al., 1986). Demisch et al. (1987) observed that a 150-mg dose of fluvoxamine given at night to healthy volunteers led to significantly increased early morning plasma levels of melatonin, whereas the administration of the same dose in the morning did not lead to an increase in melatonin during the day, suggesting that the early morning decline of melatonin in plasma is delayed after the intake of a 5-HT reuptake inhibitor the night before. Whether the former effects are mediated by beta-adrenergic receptor-linked stimulation of NAT (as the rate-limiting step in melatonin synthesis) caused by beta-adrenergic receptor subsensitivity, or by changes in the sensitivity of 5-HT receptors in the SCN (Groos & Mason, 1982), or, alternatively, by some direct effect on pineal melatonin metabolism, remains a focus of current investigation.

The Suprachiasmatic Nucleus

It is now widely accepted that the SCN of the hypothalamus is a circadian pacemaker in the mammalian brain (Moore-Ede et al., 1982). The rhythmic neural activity of the SCN appears to be an inherent property of SCN neurons since it persists after isolation of the SCN from adjacent hypothalamic tissues (Inouye & Kawamura, 1979). The SCN lies in the anterior ventral hypothalamus on either side of the third ventricle. It is thought to contain two components that function as coupled oscillators: the ventrolateral SCN and the dorso-medial SCN (Moore & Card, 1985). The former receives primary and secondary visual afferents and is the locus of entrainment to the LD cycle (Moore, 1983). The human SCN is neurochemically similar to the SCN of rats and nonhuman primates and contains the same topographical distribution of various neuropeptides (Lydic et al., 1980, 1982). In animals, the SCN is an essential component of the mechanism that regulates the circadian rhythm of sensitivity to light (Rusak & Zucker, 1979), and may also be the site of a pulse generator responsible for the generation of pulsatile hormone output (Ramirez et al., 1984; Goodman & Karsch, 1981). Circadian rhythmicity may be imparted by rhythmic SCN outputs to other inherently nonrhythmic physiological systems. An entraining effect of melatonin on mammalian circadian rhythms that is mediated by the SCN has been found in rats (Cassone et al., 1987), a species in which melatonin binding sites are consistently observed in the SCN (Vanecek et al., 1987). The finding that melatonin binding sites are located in the human SCN (Reppert et al., 1988) provides evidence that the reported effects of melatonin on human circadian rhythms may also be mediated by its direct action on the SCN.

Studies indicate that tissue within the SCN is capable of generating circadian neural rhythms and that these neural rhythms receive synchronizing information from the LD cycle (Inouye, 1984). This suggests that the effects of light on the circadian rhythm phase are not mediated solely by changes in the firing rate of SCN neurons, but rather by some other effect on the pacemaker, possibly alterations in the diurnal sensitivity of receptors and/or effects of neurotransmitters that modulate SCN activity.

Serotonin and Photoperiodicity

Entrainment or modulation of circadian pacemakers by LD cycles requires the processing of the LD information by a photoreceptor and propagation of the information to the pacemaker. The only measurable properties inherent in the oscillatory mechanism of neural pacemakers are the period and phase of the cycle. Thus, a change in the period or phase of a circadian rhythm reflects a change in the oscillatory mechanism that drives the cycle.

Several groups have reported that 5-HT shifts the phase of the rhythm generated by a neural pacemaker in the aplysia eye (Corrent et al., 1978; Nadakavukaren et al., 1986). This clock, a cytoplasmic oscillator involved in protein synthesis, manifests itself by modulating the frequency of compound action potentials originating at the cell membranes of secondary neurons in the eye (Levitan & Benson, 1981). The effect of 5-HT on these pacemaker cells is to cause an immediate and reversible decrease in the compound action potential from the eye, as well as a permanent phase shift of the oscillator (Corrent et al., 1982). Treatment with 5-HT has been found to delay the rhythm when it is applied to the rising phase and to advance it during the falling phase (Corrent et al., 1978). Any change in 5-HT receptor sensitivity in these cells would therefore have the capacity to shift the phase of the oscillator.

Increasing evidence supports the view that in higher species 5-HT is involved in mechanisms underlying particular rhythmic patterns and periodic functions. 5-HTergic mechanisms have been strongly implicated in the timing of both the REM-NREM 90–120-minute oscillatory cycles of sleep (Jouvet, 1972) and the episodic secretion of luteinizing hormone (LH) (Wuttke et al., 1978). In the freely moving cat, neuronal unit activity recorded from 5-HTergic midbrain raphe nuclei showed an elevated discharge during wakefulness and a reduced activity during sleep (Trulson & Jacobs, 1979). Significantly, both electrical and pharmacological stimulation of these same mesencephalic 5-HTergic regions inhibit pulsatile LH release (Gallo, 1980).

While it is not known whether 5-HT rhythms are directly involved with reproduction, 5-HT infused into the cerebral ventricles can alter gonadotropin secretion in rats (Hery et al., 1976) and sheep (Domanski et al., 1975). In addition, Yates and Herbert (1976) have reported that exposure of ferrets to either long or short photoperiods induces differential 5-HT rhythms in the pineal and hypothalamus, which are abolished by autonomic denervation, and that melatonin induces 5-HT rhythms characteristic of animals kept in short photoperiods. These findings have led to the proposition that localized 5-HT rhythms may be involved in the process that promotes or inhibits hypothalamic mechanisms concerned with variations in gonadotropin secretion during different photoperiods. Such differential 5-HT rhythms could allow an animal's neuroendocrine system to discriminate between photoperiods that have the greatest significance for reproductive function (Yates & Herbert, 1976).

The pineal contains large concentrations of 5-HT and has been implicated in the neural control of circadian rhythms, which themselves may be related to the genesis of annual rhythms (Sadlier, 1969). In the pineal of the rat, concentrations of 5-HT vary in phase with the photoperiod (Snyder et al., 1965). Inhibition of cerebral 5-HT synthesis prevents circadian rhythms in the concentration of LH (Hery et al., 1982), and lesions of the midbrain raphe are associated with a loss of circadian rhythmicity in plasma corticosterone levels (Dunn et al., 1983).

Loss of a distinct circadian rhythm in plasma ACTH in rodents was found after depletion of whole-brain 5-HT with parachlorophenylalanine (pCPA) (Szafarczyk et al., 1980, 1981). In these experiments, the recognizable 24-hour rhythmicity in plasma ACTH returned when 5-HTP was administered at 11:00 a.m., but not when the same dose was given at 11:00 p.m. (Szafarczyk et al., 1980), illustrating the importance of circadian variation in 5-HT sensitivity and its potential role in the regulation of the circadian secretory pattern of pituitary hormones.

Among the areas known actively to concentrate circulating hormone or to control the release of hormones from neural tissue, the SCN receives specific 5-HT projections from the dorsal raphe (Azmitia, 1978, Azmitia & Segal, 1978). In higher species, the SCN has been shown to have one of the richest densities of 5-HTergic terminals and concentrations in the brain (Azmitia & Segal, 1978a; Inouye, 1979). 5-HT–containing terminals arising from the midbrain raphe nuclei distribute in a dense plexus in the ventrolateral SCN, the area of the SCN that entrains to the LD cycle (Van den Pol & Tsujimoto, 1985). Studies have shown that monoamines inhibit SCN activity under both in vitro and in vivo conditions. For example, both the iontophoretic application of 5-HT and the stimulation of the dorsal raphe nucleus act to suppress the firing of SCN cells (Mason & Meijer, 1982; Groos & Mason, 1982), indicating that a 5-HTergic inhibition of SCN neuronal activity may be involved in the modulation of pacemaker function.

Through extracellular single-unit recordings obtained from neurons in the SCN of the rat, Mason (1986) found a diurnal variation in the response to iontophoresis of 5-HT. This variation was manifest as a two- to threefold increase in postsynaptic sensitivity to 5-HT during the subjective dark (active) phase of the circadian RA cycle. In these studies, neuronal activity in the SCN also exhibited a circadian variation in the recovery from 5-HT–induced suppression of firing. This circadian variation in recovery for SCN neurons closely follows the diurnal variation in 5-HT uptake found biochemically in the SCN (Meyer & Quay, 1976; Faradji et al., 1983). Ramirez et al. (1987) also found in rodents an increase in 5-hydroxyindoleacetic acid (5-HIAA) output in the SCN that paralleled the shift from light to dark, with highest levels during the dark phase (activity period) of the photoperiod. Significantly, 5-HIAA secretion appeared to have an inherently pulsatile nature that is superimposed on high-amplitude, possibly circadian fluctuations. Electrophysiological observations of SCN neurons demonstrate that these diurnal changes are reflected in a reduced mean discharge rate (Groos & Hendriks, 1982; Shibata et al., 1984) and a decrease in glucose utilization (Schwartz et al., 1980). Therefore, both circadian variations in 5-HT sensitivity and recovery parallel other physiological parameters associated with SCN function that show a relationship to the LD cycle.

Interestingly, animals exposed to long-term illumination (which induces circadian arrythmicity in RA behavior) showed no circadian variation in 5-HT sensitivity. This loss of a regular RA pattern, however, was accompanied by either marked subsensitivity or a two- to threefold supersensitivity to iontophoresed 5-HT (Mason, 1986). Taken together, these studies indicate that, in rats, indoleamine levels in the SCN are affected by LD cycles. A light-induced reduction of motor activity may be related to the activation of the 5-HT system. In addition, interventions that alter the state of the SCN as a circadian pacemaker also interfere with the observed diurnal variation of 5-HT sensitivity. Moreover, raphe lesions known to induce degenerative changes in the SCN alternate the amplitude of the 24-hour RA rhythm in rats by enhancing activity during the light phase (Zucker et al., 1976).

While the mechanism by which the SCN mediates the circadian sensitivity of 5-HT neurons both intrinsic to the SCN and at extrasuprachiasmatic 5-HTergic terminal areas remains to be determined, the observed diurnal variation in 5-HT receptor sensitivity could enable the SCN pacemaker to adapt to pervasive changes in photoperiod, as during the passage of seasons, and to rhythmic changes in internal metabolic conditions.

It has been proposed that this variation in 5-HT sensitivity could occur via an SCN-mediated circadian drive of raphe function (Mason, 1986) such that, during the light (sleeping phase) of the rat's circadian RA cycle, raphe discharge—and, hence, 5-HT release—would be lower than during the (active) dark phase. Mason (1986) has suggested that a disruption of raphe activity would interfere with development of the circadian adaptive changes in postsynaptic 5-HT sensitivity at the level of the SCN. Since the midbrain raphe dorsalis nucleus sends 5-HT terminals to the rostroventral area of the SCN, direct neuromodulation of this nucleus could mediate variations in 5-HT sensitivity in the SCN. Alternatively, variations in sensitivity to 5-HT could be mediated via an endogenous neuromodulator or hormonal system that is under the influence of the circadian drive from the SCN to the pineal.

The fact that melatonin binding sites have been located in the human SCN (Reppert et al., 1988) further suggests that a regulatory feedback loop exists between the pineal and the SCN. This is consistent with electron microscopic evidence that some SCN cells are clustered in direct apposition to the walls of blood capillaries (Card & Moore, 1984). These cells may act as receptors, sensing hormonal signals from the pineal.

No definitive conclusions can be drawn from a spate of animal studies linking 5-HT involvement to circadian and circannual behaviors that are associated with central pacemaker functions. However, the pronounced positive therapeutic response of patients with SAD to the 5-HT–releasing agent d-fenfluramine (O'Rourke et al., 1987) should provide the impetus to continue more selective studies of serotonin dysregulation in mood syndromes with a pattern of seasonal recurrence.

CONCLUSION

The identification of a specific form of mood disorder that can be characterized as a temporal disorder in which the timing of circannual biological rhythms is pathologically altered, and, in addition, the relief of winter depression in SAD by bright-light treatment, has suggested that some abnormality of photoperiodic regulation may be involved in the pathogenesis of this disorder.

This hypothesis is supported by evidence of abnormal melatonin concentrations and abnormal melatonin suppressibility in patients with mood disorders, and by the fact that only light of sufficient intensity to suppress melatonin in humans can also reverse the symptoms of SAD. Clinical studies with a view toward delineating the efficacy of various parameters of light treatment have begun to address some questions about the formal properties of phototherapy required to produce antidepressant effects in this condition. However, the mechanisms of photoperiodic dysfunction in depression and the cause of improvement of symptoms by phototherapy remain to be determined.

While it is possible to formulate hypothetical models by which various neuronal and neuroendocrine systems can interact to modulate seasonal changes in such diverse behavioral functions as sleeping, activity, sexual arousal, and appetite in humans, a fairly wide chasm of acquired data separates the concept of an alteration in circadian timing as etiological from the documentary evidence needed to support it. An even wider gap exists when we inquire about the methods that are available in the area of circadian and circannual measurement to convert correlational data into proof of cause and effect. Nevertheless, it is hoped that this review of the existing data on what is known about the photoperiodic response in mammals, the light-induced modification of behavioral states and rhythms, and the critical role that serotonin appears to play may be useful in future inquiries into the pathophysiology of forms of mood disorder with a seasonal pattern of recurrence.

REFERENCES

Ajika, K., & Ochi, J. (1978). Serotonergic projections to the suprachiasmatic nucleus and median eminence of the rat: Identification by fluorescence and electron microscope. *J. Anatomy, 127*, 563–576.

Akiskal, H. S., (1983). The bipolar spectrum: New concepts in classification and diagnosis. In L. Grinspoon (Ed.), *Psychiatry update* (pp. 271–292). Washington, D.C.: American Psychiatric Press.

Amerian Psychiatric Association. (1987). Diagnostic and statistical manual of mental disorders (3rd ed.).

Arendash, G. W., & Gallo, R. V. (1970). Serotonin involvement in the inhibition of episodic luteinizing hormone release: Electrical stimulation of the midbrain dorsal raphe nucleus in ovariectomized rats. *Endocrinology, 102*, 1199–1206.

Arendt, J. (1979). Radioimmunoassayable melatonin: Circulating patterns in man and sheep. In A. J. Kappers & P. Pevet (Eds.), *The pineal gland of vertebrates including man—Progress in brain research*, Vol. 52 (p. 249). Amsterdam: Elsevier/North-Holland Biomedical Press.

Aschoff, J. (1981). Annual rhythms in man. In J. Aschoff (Ed.), *Handbook of behavioral neurobiology, biological rhythms*, Vol. 4. New York: Plenum Press.

Avery, D. H., Wildshiodtz, G., Smallwood, R. G., et al. (1986). REM latency and core temperature relationships in primary depression. *Acta Psychiat. Scand., 74*, 269–280.

Azmitia, E. C. (1978). Serotonin producing neurons in the midbrain raphe nuclei. In L. L. Iverson, S. D. Iverson, & S. Snyder (Eds.), *Handbook of psychopharmacology—Chemical pathways in the brain*, Vol. 9. New York: Plenum Press.

Azmitia, E. C., & Segal, M. (1978). An autoradiographic analysis of the differential ascending projections of the dorsal and median raphe nuclei in the rat. *J. Comp. Neurol., 179*, 641–668.

Beck-Friis, J., Lyungven, J. G., Thoven, M., et al. (1985). Melatonin, cortisol and ACTH in patients with manic-depressive disorder and healthy humans with special reference to the outcome of the dexamethasone suppression test. *Psychoneuroendocrinology, 10*, 173–186.

Borbely, A. A. (1978). Effects of light on sleep and activity rhythms. *Prog. Neurobiol., 10*, 1–31.

Borbely, A. A., Tobler, I., et al. (1984). All night spectral analysis of the sleep EEG in untreated depressives and normal controls. *Psychiat. Res., 12*, 27–33.

Branchey, L., Weinberg, U., Branchey, M., et al. (1982). Simultaneous study of 24 hour pattern of melatonin and cortisol secretion in depressed patients. *Neuropsychobiology, 8*, 225–232.

Brown, R., Koscis, J. H., Caroff, S., et al. (1985). Differences in nocturnal melatonin secretion between melatonin in depressed patients and control subjects. *Am J. Psychiatry, 142*, 811–816.

Card, J. P., & Moore, R. Y. (1984). The suprachiasmatic nucleus of the golden hamster immunohistochemical analysis of cell and fiber distribution. *So. Neurosci., 13*, 415–431.

Cardinali, D. P. (1979). Models in neuroendocrinology: Neurohumoral pathways to the pineal gland. *Trends Neurosci.*, Oct., 250–253.

Carlsson, A., Svennerholm, L., & Winblau, B. (1980). Seasonal and circadian monamine variations in human brains examined postmortem. *Acta Psychiat. Scand.*, *61*(Suppl. 280), 75–85.

Carpenter, G. A., & Grossberg, S. (1985). A neural theory of circadian rhythms: Split rhythms, after-effects and motivational interaction. *J. Theor. Biol.*, *113*, 163–223.

Cassone, V. M., Roberts, M. H., & Moore, R. Y. (1987). Melatonin inhibits metabolic activity in the rat suprachiasmatic nuclei. *Neurosci. Lett.*, *81*, 29–34.

Clarke, I. J., & Cummins, J. T. (1982). The temporal relationship between gonadotropin releasing hormone (GnRH) and luteinizing hormone (LH) secretion in ovariectomized ewes. *Endocrinology, 111*, 1737–1740.

Corrent, G., McAdoo, D. J., & Eskin, A. (1978). Serotonin shifts the phase of the circadian rhythm from the aplysia eye. *Science, 202*, 977–979.

Corrent, G., McAdoo, D. J., & Eskin, A. (1982). Transmitter-like action of serotonin in phase shifting a rhythm from the aplysia eye. *Am. J. Physiol.*, *242*, 326–332.

Czeisler, C. A., Richardson, G. S., et al. (1981). Entrainment of human circadian rhythms by light-dark cycles: A reassessment. *Photochem. Photobiol.*, *34*, 239–242.

Czeisler, C. A., et al. (1986). Bright light resets the human circadian pacemaker independent of the timing of the sleep wake cycle. *Science, 233*, 667–671.

DeCoursey, P. J. (1960). Daily light sensitivity rhythm in a rodent. *Science, 131*, 33–35.

Demisch, K., Demisch, L., Nickelsen, T., & Rieth, R. (1987). The influence of acute and subchronic administration of various antidepressants on early morning melatonin plasma levels in healthy subjects: Increases following fluvoxamine. *J. Neur. Transm.*, *68*, 257–270.

Domanski, E., Przekup, F., Skubiszewski, B., & Wollinska, E. (1975). The effect and site of action of indoleamines on the hypothalamic centers involved in the control of LH release and ovulation in sheep. *Neuroendocrinology*, *17*, 265–273.

Dunn, J. D., Johnson, D. C., & Castro, A. J. (1983). The effect of raphe transection on circadian patterns of corticosterone. *Neuroendocrinol. Lett.*, *5*, 233–238.

Durkheim, E. (1897). *Le suicide* (Paris, 1952). Translated as *Suicide: A study in sociology*, J. A. Spaulding and C. Simpson. London: Routledge & Kegan Paul.

Eastwood, M. R., & Peacocke, J. (1976). Seasonal patterns of suicide, depression and electroconvulsive therapy. *Br. J. Psychiatry*, *129*, 472.

Eastwood, M. R., & Stiasny, S. (1979). Psychiatric disorder, hospital admission and season. *Arch. Gen. Psychiatry*, *35*, 469.

Egeland, J. A., & Sussex, J. N. (1985). Suicide and family loading for affective disorders. *JAMA*, *254*, 915–918.

Elliot, J. A. (1976). Circadian rhythms and photoperiodic time measurement in mammals. *Fed. Proc. Fed. Am. Soc. Exp. Biol.*, *35*, 2339–2346.

Faradji, H., Cespuglio, R., & Jouvet, M. (1983). Voltametric measurements of 5-hydroxyindole compounds in the suprachiasmatic nuclei—Circadian fluctuations. *Brain Res.*, *279*, 111–119.

Frangos, E., Athanassenas, G., Tsitourides, S., Psilolignos, P., Robos, A., Katsanou, N., & Bulgaris, C. (1980). Seasonality of the episodes of recurrent affective psychoses: Possible prophylactic interventions. *J. Affect. Dis., 2*, 239.

Gallo, R. V. (1980). Neuroendocrine regulation of pulsatile luteinizing hormone release in the rat. *Neuroendocrinology, 30*, 122–131.

Goodman, R. L., & Karsch, F. J. (1981). The hypothalamic pulse generator: A key determinant of reproductive cycles in sheep. In B. K. Follet & D. E. Follet (Eds.), *Biological clocks in seasonal reproductive cycles* (pp. 223–236). Bristol, England: J. Wright.

Groos, G., & Hendriks, J. (1982). Circadian rhythms in electrical discharge of rat suprachiasmatic neurons recorded in vitro. *Neurosci. Lett., 34*, 283–288.

Groos, G. A., & Mason, R. (1982). An electrophysiological study of the rat's suprachiasmatic nuclei: A locus for action of antidepressants. *J. Physiol., 330*, 40.

Halberg, F. (1968). Physiologic considerations underlying rhythmometry, with special reference to emotional illness. In de ajuriaguerra, J. (Ed.), *Cycles Biologiques et Psychiatrie*, Paris: Masson.

Hastings, J. H., Herbert, J., et al. (1985). Annual reproductive rhythms in mammals: Mechanisms of light synchronization. In R. J. Wurtman, M. J. Baum, & J. T. Potts, Jr. (Eds.), *The medical and biological effects of light* (pp. 123–133). New York: New York Academy of Sciences.

Hery, M., Laplante, E., & Kordon, C. (1976). Participation of serotonin in the phasic release of LH. Evidence from pharmacological experiments. *Endocrinol., 99*, 496–503.

Hery, M., Faudon, M., Dusticier, G., & Hery, F. (1982). Daily variations in serotonin metabolism in the suprachiasmatic nucleus of the rat: Influence of oestradiol implantation. *J. Endocr., 94*, 157–166.

Hippocrates: On Endemic Diseases (Air, Waters and Places). (1969). Mattuck, J. N., & Lyons, M. C. (Eds.). Cambridge: Heffer and Sons.

Illernova, H., & Vanecek, J. (1982). Two oscillator structure of the pacemaker controlling the circadian rhythm of N-acetyltransferase in the rat pineal gland. *J. Comp. Physiol., 145*, 539–548.

Inouye, S. T. (1984). Light responsiveness of the suprachiasmatic nucleus within the island with the retino-hypothalamic tract spared. *Brain Res., 294*, 263–268.

Inouye, S. T., & Kawamura, H. (1979). Persistence of circadian rhythmicity in mammalian hypothalamic "island" containing the suprachiasmatic nucleus. *Proc. Natl. Acad. Sci. U.S.A., 76*, 5961–5966.

Inouye, S. T., & Kawamura, H. (1982). Characteristics of a circadian pacemaker in the suprachiasmatic nucleus. *J. Comp. Physiol., 146*, 153–160.

Jacobsen, F. M., Mueller, E. A., Sack, D. A., & Rosenthal, N. E. (1987). Subjective and physiological responses of SAD patients and controls to intravenous m-CPP. Paper presented at the 42nd annual meeting of the Society of Biological Psychiatry, Chicago, May.

Jouvet, M. (1972). The role of monoamines and acetylcholine-containing neurons in the regulation of the sleep-waking cycle. *Ergeb. Physiol., 64*, 166–307.

Klein, D. C. (1985). Photoneural regulation of the mammalian pineal gland. In F. Pittman (Ed.), *Photoperiodism, melatonin and the pineal.* (Ciba Foundation Symposium 17) (pp. 38–56).

Klein, D. C., & Weller, J. L. (1972). Rapid light-induced decrease in pineal serotonin N-acetytransferase activity. *Science, 177*, 532–533.

Kraepelin, E. (1921). *Manic-depressive insanity and paranoia.* Translated by R. M.
Barclay (G. M. Robertson, Ed.), Edinburgh: E. & S. Livingston.

Kripke, D. (1983). Phase advance theories for affective illness. In T. A. Wehr &
F. K. Goodwin (Eds.), *Circadian rhythms in psychiatry* (pp. 41–47). Pacific
Grove, CA: Boxwood Press.

Kripke, D. F. (1984). Critical interval hypotheses for depression. *Chronobiol. Int.,
1*, 73–80.

Kripke, D. F., Mullaney, D. J., Atkinson, M. L., & Wolf, S. (1978). Circadian
rhythm disorders in manic-depressives. *Biol. Psychiatry, 13*, 335–351.

Kupfer, D. J., & Reynolds, R. F. (1983). Neurophysiological studies of depression:
State of the art. In J. Angst (Ed.), *The origins of depression* (pp. 235–252).
Berlin: Heidelberg.

Lester, D. (1979). Seasonal variation in suicidal deaths. *Br. J. Psychiatry, 118*, 627–
628.

Levitan, I. B., & Benson, J. A. (1981). Neuronal oscillators in aplysia: Modulation
by serotonin and cyclic AMP. *Trends Neurosci., 4*, 38–41.

Lewy, A. J., Sack, R. L., et al. (1983). The use of bright light in the treatment of
chronobiologic sleep and mood disorder. The phase response-curve. *Psychopharm. Bull., 19*, 523–525.

Lewy, A. J., Sack, R. L., & Singer, C. M. (1984). Assessment and treatment of
chronobiologic disorders using plasma melatonin levels and bright light exposure: The clock-gate model and phase response curve. *Psychopharmacol. Bull.,
20*, 561–565.

Lewy, A. J., Sack, R. L., & Singer, C. M. (1985). Immediate and delayed effects of
bright light on human melatonin production. *Ann. N. Y. Acad. Sci., 453*, 253–
259.

Lewy, A. J., Wehr, T. A., et al. (1980). Light suppresses melatonin secretion in humans. *Science, 210*, 1267–1269.

Lewy, A. J., Wehr, T. A., et al. (1981). Manic-depressive patients may be supersensitive to light. *Lancet, 8216*, 383–384.

Lewy, A. J., Sack, R. L., & Singer, C. M. (1986). Bright light, melatonin, and biological rhythms. *Psychopharm. Bull., 21*, 368–372.

Lewy, A. J., Sack, R. L., & Singer, C. M. (1985). Treating phase-typed chronobiologic sleep and mood disorders using appropriately timed bright artificial
light. *Psychopharm. Bull., 21*, 368–372.

Lewy, A. J., Sack, R. L., Singer, C. M., & White, D. M. (1987a). The phase shift
hypothesis of bright light. Therapeutic mechanism of action: Theoretical considerations and experimental evidence. *Psychopharm. Bull., 23*, 349–353.

Lewy, A. J., Sack, R. L., Miller, S., & Hoban, T. M. (1987b). Antidepressant and
circadian phase-shifting effects of light. *Science, 235*, 352–354.

Lewy, A. J., Sack, R. L., Singer, C. W., White, D. M., & Hoban, T. M. (1988).
Winter depression and the phase-shift hypothesis for bright light's therapeutic
effects: History, theory and experimental evidence. *J. Biol. Rhythms, 3*, 121–
134.

Lydic, R., Albers, H. E., Tepper, B., & Moore-Ede, M. C. (1982). Three-dimensional structure of the mammalian suprachiasmatic nucleus: A comparative study of five species. *J. Comp. Neurol.*, *204*, 225-237.

Lydic, R., Schoene, W. C., Czeisler, C. A., & Moore-Ede, M. C. (1980). Suprachiasmatic region of the human hypothalamus: Homolog to the primate circadian pacemaker? *Sleep*, *2*, 355-361.

Mason, R. (1986). Circadian variation in sensitivity of suprachiasmatic and lateral geniculate neurones to 5-hydroxytryptamine in the rat. *J. Physiol.*, *377*, 1-13.

Mason, R., & Meijer, J. (1982). Enhanced responsiveness of rat suprachiasmatic nucleus (SCN) neurons to 5-hydroxytryptamine (5-HT) following chronic imipramine treatment. *J. Physiol.*, *332*, 105-106.

Menaker, M. (1979). Aspects of the physiology of circadian rhythmicity in the vertebrate nervous system. In F. O. Schmitt & F. G. Worden (Eds.), *The neurosciences: Third study program* (pp. 479-489). Cambridge, MA: MIT Press.

Mendlewicz, J., Branchey, L., et al. (1980). The 24-hour profile of plasma melatonin in depressed patients before and after treatment. *Psychopharm.*, *4*, 49-55.

Meyer, D. C., & Quay, W. B. (1976). Hypothalamic and suprachiasmatic uptake of serotonic in vitro: Twenty-four hour changes in male and proostrous female rats. *Endocrinology*, *98*, 1160-1165.

Milstein, V., Small, J. G., Shelbourne, D., & Small, I. F. (1976). Manic depressive illness: Onset, diurnal temperature and season of birth. *Dis. Nerv. System.*, *37*, 373.

Moore, R. Y. (1983). Organization and function of a central nervous system circadian oscillator. The suprachiasmatic hypothalamic nucleus. *Fed. Proc.*, *42*, 2783-2787.

Moore, R. Y., & Card, J. P. (1985). Visual pathways and the entrainment of circadian rhythms. In R. J. Wurtman, M. J. Baum, & J. T. Potts, Jr. (Eds.), *The medical and biological effects of light* (pp. 123-133). New York: New York Academy of Sciences.

Moore-Ede, M., & Sulzman, W. S. (1981). Internal temporal order. In J. Aschoff (Ed.), *Handbook of behavioral neurology, vol. 4, Biological rhythms* (pp. 215-241). New York: Plenum Press.

Moore-Ede, M. C., Sulzman, W. S., & Fuller, C. A. (1982). *The clocks that time us* (pp. 152-200). Cambridge, MA: Harvard University Press.

Moore-Ede, M. C., Sulzman, W. S., et al. (1976). Internal organizations of the circadian timing system in multicellular animals. *Am. Soc. Exp. Biol.*, *35*, 2333-2358.

Murphy, D. L., Garrich, N. A., Tamarkin, L., Taylor, P. L., & Markeg, S. P. (1986). Effects of antidepressants and other psychotropic drugs on melatonin release and pineal gland function. In R. J. Wurtman & F. Waldhauser (Eds.), *Melatonin in humans, Proceedings*, First International Conference on Melatonin in Humans, Vienna, Austria, November 7-9, 1985. New York: Springer [*J. Neural Trans.*, *21* (Suppl), 261-277].

Myers, D. H., & Davies, P. (1978). The seasonal incidence of mania and its relationship to climatic variables. *Psychol. Med.*, *8*, 433.

Nadakavukaren, J. J., Lickey, M. E., & Jordan, W. P. (1986). Regulation of the circadian clock in the aplysia eye: Mimicry of neural action by serotonin. *J. Neurosci.*, *6*, 14–21.

Namboodiri, M. A. A., Sugden, D., Klein, D. C., Tamarkin, L., & Medford, I. N. (1985). Serum melatonin and pineal indolamine metabolism in a species with a small day/light N-acetytansferase rhythm. *Comp. Biochem. Physiol. B. Comp. Biochem.*, *80*, 731–736.

O'Rourke, D. A., Wurtman, J. J., Brzezinski, A., Nader, T. A., & Chew, B. (1987). Serotonin implicated in the etiology of seasonal affective disorder. *Psychopharmacol. Bull.*, *23*, 258–360.

Papousek, M. (1975). Chronobiological aspects of cyclothymia. *Fortschr. Neurol. Psychiatr.*, *43*, 381–440.

Pengelley, E. T., & Asmundson, S. J. (1974). Circannual periodicity in hibernating mammals. In E. Pengelley (Ed.), *Circannual clocks: Annual biological rhythms*. New York: Academic Press.

Pinel, P. (1806). *A treatise on insanity*. Translated by D. D. David. London: Cadell & Davies.

Pittendrigh, C. S. (1961). On temporal organization in living systems—The handiwork of Darwin's demon. Lecture delivered at Princeton University, January 19, 1961.

Ramirez, V. D., Feder, H. H., & Sawyer, C. H. (1984). The role of LH secretion: A critical inquiry. In L. Maritini & W. F. Ganong (Eds.), *Frontiers in neuroendocrinology* (pp. 27–84). New York: Raven Press.

Ramirez, A. D., Ramirez, V. D., & Meyer, D. C. (1987). The nature and magnitude of in vivo 5-hydroxyindoleacetic acid output from 5-hydroxytryptamine terminals is related to specific regions of the suprachiasmatic nucleus. *Neuroendocrinology*, *46*, 430–438.

Rasmussen, D. D. (1986). Physiological interactions of the basic rest-activity cycle of the brain: Pulsatile luteinizing hormone secretion as a model. *Psychoneuroendocrinology*, *11*, 389–405.

Rasmussen, D. D., Liu, J. H., Wolf, P. L., & S. S. C. Yen (1983). Regulation of gonadotropin-releasing hormone release from the human fetal hypothalamus in vitro. *J. Clin. Endocrinol. Metab.*, *57*, 881–884.

Reiter, R. J. (1983). Seasonal reproductive events related to the pineal gland. In J. Axelrod, F. Fraxhim, & G. P. Velo (Eds.), *The pineal gland and its endocrine role* (pp. 303–316). New York: Plenum Press.

Reppert, S. M., Perlow, M. J., Ungerleider, L. G., Mishkin, M., et al. (1981). Effects of damage to the suprachiasmatic area of the anterior hypothalamus on the daily melatonin and cortisol rhythms in the rhesus monkey. *J. Neurosci.*, *1*, 1414–1425.

Reppert, S. M., Weaver, D. R., Rivkees, S. A., & Stopa, E. G. (1988). Putative melatonin receptors in a human biological clock. *Science*, *242*, 78–80.

Rosenthal, N. E., Genhart, M., Jacobsen, F. M., Skwerer, R. G., & Wehr, T. A. (1987). Disturbances of appetite and weight regulation in seasonal affective disorder. *Ann. N.Y. Acad. Sci.*, *499*, 216–230.

Rosenthal, N. E., Sack, D. A., Carpenter, C. D., Perry, B. L., Mendelson, W. B., Tamarkin, L., & Wehr, T. A. (1985). Antidepressant effects of light in seasonal affective disorder. *Am. J. Psych.*, *143*, 163–170.

Rosenthal, N. E., Sack, D. A., James, S. P., Perry, B. L., Mendelson, W. B., Tamarkin, L., & Wehr, T. A. (1985). Seasonal affective disorder and phototherapy. *Ann. N.Y. Acad. Sci.*, *453*, 260–268.

Rosenthal, N. E., Sack, D. A., Gillin, J. C., & Lewy, A. J. (1984). Seasonal affective disorder. *Arch. Gen. Psych.*, *41*, 72–80.

Rosenthal, N. E., Skwerer, R. G., Sack, D. A., et al. (1987). Biological effects of morning plus-evening bright light treatment of seasonal affective disorder. *Psychopharm. Bull.*, *23*, 3.

Rusak, B., & Zucker, I. (1979). Neural regulation of circadian rhythms. *Physiol. Rev.*, *59*, 449–526.

Sack, D. A., James, S. P., Rosenthal, N. E., et al. (1988). Deficient nocturnal surge of TSH secretion during sleep and sleep deprivation in rapid-cycling bipolar illness. *Psychiatry Res.*, *23*, 179–191.

Sadlier, R. M. F. S. (1969). *The ecology of reproduction in wild and domestic mammals*. London: Methuen.

Schulz, H., & Lund, R. (1985). On the origins of early REM episodes in the sleep of depressed patients: A comparison of three hypotheses. *Psychiat. Res.*, *16*, 65–77.

Schwartz, W. T., Davidson, L. C., & Sanita, C. B. (1980). In vivo metabolic activity of a putative circadian oscillator, the rat suprachiasmatic nucleus. *J. Comp. Neurol.*, *189*, 157–167.

Shibata, S., Lion, S. Y., Ueki, S., Oomura, Y. (1984). Influence of environmental light-dark cycle and enucleation on activity of suprachiasmatic nucleus in slice preparation. *Brain. Res.*, *302*, 75–81.

Siever, L. J., & Davis, K. L. (1985). Overview: Toward a dysregulation hypothesis of depression. *Am J. Psychiatry*, *142*, 1017–1031.

Skwerer, R. G., Jacobsen, F. M., Duncan, C. C., Kelley, K. A., et al. (1988). Neurobiology of seasonal affective disorder and phototherapy. *J. Biol. Rhythms*, *3*, 135–154.

Snyder, S. H., Zweig, M., Axelrod, J., & Fisher, J. E. (1965). *Proc. Nat. Acad. Sci. U.S.A.*, *53*, 301–305.

Souetre, E., Salvati, E., Belgou, J. L., Douillet, P., et al. (1987). Seasonality of suicides: Environmental, sociological and biological covariations. *J. Affect. Dis.*, *13*, 215–225.

Souetre, E., Salvati, E., Wehr, T., Sack, D., et al. (1988). Twenty-four-hour profiles of body temperature and plasma TSH in bipolar patients during depression, during remission and in normal controls. *Am. J. Psych.*, *145*, 1133–1136.

Szafarczyk, A., Alonso, G., & Malatal, G. (1980). Serotonergic system and circadian rhythms of ACTH and corticosterone. *Am. J. Physiol.*, *239*, 482–489.

Szafarczyk, A., Ixart, G., Alonso, G., Malaval, F., Nouguier-Soule, J., & Assenmacher, I. (1981). Effects of raphe lesions on circadian ACTH, corticosterone and motor-activity rhythms in free running blinded rats. *Neurosci. Lett.*, *23*, 92–97.

Teicher, M. H., Lawrence, J., Barker, N., et al. (1988). Increased activity and phase delay in circadian activity motility rhythms in geriatric depression. *Arch. Gen. Psych.*, *45*, 913–917.

Terman, M., & Terman, J. (1985). A circadian pacemaker for visual sensitivity. In

R. J. Wurtman, M. J. Baum, & J. T. Potts, Jr. (Eds.), *The medical and biological effects of light*. New York: New York Academy of Sciences.

Thompson, C., & Issacs, G. (1988). Seasonal affective disorder—A British sample. *J. Affect. Dis.*, *14*, 1–11.

Thompson, C., Mezey, G., Corn, T., Franey, C., English, J., Arendt, S. A., Checkley. (1985). The effect of desipramine upon melatonin and cortisol secretions in depressed and normal subjects. *Br. J. Psychiatry*, *147*, (4), 389–393.

Trulson, M. E., & Jacobs, B. L. (1979). Raphe unit activity in freely moving cats: Correlation with level of behavioral arousal. *Brain Res.*, *163*, 135–150.

Van den Pol, A., & Tsujimoto, K. L. (1985). Neurotransmitters of the hypothalamic suprachiasmatic nucleus: Immunocytochemical analysis of 25 neuronal antigens. *Neuroscience*, *15*, 1049–1086.

Van de Kar, L. D., & Lorens, S. A. (1979). Differential serotonin innervation of individual hypothalamic nuclei and other forebrain regions by the dorsal and median raphe nuclei. *Brain Res.*, *162*, 45–54.

Vanecek, J., Pavlik, A., & Illernova, H. (1987). Hypothalamic melatonin receptor sites revealed by autoradiography. *Brain Res.*, *435*, 359–362.

Vaughn, M. K. (1981). The pineal gland—A survey of its antigonadotropic substances and their actions. In S. M. McCann (Ed.), *International review of physiology—Endocrine physiology III*, vol. 24 (pp. 41–95). Baltimore, MD: University Park Press.

Voisin, P., Namboodiri, M. A. A., & Klein, D. C. (1984). Arylamine N-acetyltransferase and arylalkylamine N-acetyltransferase in the mammalian pineal gland. *J. Biol. Chem.*, *254*, 10913–10918.

Von Zerssen, D., Barthelems, H., Dirlich, G., et al. (1985). Circadian rhythms in endogenous depression. *Psychiatry Res.*, *16*, 51–63.

Walter, S. D. (1977). Seasonality of mania: A reappraisal. *Br. J. Psychiatry*, *131*, 345.

Wehr, T. A., Jacobsen, F., Sack, D. A., Arendt, J., Tamarkin, L., & Rosenthal, N. E. (1985). The efficacy of phototherapy in seasonal affective disorder appears not to depend on its timing or its effect on melatonin secretion. *Arch. Gen. Psychiatry*, 43, 870.

Wehr, T. A., Sack, D. A., & Rosenthal, N. E. (1987). Seasonal affective disorder with summer depression and winter hypomania. *Am. J. Psychiatry*, *144*, 1602–1603.

Wehr, T. A., & Rosenthal, N. E. (1989). Seasonality and affective illness. *Am. J. Psychiatry*, *146*, 829–837.

Weitzman, E. D., Czeisler, C. A., & Moore-Ede, M. C. (1979). Sleep-wake, neuroendocrine and body temperature circadian rhythms under entrained and non-entrained (free-running) conditions in man. In M. Suda, O. Hayaishi, & H. Nakaguwa (Eds.), *The NATO Foundation. Biological rhythms and their central mechanism*. Amsterdam: Elsevier/North-Holland Biomedical Press.

Wever, R. (1974). Influence of light on human circadian rhythms. *Nordic Council Arct. Med. Res. Rep.*, *10*, 33–47.

Wuttke, W., Hancke, J. L., Hohn, K. G., & Baumgarten, H. G. (1978). Effect of intraventricular injection of 5,7-dihydroxytryptamine on serum gonadotropins and prolactin. *Ann. N.Y. Acad. Sci.*, *305*, 423–436.

Yates, C. A., & Herbert, J. (1976). Differential circadian rhythms in pineal and hypothalamic 5-HT induced by artificial photoperiods or melatonin. *Nature, 262,* 219–220.

Zucker, I., Rusak, B., & King, R. C., Jr. (1976). Neural basis for circadian rhythms in rodent behavior. In A. H. Rieser & R. F. Thompson (Eds.), *Advances in psychobiology* (pp. 35–74). New York: Wiley.

12

Serotonergic Parameters of Aggression and Suicide

ALAN APTER
SERENA-LYNN BROWN
MARTIN L. KORN
HERMAN M. van PRAAG

THE IMPORTANCE OF THE CONCEPT OF AGGRESSION IN PSYCHIATRY

Aggression as a psychiatric concept requires examination in broad evolutionary terms. It is a complex phenomenon that serves many functions in human and animal life. Ethologists have noted that there are a number of similarities between threat and attack patterns in chimpanzees and humans (Hamburg, 1971), and have pointed out that aggressive behavior increases access to resources, helps resolve conflicts among individuals having hierarchical relationships with one another, mobilizes energy for mating competition, and increases the chances of successful courtship and mating (Tinbergen, 1953; Feshbach, 1964; Lorenz, 1966). Thus, aggression can be seen as an adaptive response under specific conditions, increasing the chances of individual survival as well as the likelihood of genetic representation in future generations. This is referred to by ethologists as "inclusive fitness" (Plutchik et al., 1986).

So fundamental is aggression to animal behavior that most species have developed display behaviors to indicate its presence. For example, Leyhausen has identified various typical aggressive and fearful postures used by cats (Hinde, 1966). Similar patterns have been described in dogs, birds, and fish (Morris, 1954; Hinde, 1966; Eibl-Eibesfeldt, 1971).

Neuroanatomical and neurophysiological research have shown that affect and emotion are modulated by the limbic system. Brain loci that are believed to organize specific patterns of aggressive behavior include the lateral hypothalamus, the ventral tegmental area, the centromedial amygdala, the

284

midbrain central grey area, and the central and anterior portions of the septum (Miller, 1957; Adams, 1979; Valzelli, 1981; Brain, 1984; Kling, 1986). Elliott (1987) has pointed out that activating and inhibitory areas of the neuronal network appear in close proximity, so that one can see either assaultive or rageful behavior or inhibition of aggression by stimulation of different narrowly specified portions of the same neuroanatomical area, such as the amygdala, in both humans and monkeys.

Elliott (1987) has also described several distinct types of human aggressive behavioral syndromes, along with evidence that these syndromes may have an organic basis. He suggests that compulsive aggression may be associated with lesions of the hypothalamus, cingulate gyrus, and orbitofrontal and temporal lobes. Out of 286 cases of episodic dyscontrol syndrome studied by Elliott, he reports that 102 cases developed following a specific brain insult, with the remaining 184 associated with childhood minimal brain dysfunction, perinatal problems, epilepsy, other persistent convulsions, or encephalitis during early years. Finally, he suggests that antisocial personality disorder may have an organic etiology. Specifically, he cites evidence from animal research that a certain form of animal "psychopathic behavior" is seen when monkeys and other animals are isolated in early life and are subjected to social and sensory deprivation. Because of histological and other organic abnormalities seen in the brains of these animals at autopsy, Elliott speculates that such behavior in humans, seen in antisocial personality disorder, may arise from abnormalities in postnatal brain development (involving such processes as myelination), since this has been shown to be dependent on appropriate external stimulation.

Neurotransmitter systems are also thought to play an important role in the expression of aggression (Raleigh & McGuire, 1980). Evidence suggests that serotonin (5-hydroxytryptamine, or 5-HT), norepinephrine (NE), dopamine (DA), and acetylcholine may all be involved in the initiation and maintenance of aggressive behaviors in animals, and there are some recent data suggesting the involvement of serotonin and the catecholamines (CAs) in human aggression (Raleigh & McGuire, 1980; Valzelli, 1981; van Praag, 1984; King, 1986).

Aggressivity may also be related to genetically transmitted factors. Agonistic behavior has been shown to be heritable in mice and dogs (Fuller, 1986). Maxson and Trattner (1981), and Selmanoff and Ginsberg (1981) have selectively bred a line of aggressive mice in which aggressivity cosegregates with the Y chromosome. The combination of genetic and biochemical studies may be a fruitful avenue for elucidating underlying mechanisms of aggression. For instance, Ciaranello et al. (1974) have demonstrated that inheritance of high concentrations of adrenal or CAergic enzymes is highly correlated with aggressive behavior in mice, and segregates as a single Mendelian recessive gene (Ciaranello, 1979), and Orenberg et al. (1975) have shown that genetic transmission of brain cyclic adenosine monophosphate (cAMP) is closely correlated with aggressive behavior in mice (Elliott et al., 1987).

Human studies of personality and temperament have indicated significant genetic components for assertiveness, extroversion, and dominance (Loehlin & Nichols, 1976; Loehlin et al., 1981), while other studies have also suggested a genetic component to aggressive behavior (Fuller & Thompson, 1978; Goldsmith, 1983; Wimer & Wimer, 1985).

It should be noted, however, that Palmour (1983) has pointed out that one major problem with human genetic studies of aggression is that investigators have equated criminality with aggressive behavior, without taking ability or inability to control aggressive impulses into account. There is, in fact, a large body of literature concerning the possible association between criminal behavior/aggression and the chromosomal abnormality 47,XYY in men. However, while a number of studies have demonstrated such a correlation, some investigators have shown no association between individuals with this genetic abnormality and higher levels of aggression or criminal activity (Kessler et al., 1977; Vogel & Motulsky, 1979).

Finally, Palmour (1983) has conducted a series of studies on Lesch-Nyhan disease, an X-linked recessive disorder associated with compulsive self-mutilatory behavior. This disease is characterized by deficiency of the enzyme hypoxanthine phosphoribosyltransferase (HPRT), and by excessive purine synthesis. She has succeeded in inducing self-mutilatory behavior in rats through the use of a variety of agents, including DA agonists, and is currently looking at the possible role of the DAergic system in this type of self-directed aggressive behavior.

Apart from its bioevolutionary importance to psychiatry, an understanding of aggression is also important in everyday clinical practice. Tardiff and Sweillam (1980), in surveying admissions to New York State psychiatric hospitals, reported that approximately 10% of patients had engaged in aggressive or assaultive behaviors in the two weeks prior to admission, and other studies of individual hospital psychiatric populations have reported that up to 40% of psychiatric patients had engaged in such behavior before being admitted (Rossi et al., 1985; Binder & McNeil, 1986). Acts of violence by psychiatric patients are common, and as a result, restraint and seclusion procedures, as well as medications, are used routinely in most hospitals to calm patients. Surveys of seclusion practices have indicated that, at one major urban acute service hospital, 26% of inpatients are secluded during their hospital stay, primarily for assaultive behavior (Plutchik et al., 1976). In addition, there are reports that up to 40% of psychiatrists may have been physically attacked at least once by patients

(Madden et al., 1976), and some work has been done demonstrating the need for training programs to enhance clinician confidence in coping with possible patient aggression (Thackrey, 1987).

The role of aggression, both inwardly and outwardly directed, in the various major psychiatric disorders has not yet been addressed in any systematic manner. Thus, both because of obvious moral, legal, and sociological issues, and because of its prevalence among psychiatric patients, the study of aggression is emerging as an increasingly important area of psychiatric research.

CLINICAL RELATIONSHIP BETWEEN SUICIDALITY AND AGGRESSION

The importance of suicidology for psychiatry needs no elaboration. However, the "epidemic" of suicidal behavior in the young in recent years (Shaffer & Fisher, 1981) has made this a major public health issue, as well. Suicide, homicide, and car accidents are now the leading causes of death in the 15–24-year-old age group (Pfeffer, 1986). Prevention programs have proved ineffective, and may even be dangerous (Eisenberg, 1986), as there is some debate as to whether they might cause an increase in suicide attempts, probably via a "Werther" effect in which individuals imitate others' suicidal behavior (Gould & Shaffer, 1986).

The relationship between suicide and aggression has long been recognized by psychoanalysts, and has been best formulated by Menninger (1933), who proposed that a dynamic triad underlies all aggressive behavior, whether directed inward or outward: the wish to die, the wish to kill, and the wish to be killed. These are all seen as derivatives of Freud's concept of *thanatos*, or the death instinct.

There are many reports in the daily press of murderers who commit suicide. Roughly one out of four patients with a history of violent actions has made a suicide attempt (Skodal & Karasu, 1978; Tardiff & Sweillam, 1980). Inamdar et al. (1982), reporting on the prevalence of violent and suicidal behavior in a sample of 51 hospitalized adolescents, found that 66.7% had been violent, 43.1% had been suicidal, and 27.5% had been both. According to various authors, from 7% to 48% of those patients with a history of violent behavior have also made suicide attempts in the past. This is reported to be true for adults (Skodal & Karasu, 1978) and for prepubertal children (Pfeffer et al., 1986). Similar findings have been reported in prisoners (Plutchik et al., 1976; Climent et al., 1977).

Looking at the issue in terms of patients who are predominantly suicidal, Tardiff and Sweillam (1980) found that of a large group of suicidal patients admitted to mental hospitals, 14% of males and 7% of females were assaultive at the time of or just prior to admission. Similarly, on the basis of detailed studies of psychotic patients, Kermani (1981) has identified what he calls the "violent depressive type," who has a long history of suicide attempts, as well as a history of violence. It has likewise been reported that female suicide attempters show more hostility and engage in more arguments and have more friction with friends and relatives than a comparable group of nonsuicidal depressed women. Hospitalized depressed patients with a history of self-destructive acts have also been found to have high levels of hostility and violence as measured by their need for seclusion and restraint (Weissman et al., 1973).

In a group of 100 psychiatric inpatients with mixed diagnoses, Plutchik et al. (1986) found that about 40% had made past suicide attempts, 42% had engaged in past violent behavior, and 23% had histories of both types of behavior. These investigators measured 30 variables in this group of patients, including such parameters as life problems, hopelessness, styles of coping, and depression. Almost every one of these 30 variables turned out to be a significant predictor of both suicide risk and violence risk. These results strongly support the idea of a close link between suicide risk and violence risk regardless of diagnosis.

In summary, then, there seems to be a significant relationship between aggression and suicidality among both psychiatric patients and people who have never been treated psychiatrically. Such a relationship has been noted and commented upon by a number of investigators, but as yet has not been further teased out. We suggest that this relationship may be critical to the understanding of both suicidality and violence, and requires extensive further study.

SEROTONIN AND SUICIDALITY

5-hydroxyindoleacetic acid (5-HIAA) is the major metabolite of serotonin (5-HT). Low baseline and postprobenecid cerebrospinal fluid (CSF) 5-HIAA is thought to be indicative of lowered 5-HT metabolism in the central nervous system (CNS) (van Praag, 1986). Decreased levels of CSF 5-HIAA in depressed individuals provided the first evidence suggesting disordered 5-HT metabolism in depressive disorder. This finding has been reported by most, though not by all, investigators, under both baseline conditions and after probenecid loading (van Praag, 1982). Such decreased levels of CSF 5-HIAA are found mostly in patients with major depression, melancholic subtype. However, it should be noted that, in most studies, no more than 30–40% of patients with melancholic depression showed this finding, suggesting the possibility of biological subtypes of melancholic depression, and spurring further research in this area.

A good deal of further investigation of CSF 5-HIAA in depression and in other psychiatric disorders, showing lowered CSF 5-HIAA associated with suicidality regardless of psychiatric diagnosis, led to the hypothesis that such 5-HT disturbances (as reflected by lowered CSF 5-HIAA) may not be related to a particular subtype of depression per se (the nosological approach), but rather to particular psychopathological dimensions often associated with depression (the functional or dimensional approach) (van Praag et al., 1987). One such dimension that our group has focused upon has been suicidality (van Praag, 1986; van Praag et al., 1987).

The risk of suicide attempts in depressed patients has been found to be unevenly distributed (van Praag & Plutchik, 1988). Some patients resort to such attempts, but the majority do not, and there seems to be no direct relationship between degree of depression and degree of suicidality, suggesting different biological markers for depression and suicidality. This is supported by the fact that, in a group of depressed patients with a lifetime history of at least one suicide attempt, the attempt frequency was shown to be skewed, with a minority of patients being responsible for the majority of attempts. The depressed multiple-suicide attempters were also most likely to have decreased CSF 5-HIAA (van Praag & Plutchik, 1988).

Decreased CSF 5-HIAA has been demonstrated in depressed patients after inpatient hospital admission for a suicide attempt (Oreland et al., 1981; van Praag, 1982; Banki & Arato, 1983; Banki et al., 1984). It has also been found in patients with a lifetime history of suicidal behavior (Agren, 1980), as well as in subjects with suicidal ideation (Agren, 1983; Palanappian et al., 1983; Lopez-Ibor et al., 1985). It should be noted, however, that one study has reported both increased and decreased CSF 5-HIAA levels in patients with suicidal ideation (Agren, 1983). Interestingly, low CSF 5-HIAA in suicide attempters has also been reported to be correlated with lowered CSF magnesium levels (Banki et al., 1985).

Traskman et al. (1981) did a one-year follow-up study of a cohort of 119 depressed patients, 46 of whom had been admitted to the hospital for a suicide attempt. Within this group of 46, 30 patients had low CSF 5-HIAA levels at index admission. One year after discharge, six of these low CSF 5-HIAA patients had committed suicide but none of the other 89 patients with low CSF 5-HIAA had done so. Thus, these data suggest that one might be able to obtain prospective information by measuring CSF 5-HIAA. Commensurate with this, it has also been reported that depressives with low CSF 5-HIAA may have lower response rates to antidepressant medication (van Praag et al., 1973a).

Three negative studies have been published, of which two are from the same group. Roy et al. (1985,1986) reported low CSF homovanillic acid (HVA), the primary metabolite of DA, but normal CSF 5-HIAA in depressed patients with a past history of suicide attempts. In the first study

(Roy et al., 1985), most of the subject population was diagnosed as having bipolar disorder, as compared with the majority of studies done in this area, which have been conducted with unipolar patients, which may account for this finding (Agren, 1983). Moreover, CSF 5-HIAA levels in control subjects were much lower than those reported by Asberg's group (Asberg et al., 1976), suggesting that the two samples may not be comparable (van Praag, 1986). In the third negative study (Westergaard et al., 1978), a mixed group of unipolar, bipolar, and newly diagnosed depressives was studied, but the criteria for suicidality were not reported. None of these studies addressed the issue of violent versus nonviolent suicide attempts.

Further evidence suggesting a correlation between low CSF 5-HIAA and suicidality, rather than between low CSF 5-HIAA and depression, comes from the fact that nondepressed suicide attempters have also been shown to have low CSF 5-HIAA. Patients with personality disorders who have attempted suicide show low CSF 5-HIAA (Brown et al., 1979, 1982), as do schizophrenics who have made suicide attempts because of command hallucinations (Ninan et al., 1984). Similarly, Traskman (1981) reported on a group of both depressed and nondepressed suicide attempters, all of whom had decreased CSF 5-HIAA. Oreland et al. (1981) confirmed these findings in suicidal patients with minor depressive illnesses, anxiety states, personality disorders, and drug or alcohol addictions. No negative studies have been reported in nondepressed suicide attempters.

Finally, Stanley et al. (1982) and Stanley and Mann (1983) have reported a decrease in presynaptic ^{3}H-imipramine binding sites (thought to be associated with the 5-HT uptake site and to provide an index for central 5-HT function) in the hippocampus and occipital cortex of suicide victims. These findings, however, were not replicated by Meyerson et al. (1982). Gross-Isseroff et al. (1989) have found region-specific differences in ^{3}H-imipramine binding in postmortem brains of suicide victims, with increased binding in the hippocampus and the dentate gyrus and decreased binding in the postcentral cortical gyrus, insular cortex, and claustrum. However, Cheetham et al. (1988) could find no difference in binding of ^{3}H-ketanserin to 5-HT$_2$ receptor sites in the brains of 19 depressed suicide victims as compared with matched normal controls. Such studies provide mixed data, with some slight evidence of decreased 5-HT metabolism in suicide attempters. There are a number of serious problems with postmortem brain studies, however, as discussed in Chapter 5 of this volume, and a great deal of work remains to be done in this area.

SEROTONERGIC LINKS BETWEEN SUICIDALITY AND AGGRESSION

In a study of 44 patients with endogenous depression and 24 with reactive depression, Asberg et al. (1976) found a high correlation between decreased CSF 5-HIAA and history of suicide attempts, particularly those that had a violent component, during the index illness. This finding has been confirmed by most, but not all, investigators (van Praag et al., 1970, 1973a, 1973b; Oreland et al., 1981; Traskman et al., 1981; Agren, 1983; Banki & Arato, 1983; Roy-Byrne et al., 1983). Agren (1980) also found that, in depressed patients, low CSF 5-HIAA correlated not only with suicidal ideation, but also with overt anger, and has suggested that this might provide evidence in support of the hypothesis that depressives with low CSF 5-HIAA are more prone to violent suicidal acts than depressives without low CSF 5-HIAA.

Depressives with low CSF 5-HIAA appear to be not only more suicidal, but also more aggressive. Van Praag (1986) compared two groups of melancholic patients on several aggression measures, as well as on CSF 5-HIAA levels. Depressives were divided into two groups, one with normal and the other with low postprobenecid CSF 5-HIAA levels. It was found that the latter group had made more suicide attempts and demonstrated higher hostility ratings on several measures than the former group.

Interestingly, van Praag (1983), Banki et al. (1984), and Ninan et al. (1984) have all reported significantly lower concentrations of CSF 5-HIAA in suicidal (nondepressed) schizophrenic patients, with a correlation between recent suicide attempts and lower 5-HIAA, thus suggesting that the psychopathological correlate of decreased CSF 5-HIAA might involve suicidality across psychiatric diagnoses. However, it should be noted that Roy et al. (1985) could not replicate these findings, nor could Pickar et al. (1987), although these latter investigators did show a relationship between lower CSF 5-HIAA and higher hostility and uncooperativeness ratings in drug-free schizophrenics. In addition, Brown et al. (1982) reported that a history of aggressive behavior, a history of suicide attempts, and low CSF 5-HIAA were all significantly positively correlated among patients with personality disorders, while Rydin et al. (1982) showed that depressed and/ or suicidal patients with low CSF 5-HIAA had higher hostility scores and a lower anxiety tolerance than their counterparts with normal CSF 5-HIAA values.

SEROTONERGIC CORRELATES OF OUTWARDLY DIRECTED AGGRESSION

The study of aggression in both humans and animals has been hampered by the lack of a set of uniform definitions and by the variation in the display of aggressive behavior that depends on the social context in which it is expressed. Moyer (1976) has delineated seven types of aggressive behaviors and has hypothesized that a different neuroanatomical and neuropharmacological substratum underlies each of these subtypes. While such categories are important in understanding aggressive behavior in animals, it has been pointed out by Cochrane (1975) and by Marini and Sheard (1977) that the study of aggression in humans is more complicated than in animals, since a variety of psychological factors, including unconscious defense mechanisms, and environmental and social variables must also be taken into account.

In general, data from studies of the role of 5-HT in human aggression suggest that aggression and hostility can be associated with decreased 5-HT function. Brown et al. (1979) looked at 26 military men with personality disorders who were being evaluated for suitability for further service. CSF 5-HIAA showed a significant negative correlation with past history of aggressive behavior, whereas CSF 3-methoxy-4-hydroxyphenethylene glycol (MHPG), the primary CNS metabolite of NE, showed a significant correlation with such behavior. Those subjects who received a diagnosis of personality disorder associated with impulsive behavior had lower CSF 5-HIAA and higher CSF MHPG than those who did not. In a second study, Brown et al. (1982) demonstrated significant negative correlations between CSF 5-HIAA and both aggression scores on the MMPI and a history of suicide attempts in 12 individuals diagnosed as having borderline personality disorder. These data support the concept of decreased 5-HT levels in aggression, and indicate the possibility of increased NE levels in these aggressive individuals.

Similarly, Lidberg et al. (1984) reported case histories of three individuals who had a history of aggression against family members, all of whom eventually murdered a child. All three had low CSF 5-HIAA levels. Lidberg et al. (1985) also compared 16 men who had committed homicide, 22 men who had attempted suicide, and 39 controls. CSF 5-HIAA levels were lower in the suicidal men, especially in those who had used violent means and those who had killed a sexual partner (i.e., crimes of passion involving impulsivity and intense affect). Linnoila et al. (1982) found that impulsive murderers had lower CSF 5-HIAA levels than nonimpulsive murderers and multiple murderers had lower CSF 5-HIAA levels than single murderers. Other monoamine metabolites were also decreased in these impulsive murderers, but not significantly so. These studies have provided evidence that it may not be the aggressive behavior per se, but rather a lack of impulse control, that constitutes the behavioral correlate of deficient 5-HT metabolism.

Linnoila (1986) found that 20 arsonists had lower CSF 5-HIAA levels than both habitual offenders and normal controls, supporting the hypothesis that poor impulse control may be the key variable associated with decreased 5-HT metabolism in criminal offenders (Virkkunen et al., 1987).

Bioulac et al. (1980) showed that criminals with the 47,XYY syndrome (0.1% of the general population, but found in a disproportionately high percentage among the criminal population) also had significantly lower CSF 5-HIAA levels than normal controls. Treatment with the 5-HT precursor 5-HTP for five months led to clinical improvement, with a dramatic increase in CSF 5-HIAA levels in these individuals. Decreased CSF 5-HIAA has also been demonstrated in mentally retarded patients who exhibit aggression toward others (Greenberg & Coleman, 1976). O'Neil et al. (1986) have reported a case study of a retarded man with Cornelia de Lange syndrome, intense aggressive behavior toward others, and low blood 5-HT levels in whom treatment with trazodone and tryptophan resulted in an increase in blood 5-HT levels and a decrease in aggressive behavior. Finally, in contrast to the above results, it should be noted that Pliszka et al. (1987) have reported that violent delinquent boys have higher whole-blood 5-HT levels than nonviolent offenders and depressed/anxious adolescents.

Animal studies have also provided a preponderance of evidence demonstrating that potentiation of 5-HT function decreases aggression in mice and muricidal rats, while decreasing 5-HT function increases aggression in mice (Yen et al., 1959; Koe & Weissman, 1966; Kulkarni, 1968; Sheard, 1969; Hodge & Butcher, 1974; Kantak et al., 1980), thus suggesting the importance of 5-HTergic mechanisms in the mediation of aggression in these animal models (Hodge & Butcher, 1974; Valzelli, 1984). It has been proposed that specific aggressive behaviors are exhibited by animals when a critical balance between the monoaminergic systems is disturbed (Lycke et al., 1969; Eichelman & Thoa, 1973; Hodge & Butcher, 1975; Valzelli, 1984). Hodge and Butcher (1974) have suggested that the decreased aggression they have shown in mice following 5-HTP administration may be due to a combination of reduced levels of NE and/or DA and increased 5-HT levels. There are other data that support this hypothesis, such as work by Ellison and Bresler (1974) demonstrating an increase in shock-induced aggression after rats are given 6-hydroxydopamine and parachlorophenylalanine (pCPA), with consequent reductions in both CA and 5-HT levels, but not after reduction of the CA level alone. However, there are contradictory reports of increased aggression in mice after increasing DA levels through either viral encephalitis or administration of L-dopa, and decreasing 5-HT levels with pCPA (Lycke et al., 1969). These investigators also suggest that aggression may be caused by a disturbed balance between the 5-HTergic and CAergic systems.

Finally, Eichelman (1987) has suggested that the antiaggressive effects of lithium shown in both humans and rats may be moderated through the 5-HT system, since lithium is known to increase brain uptake of tryptophan, the primary dietary precursor of 5-HT, and is thought to increase brain neurotransmission of 5-HT.

CONCLUSION

The available evidence appears to indicate that low CSF 5-HIAA (both baseline and postprobenecid), indicative of decreased 5-HT metabolism in the brain, is related in some way to suicidal behavior, irrespective of syndromal or nosological diagnosis. At the same time, research in the area of outwardly directed aggression has also consistently demonstrated a negative correlation between CSF 5-HIAA levels and violence across subject populations. The nature of this relationship, encompassing low 5-HT metabolism, suicidality, and aggression, remains to be determined more fully.

For instance, we have shown that depressed patients with low CSF 5-HIAA have an increased frequency of both suicide attempts and outwardly directed aggressive behavior (van Praag, et al., 1986). This certainly provides evidence to suggest that dysregulation of aggression may be a dimension in depression, and that lowered central 5-HT metabolism thus may more accurately reflect aggression dysregulation rather than a specific 5-HTergic dysfunction directly related to the nosological category of depression itself.

Although there is some pharmacological evidence that raising brain 5-HT levels reduces aggressive behavior (see above), the relationship may be considerably more complicated than a simple linear one. Aggression is far from being a simple unidimensional psychological concept, and thus it makes such data more difficult to interpret. For instance, anxiety, another important psychopathological dimension that has never been controlled for in studies of suicide and aggression, is also associated with dysregulation of 5-HT (see Chapter 6 in this volume). Impulsivity, another psychological dimension that is often involved in suicidal and aggressive behavior, may also be associated with abnormalities in 5-HT metabolism (Plutchik et al., 1986). Much future work remains to be done on teasing apart these psychological variables in the area of aggression dysregulation, and examining the role of biological abnormalities in each. We have begun such work recently, examining predictors of suicide and violence in psychiatric patients with a variety of diagnoses. In this diverse population, we have shown that trait anxiety is highly correlated with both violence and suicidal risk, and, in fact, can be used to differentiate patients admitted to a hospital for suicide attempts from other patients (Apter et al., 1989). Such findings provide more evidence for an intercorrelation between the psychopathological dimensions of aggression dysregulation and increased anxiety (both of which have been shown to involve 5-HT disturbances), and thus for the theory that biological markers such as dysregulation of 5-HT metabolism must be conceived of in dimensional rather than nosological terms.

Yet another question that remains to be resolved involves the role of the state/trait dimension in aggression dysregulation. Abnormal CSF 5-HIAA findings may relate to personality traits that predispose towards aggressive or suicidal behavior during periods of stress (Traskman-Bendz et al., 1984). Deficient impulse control could be such a trait.

To answer these questions, continuing research into the relationships among these various psychological dimensions and personality traits and 5-HT biological markers must be undertaken. For instance, the nature of the relationship between anxiety and aggression needs to be explored. Some such relationships may be primary in nature, but others may be secondary or derivative phenomena. Clinical psychopharmacological studies must be undertaken to determine whether the use of medications that more selectively increase central 5-HT availability might be effective in the treatment of individuals with disturbances in the regulation of aggression. Also, a number of 5-HTergic parameters other than CSF 5-HIAA must be examined in disorders of aggression in order to pinpoint the nature of the specific relationship between 5-HT dysfunction and aggression more clearly. Only after a considerable amount of further investigation in this area will we be able to develop rational management programs for patients with different forms of pathological aggression.

REFERENCES

Adams, D. B. (1979). Brain mechanisms for offense, defense and submission. *Behav. Brain Sci.*, *2*, 201–241.

Agren, H. (1980). Symptom patterns in unipolar and bipolar depression correlating with monoamine metabolites in the cerebrospinal fluid. 1. General patterns. *Psychiatry Res.*, *3*, 211–223.

Agren, H. (1980). Symptom patterns in unipolar and bipolar depression correlated with monoamine metabolites in the cerebrospinal fluid. 2. Suicide. *Psychiatry Res.*, *3*, 225–236.

Agren, H. (1983). Life at risk: Markers of suicidality in depression. *Psychiatr. Dev.*, *1*, 87–103.

Apter, A., van Praag, H. M., Plutchik, R., Sevy, S., Korn, M. L., & Brown, S. L. (1989). The relationship between a serotonergically-linked series of psychological dimensions. Presented at the American Psychiatric Association, San Francisco, Calif.

Asberg, A., Traskman, L., & Thoren, P. (1976). 5HIAA in cerebrospinal fluid: A biochemical suicide predictor? *Arch. Gen. Psychiatry*, *33*, 1193–1197.

Banki, C. M., & Arato, M. (1983). Amine metabolites, neuroendocrine findings, and personality dimensions as correlates of suicidal behavior. *Psychiatry Res.*, *10*, 253–261.

Banki, C. M., Arato, M., Papp, Z., & Kurcz, M. (1984). Biochemical markers in suicidal patients: Investigations with cerebrospinal fluid amine metabolites and neuroendocrine tests. *J. Affect. Dis.*, *6*, 342–350.

Banki, C. M., Vojnik, M., Papp, Z., & Arato, M. (1985). Cerebrospinal fluid magnesium and calcium related to amine metabolites, diagnosis and suicide attempts. *Biol. Psychiatry*, *20*, 163–171.

Binder, R. L., & McNeil, D. E. (1986). Victims and families of violent psychiatric patients. *Bull. Am. Acad. Psychiatry Law*, *142*, 131–139.

Bioulac, B., Benezich, M., Renaud, B., Noel, B., & Roche, D. (1980). Serotonergic functions in the 47-XYY syndrome. *Biol. Psychiatry*, *15*, 917–923.

Brain, P. F. (1984). Biological explanations of human aggression and the resulting therapies offered by such approaches: A critical evaluation. In R. J. Blanchard & D. J. Blanchard (Eds.), *Advances in the study of aggression, Vol. 1* (pp. 63–102). New York: Academic Press.

Brown, G. L., Goodwin, F. K., Ballenger, J. C., Goyer, P. F., & Major, L. F. (1979). Aggression in humans correlates with cerebrospinal fluid amine metabolites. *Psychiatry Res.*, *1*, 131–139.

Brown, G. L., Goodwin, F. K., & Bunney, W. E. (1982). Human aggression and suicide: Their relationship to neuropsychiatric diagnoses and serotonin metabolism. In B. T. Ho, J. C. Schoolar, & E. Usdin (Eds.), *Advances in biochemical psychopharmacology: Serotonin in biological psychiatry, Vol. 34* (pp. 287–307). New York: Raven Press.

Cheetham, S. C., Crompton, M. R., Katona, C. L., & Horton, R. W. (1988). Brain 5-HT2 receptor binding sites in depressed suicide victims. *Brain Res.*, *443*, 272–280.

Ciaranello, R. (1979). Genetic regulation of the catecholamine synthesizing amines. In J. G. M. Shire (Ed.), *Genetic variation in hormone systems, Vol. 2* (pp. 49–61). Boca Raton, FL: CRC Press.

Ciaranello, R., Lipsky, A., & Axelrod, J. (1974). An association between fighting behavior and catecholamine biosynthetic enzyme activity in two inbred mouse sublines. *Proc. Nat. Acad. Sci. U.S.A.*, *71*, 3006–3008.

Climent, C., Plutchik, R., & Ervin, F. R. (1977). Parental loss, depression, and violence. *Acta Psychiatr. Scand.*, *55*, 261–268.

Cochrane, N. (1975). Assessing the aggressive component in personality: I. Problems. *Br. J. Med. Psychol.*, *48*, 9–14.

Davis, B. A., Yu, P. H., Bolton, A. A., Wermoth, J. S., & Addington, B. (1983). Correlative relationship between biochemical activity and aggressive behavior. *Prog. Neuropsychopharmacol. Biol. Psychiatry*, *7*, 529–535.

Eibl-Eibesfeldt, E. (1971). *Love and hate.* New York: Holt, Rinehart & Winston.

Eichelman, B.S. (1987). The neurochemical bases of aggressive behavior: Significant insights in neurochemical research. *Psychiatr. Ann.*, *17*, 371–374.

Eichelman, B. S., & Thoa, N. B. (1973). The aggressive monoamines. *Biol. Psychiatry*, *2*, 143–163.

Eisenberg, L. (1986). Does bad news about suicide beget suicide? *N. Engl. J. Med.*, *315*, 705–707.

Elliott, F. (1987). Neuroanatomy and neurology of aggression. *Psychiatr. Ann.*, *17*, 385–388.

Ellison, G. D., & Bresler, D. E. (1974). Tests of emotional behavior in rats following depletion of norepinephrine, of serotonin, or of both. *Psychopharmacologia (Berlin), 34,* 275–288.

Feshbach, S. (1964). The function of aggression and the regulation of aggressive drives. *Psychol. Rev., 71,* 257–272.

Fuller, J. L. (1986). The genetics of alcohol consumption in animals. *Soc. Biol., 32,* 310–321.

Fuller, J. L., & Thompson, W. R. (1978). *Foundations of behavior genetics.* St. Louis, MO: Mosby.

Goldsmith, H. H. (1983). Genetic influences on personality from infancy to adulthood. *Child Dev., 54,* 331–355.

Gould, M. S., & Shaffer, D. (1986). The impact of suicide in television movies: Evidence of imitation. *N. Engl. J. Med., 315,* 690–694.

Greenberg, A. S., & Coleman, D. (1976). Depressed 5-hydroxyindole levels associated with hyperactivity and aggressive behavior. *Arch. Gen. Psychiatry, 33,* 331–336.

Gross-Isseroff, R., Israeli, M., & Biegon, A. (1989). Autoradiographic analysis of tritiated imipramine binding in the human brain post mortem: Effects of suicide. *Arch. Gen. Psychiatry, 46,* 237–241.

Hamburg, D. A. (1971). Aggressive behavior of chimpanzees and baboons in natural habitats. *J. Psychiatr. Res., 8,* 385–398.

Hinde, R. A. (1966). *Animal behavior: A synthesis of ethology and comparative psychology.* New York: McGraw-Hill.

Hodge, G. K., & Butcher, L. L. (1974). 5-hydroxytryptamine correlates with isolation induced aggression in mice. *Eur. J. Pharmacol., 28,* 326–337.

Inamdar, S. E., Lewis, D. O., Siomopolous, G., Shanock, S. S., & Lamella, M. (1982). Violent and suicidal behavior in psychotic adolescents. *Am. J. Psychiatry, 139,* 932–935.

Kantak, K. N., Hegstrand, L. R., & Eichelman, B. (1980). Dietary tryptophan modulation and aggressive behavior in mice. *Pharmacol. Biochem. Behav., 12,* 675–679.

Kermani, E. J. (1981). Violent psychiatric patients: A study. *Am J. Psychother., 35,* 215–255.

Kessler, S., Elliot, G. R., Orenberg, E. K., & Barkas, J. D. (1977). A genetic analysis of aggressive behavior in two strains of mice. *Behav. Genet., 7,* 313–321.

King, R. (1986). Motivational diversity and mesolimbic dopamine: A hypothesis concerning temperament. In R. Plutchik & H. Kellerman (Eds.), *Biological foundations of emotion* (pp. 363–380). New York: Academic Press.

Kling, A. S. (1986). The anatomy of aggression and affiliation. In R. Plutchik & H. Kellerman (Eds.), *Biological foundations of emotion* (pp. 237–264). New York: Academic Press.

Koe, B. B., & Weisman, A. (1966). Chlorphenylalanine: A specific depleter of brain serotonin. *J. Pharmacol. Exp. Ther., 154,* 499–516.

Kulkarni, A. S. (1968). Muricidal block produced by 5-hydroxytryptophan and various drugs. *Life Sci., 7,* 125.

Lidberg, L., Asberg, M., & Sundquist-Stensman, U. B. (1984). 5-hydroxyindole-acetic acid in attempted suicides who kill their children. *Lancet, 2,* 928.

Lidberg, L., Tuck, J. R., Asberg, M., Scalia-Tomba, G. P., & Bertilsson, L. (1985). Homicide, suicide and CSF 5HIAA. *Acta Psychiatr. Scand., 71,* 230–236.

Linnoila, M., Virkkunen, N., & Roy, A. (1986). The biochemical aspects of aggression in man. *Clin. Neuropharmacol., 9*(Suppl. 4), 377–379.

Linnoila, M., Virkkunen, N., Scheinin, M., Nuutila, A., Rimon, R., & Goodwin, F. K. (1982). Low cerebrospinal fluid 5-hydroxyindoleacetic acid concentration differentiates impulsive from nonimpulsive violent behavior. *Life Sci., 33,* 2609–2614.

Loehlin, J. C., & Nichols, R. C. (1976). *Heredity, environment and personality: A study of 850 twins.* Austin, TX: University of Texas Press.

Loehlin, J. C., Thorn, J. N., & Williams, L. (1981). Personality resemblance in adoptive families. *Behav. Genet., 11,* 309–331.

Lopez-Ibor, J. J., Saiz-Ruiz, J., & Perez de los Cobos, J. C. (1985). Biological correlations of suicide and aggressivity in major depressions (with melancholia): 5-Hydroxyindoleacetic acid and cortisol in the cerebrospinal fluid. Dexamethasone suppression test and response to 5 hydroxytryptophan. *Neuropsychobiology, 14,* 67–74.

Lorenz, K. (1966). *On aggression.* New York: Harcourt Brace.

Lycke, E., Modig, K., & Roos, B. E. (1969). Aggression in mice associated with changes in the monoamine metabolism of the brain. *Experientia, 25,* 951.

Madden, D. J., Lion, J. R., & Penna, M. W. (1976). Assaults on psychiatrists by patients. *Am J. Psychiatry, 133,* 422–425.

Marini, J. L., & Sheard, M. H. (1977). Anti-aggressive effect of the lithium ion in man. *Acta Psychiatr. Scand., 55,* 269–286.

Maxson, S. C. & Trattner, A. (1981). The interaction of genotype and fostering in the development of behavior of DBA and C-57 mice. *Behav. Genet., 11,* 153–165.

Menninger, K. (1933). *Man against himself.* New York: Harcourt Brace.

Meyerson, L. R., Wennogle, L. P., Abel, M. S., Coupet, J., Lippa, A. S., Rauh, C. E., & Beer, B. (1982). Human brain receptor alternations in suicide victims. *Pharmacol. Biochem. Behav., 17,* 159–163.

Miller, M. E. (1957). Experiments on motivation. *Science, 126,* 1271–1278.

Morris, D. J. (1954). The reproductive behavior of the zebra fish [peophila guttata] with special reference to pseudofemale behavior and displacement activities. *Behavior, 6,* 271–322.

Moyer, K. E. (1976). *The psychobiology of aggression.* New York: Harper & Row.

Ninan, P. T., van Kammen, D. P., Sheinann, M., Linnoila, M., Bunney, W. E., & Goodwin, F. K. (1984). CSF 5HIAA levels in suicidal schizophrenic patients. *Am. J. Psychiatry, 141,* 566–569.

O'Neil, M., Page, N., & Eichelman, B. (1986). Tryptophan-trazodone treatment of aggressive behavior. *Lancet, 2,* 859–860.

Oreland, L., Wiberg, A., Asberg, M., Traskman, L., Sjostrand, L., Thoren, T., Bertilsson, L., & Tybring, G. (1981). Platelet MAO activity and monoamine metabolites in cerebrospinal fluid in depressed and suicidal patients and in healthy controls. *Psychiatry Res.*, *4*, 21–29.

Orenberg, E. K., Renson, J., & Elliot, G. R. (1975). Genetic determination of aggressive behavior and brain cyclic AMP. *Psychopharmacol. Comm.*, *1*, 99–107.

Ostroff, R., Giller, E., Bonese, K., Ebersole, E., Harkness, L., & Mason, J. (1982). Neuroendocrine risk factors of suicidal behavior. *Am. J. Psychiatry*, *139*, 1323–1325.

Palanappian, V., Rachamandran, V., & Somasudaram, O. (1983). Suicidal ideation and biogenic amines in depression. *Indian J. Psychiatry*, *25*, 286–292.

Palmour, R. M. (1983). Genetic models for the study of aggressive behavior. *Prog. Neuropsychopharmacol. Biol. Psychiatry*, *7*, 513–517.

Pfeffer, C. R. (1986). *The suicidal child*. New York: Basic Books.

Pickar, D., Roy, A., Breier, A., Doran, A., Wolkowitz, O., Collison, J., & Agren, H. (1987). Suicide and aggression in schizophrenia. Neurobiologic correlates. *Ann. N.Y. Acad. Med.*, *487*, 189–196.

Pliszka, S. R., Rogeness, G. A., & Renner, P. (1987). Higher whole blood serotonin in aggressive juvenile delinquents. Paper presented at the American Academy of Child Psychiatry, Washington, D. C.

Plutchik, R., Climent, C., & Ervin, F. R. (1976). Research strategies for the study of human violence. In W. L. Smith & A. Kling (Eds.), *Issues in brain and behavior control* (pp. 69–94). New York: Spectrum.

Plutchik, R., van Praag, H. M., & Conte, H. R. (1986). Suicide and violence risk in psychiatric patients. Paper presented at the American Psychiatric Association, Washington, D. C.

Raleigh, M. J., & McGuire, M. T. (1980). Biosocial pharmacology. *McLean Hosp. J.*, *2*, 73–84.

Rossi, A. M., Jacobs, M., Monteleone, M., Olson, R., Surber, R. W., Winkler, E. L., & Wommack, A. (1985). Characteristics of psychiatric patients who engage in assaultive or other fear-inducing behaviors. *J. Nerv. Ment. Dis.*, *174*, 154–160.

Roy, A., Agren, H., Pickar, D., Linnoila, M., Doran, A. R., Cutler, N. R., & Paul, S. M. (1986). Reduced cerebrospinal fluid concentrations of homovanillic acid and homovanillic acid to 5-hydroxyindoleacetic acid ratios in depressed patients. Relationship to suicidal behavior and dexamethasone nonsuppression. *Am. J. Psychiatry*, *143*, 1539–1545.

Roy, A., Ninan, P. H., Mazonson, A., Pickar, D., van Kammen, D., Linnoila, M., & Paul, S. M. (1985). CSF monoamine metabolites in chronic schizophrenic patients who attempt suicide. *Psych. Med.*, *15*, 325–340.

Roy-Byrne, P., Post, R. M., Rubinow, D. R., Linnoila, M., Savard, R., & Davis, D. (1983). CSF 5HIAA and personal and family history of suicide in affectively ill patients: A negative study. *Psychiatry Res.*, *10*, 263–274.

Rydin, E., Schalling, D., & Asberg, M. (1982). Rorschach ratings in depressed and suicidal patients with low levels of 5HIAA in cerebrospinal fluid. *Psychiatry Res.*, *7*, 229–243.

Selmanoff, V. K., & Ginsberg, G. B. E. (1981). Genetic variability in aggression and endocrine function in inbred strains of mice. In P. F. Brain & D. Benton (Eds.),

Multidisciplinary approaches to aggression research. New York: Elsevier North-Holland Biomedical Press.

Shaffer, D., & Fisher, P. (1981). The epidemiology of suicide in children and young adolescents. *J. Am. Acad. Child Psychiatry, 20*, 545–565.

Sheard, M. (1969). The effect of p-chlorophenylalanine on behavior in rats: Relation to brain serotonin and 5-hydroxyindoleacetic acid. *Brain Res., 15*, 524.

Skodol, A. E., & Karasu, T. B. (1978). Emergency psychiatry and the assaultive patient. *Am. J. Psychiatry, 135*, 202–205.

Stanley, M., & Mann, J. J. (1983). Increased serotonin-2 binding sites in frontal cortex of suicide victims. *Lancet, 1*, 214–216.

Stanley, M., Virgilio, J., & Gershon, S. (1982). Tritiated imipramine binding sites are decreased in the frontal cortex of suicides. *Science, 216*, 1337–1339.

Tardiff, K., & Sweillam, A. (1980). Assault, suicide and mental illness. *Arch. Gen. Psychiatry, 37*, 164–169.

Thackrey, M. (1987). *Therapeutics for aggression. Psychological and physical crisis intervention*. New York: Human Sciences Press.

Tinbergen, N. (1953). *Social behavior in animals*. New York: Wiley.

Traskman, L., Asberg, M., Bertilsson, L., & Sjostrand, L. (1981). Monoamine metabolites in CSF and suicidal behavior. *Arch. Gen. Psychiatry, 38*, 631–636.

Traskman-Bendz, L., Asberg, M., Bertilsson, L., & Thoren, P. (1984). CSF monoamine metabolites of depressed patients during illness and recovery. *Acta Psychiatr. Scand., 69*, 333–342.

Valzelli, L. (1981). *The psychobiology of aggression and violence*. New York: Raven Press.

Valzelli, L. (1984). Reflections on experimental and human pathology of aggression. *Prog. Neuropsychopharmacol. Biol. Psychiatry, 8*, 311–325.

van Praag, H. M. (1982). Neurotransmitters and CNS disease: Depression. *Lancet, 2*, 1259–1264.

van Praag, H. M. (1983). CSF 5HIAA and suicide in nondepressed schizophrenics. *Lancet, 2*, 977–978.

van Praag, H. M. (1984). Monoamines and depression: The present state of the art. In R. Plutchik & H. Kellerman (Eds.), *Biological foundations of emotion* (pp. 335–361). New York: Academic Press.

van Praag, H. M. (1986). Biological suicide research: Outcome and limitations. *Biol. Psychiatry, 21*, 1305–1323.

van Praag, H. M., Korf, J., & Schut, T. (1973a). Cerebral monoamines and depression. An investigation with the probenecid technique. *Arch. Gen. Psychiatry, 28*, 827–831.

van Praag, H. M., Flentge, F., Korf, J., Dols, L. C. W., & Schut, T. (1973b). The influence of probenecid on the metabolism of serotonin, dopamine and their precursors in man. *Psychopharmacologia, 33*, 141–151.

van Praag, H. M., Kahn, R., Asnis, G. M., Wetzler, S., Brown, S. L., Bleich, A., & Korn, M. L. (1987). Denosologization of biological psychiatry, or the specificity of 5-HT disturbances in psychiatric disorders. *J. Affect. Dis., 13*, 1–8.

van Praag, H. M., Korf, J., & Puite, J. (1970). 5-Hydroxyindoleacetic acid levels in the cerebrospinal fluid of depressive patients treated with probenecid. *Nature*, *225*, 1259-1260.

van Praag, H. M., & Plutchik, R. (1988). Increased suicidality in depression: Group- or subgroup-characteristic? *Psychiatry Res.*, *26*, 273-278.

van Praag, H. M., Plutchik, R., & Conte, H. (1986). The serotonin hypothesis of (auto)aggression. Critical appraisal of the evidence. *Ann. N.Y. Acad. Sci.*, *487*, 150-167.

Virkkunen, M., Nuutila, A., Goodwin, F. K., & Linnoila, M. (1987). Cerebrospinal fluid monoamine metabolite levels in male arsonists. *Arch. Gen. Psychiatry*, *44*, 241-247.

Vogel, F., & Motulsky, A. G. (1979). *Human genetics*. New York: Springer Verlag.

Weissman, M., Fox, K., & Klerman, G. L. (1973). Hostility and depression associated with suicide attempts. *Am J. Psychiatry*, *130*, 450-455.

Westergaard, P., Sorensen, T., Hoppe, E., Rafaelson, O. J., Yates, C. M., & Nicolau, N. (1978). Biogenic amine metabolites in cerebrospinal fluid of patients with affective disorders. *Acta Psychiatr. Scand.*, *58*, 88-96.

Wimer, R. E., & Wimer, C. C. (1985). Animal behavior genetics: A search for the biological foundations of behavior. *Ann. Rev. Psychol.*, *36*, 171-218.

Yen, C. Y., Stanger, R. L., & Millman, N. (1959). Ataraxic suppression of isolation induced aggressive behavior. *Arch. Int. Psychodynam.*, *123*, 179.

13

Beyond Serotonin
A Multiaminergic Perspective on Abnormal Behavior

HERMAN M. VAN PRAAG
SERENA-LYNN BROWN
GREGORY M. ASNIS
RENE S. KAHN
MARTIN L. KORN
JILL M. HARKAVY-FRIEDMAN
SCOTT WETZLER

FUNCTIONAL PSYCHOPATHOLOGY: A LOOK BACKWARD

From the very beginning, biological psychiatry has fallen under the spell of nosology, a way of looking at behavioral disorders as distinct, clearly separable entities, each with its own symptomatology, causation, outcome, and treatment. Finding a marker for, and eventually the cause of, for instance, schizophrenia, depression, or panic disorder has been, and still is, the major goal of biological psychiatric research. The introduction of the third edition of the *Diagnostic and Statistical Manual of Mental Disorders* (DSM-III) in 1980 forcefully reinforced biological psychiatry's nosological orientation.

For many years now, we have advocated and pursued another route, marked by what we have called a functional approach to psychopathology (van Praag & Leijnse, 1965; van Praag et al., 1975, 1987c). Most parsimoniously formulated, this concept holds three tenets:

1. The basic units of classification in psychopathology are not syndromes or nosological entities, but psychological dysfunctions, such as disturbances in perception, cognition, memory, or information proc-

302

essing, among many others. *They* are the elementary constituents of which psychiatric syndromes are made.

2. Nosological classification of a given psychiatric disorder is the first step in diagnosis. The next step is dissection of the syndrome into its component parts—that is, the psychological dysfunctions and their subsequent measurement.

3. In biological psychiatric research, correlations between biological and psychological dysfunctions should be sought.

Analogies with two-tier diagnosing can be found in other areas of medicine. Myocardial infarction, for example, is a nosological diagnosis that is routinely complemented by an analysis of its functional sequelae on, for instance, heart rate and rhythm, conductance, and output. Treatment is predicated on the functional analysis, not on the nosological diagnosis.

We have pursued the functional approach in psychiatry for many years and believe this route to be quite productive, as illustrated in the following.

THE ROLE OF DOPAMINE IN ABNORMAL BEHAVIOR

In the late 1960s, we reported on the occurrence of dopamine (DA) disturbances in depression, most notably in vital depression (major depression, melancholic type, here called "melancholic depression") (van Praag & Korf, 1971a). In some patients, the probenecid-induced accumulation of the major DA metabolite homovanillic acid (HVA) in cerebrospinal fluid (CSF) was decreased, indicating a lowered DA metabolism in the central nervous system (CNS), particularly in the nigro-striatal DA system, the region that is predominantly represented by CSF HVA. Guided by Parkinson's disease, with its severe disturbances in motor functioning and profound DA depletion, we searched for correlations between lowered CSF HVA and motor retardation. In comparing groups of depressed patients with and without pronounced motor retardation and lack of initiative, the HVA accumulation after probenecid appeared to be twice as low in the retarded patients as in the nonretarded depressives and in a control group. Similar findings have been reported by other investigators (Papeschi & McClure, 1971; Banki, 1977a; Banki et al., 1981).

If lowered DA metabolism in the nigrostriatal system underlies retardation and inertia, increasing DA availability could be expected to exert an activating and energizing effect. We used L-dopa to boost DA metabolism, since we had demonstrated in humans that this drug increases DA metabolism substantially, while having little impact on norepinephrine (NE) metabolism. Moreover, the increase in DA metabolism persists (van Praag & Lemus, 1986) (Figure 13-1).

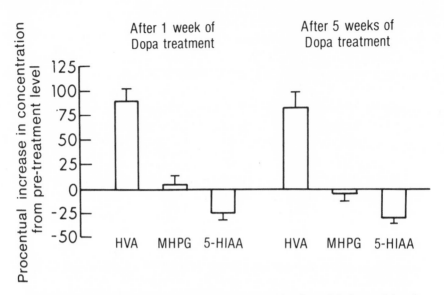

Figure 13-1. L-dopa (mean, 290 mg/day) in combination with the peripheral decarboxylase inhibitor MK 486 (150 mg/day) induced in five controls a significant increase in postprobenecid CSF HVA. The concentration of MHPG did not change significantly, while postprobenecid 5-HIAA decreased slightly but consistently (in all individuals). CSF concentrations were measured before treatment and after one week and five weeks of L-dopa treatment. The changes persisted over time.

L-dopa (at an average dose of 260 mg/day), in combination with a peripheral decarboxylase inhibitor, was first studied in a group of biochemically undifferentiated, melancholically depressed patients and found to be lacking in overall therapeutic effects. Subsequently, we compared the effect of L-dopa (290 mg/day) and a peripheral decarboxylase inhibitor in melancholic patients with lowered postprobenecid CSF HVA and in melancholic patients with normal HVA response. Motor retardation and inertia were significantly more pronounced in the former group. L-dopa was shown to improve motor functioning and level of initiative in the low HVA group and to normalize the HVA level (Figure 13-2). Mood and hedonic functioning were not significantly influenced. Anxiety levels rose slightly, but significantly. In the group with normal HVA response, L-dopa failed to exhibit therapeutic effects (van Praag & Korf, 1975).

We repeated the latter experiment in a different group of patients, using L-tyrosine instead of L-dopa (van Praag, 1986b). In contrast to L-dopa, L-tyrosine, the precursor of the catecholamines (CAs) DA and NE, significantly increases CSF 3-methoxy-4-hydroxyphenethylene glycol (MHPG;

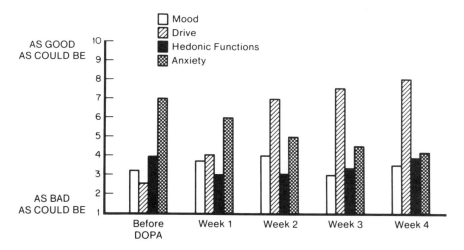

Figure 13-2. L-dopa (average 260 mg/day) in combination with a peripheral decarboxylase inhibitor was administered for four weeks to 10 patients with major depression, melancholic type, pronounced motor retardation, and low postprobenecid CSF HVA. Motor retardation and inertia ("drive") improved significantly. Mood and hedonic functioning were not significantly influenced. Postprobenecid CSF HVA was normalized. In melancholic patients with normal HVA response and without motor retardation, L-dopa was ineffectual and no better than placebo (van Praag & Korf, 1975; van Praag & Lemus, 1986).

the principal metabolite of NE) in humans, indicating increased NE metabolism. CSF HVA, on the other hand, rises only slightly, suggesting that tyrosine's impact on DA metabolism (in the nigro-striatal system) is less pronounced than that of L-dopa. (See Figure 13-3.)

Again studying melancholic patients with and without lowered CSF HVA accumulation after probenecid, we observed no therapeutic effect of tyrosine on motor retardation and inertia in either group (Figure 13-4). Normalization of CSF HVA did not occur either.

Based on these findings, we hypothesized that diminished DA metabolism in the nigro-striatal system underlies decreased motor activity and lowered level of initiative, irrespective of nosological diagnosis (van Praag et al., 1975). In accordance with this hypothesis is the observation by Lindstrom (1985) that low CSF HVA is seen in schizophrenics with pronounced lassitude and slowness of movement.

When one attempts to link the DA system to the ability to carry out goal-directed behavior, one has to take into account the fact that such behavior is a composite of different components. First, an initial stimulus is needed. This can be an instinctual drive, such as hunger, thirst, or sex; an emotion,

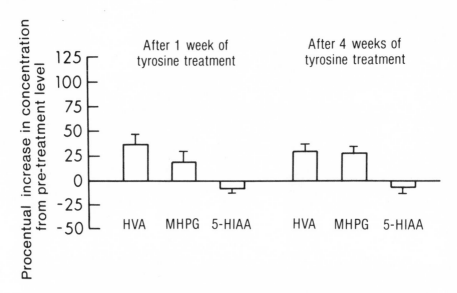

Figure 13-3. L-tyrosine (100 mg/kg/day) given to five controls induced a significant increase in CSF MHPG. CSF HVA increased significantly as well, but in a much less pronounced manner than after L-dopa administration (see Figure 13-1). CSF 5-HIAA did not change significantly. CSF concentrations were measured after probenecid loading, before treatment, and after one and four weeks of L-tyrosine treatment. The changes persisted over time. Lumbar punctures were performed two hours after a dose of L-tyrosine (van Praag & Lemus, 1986).

such as anger; or a cognitive set (e.g., the realization of having to prepare for a test). Next, the goals for appropriate response to the stimulus have to be selected—for example, finding food to satisfy hunger, displaying aggressive behavior to reduce anger, or going to a library to study, in the case of a student facing an upcoming test. Subsequently, the behavior to attain these goals has to be initiated and sustained. Finally, signals should be set in operation when the mission has been accomplished so that the behavior can be terminated. The term "drive" is used to indicate an initial stimulus of an instinctual nature. It is also used for the entire process of initiation and completion of goal-directed behavior. For the sake of brevity, we use the term in the latter sense in this chapter.

The sequence leading to goal-directed behavior can be disturbed at any junction. The human data suggest that DA is involved in the mobilization, facilitation, and sustenance of goal-directed behavior. The large pool of animal data available is in accord with this conclusion (Crow & Deakin, 1985; Freed & Yamamoto, 1985; Ashton, 1987).

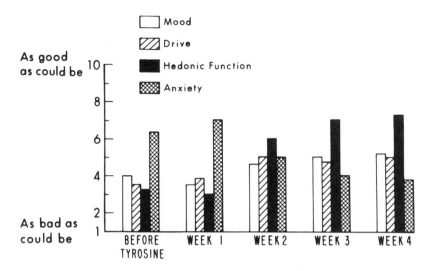

Figure 13-4. In 10 patients with major depression, melancholic type, L-tyrosine (100 mg/kg/day for 4 weeks) did not change the overall Hamilton score. Discrete components of the syndrome, however, did change significantly. Hedonic functioning improved while anxiety levels increased. Placebo did not change these psychopathological dimensions. (Unpublished observations).

THE ROLE OF SEROTONIN IN ABNORMAL BEHAVIOR

5-HT Depression

Disturbances in central serotonin (5-hydroxytryptamine; 5-HT) metabolism were first reported in depression. They were inferred to exist based on the finding of lowered postprobenecid minus baseline levels of 5-hydroxyindoleacetic acid (5-HIAA, the major degradation product of 5-HT) in the CSF of depressed individuals, indicating diminished 5-HT metabolism in the CNS (van Praag et al., 1970).

Subsequently, disturbances in other systems indicative of central 5-HTergic functioning were observed. Studies of blood platelets, considered to be a model of central 5-HTergic nerve endings, found disturbances in platelet 5-HT, such as deviations in 5-HT content and uptake and in the density of imipramine receptors. Furthermore, disturbances in the ratio of the plasma concentration of tryptophan to the competing amino acids were found. This ratio determines the influx of tryptophan into the CNS, and, CNS availability of tryptophan in its turn, is an important determinant of 5-HT synthesis rate. Moreover, several neuroendocrine challenge tests also indicated disturbances in 5-HTergic functioning. Finally, psychopharmacological experiments with indirect 5-HT agonists [e.g., the 5-HT precursor 5-

hydroxytryptophan (5-HTP), the selective 5-HT uptake inhibitors, and the 5-HT precursor 5-hydroxy–tryptophan (5-HTP)] and the 5-HT antagonists, such as parachlorophenylalanine [(pCPA), a 5-HT synthesis inhibitor] suggested that manipulation of central 5-HT can effect mood changes (see Chapter 5 of this volume).

The data most clearly and directly related to central 5-HT metabolism are derived from CSF studies, although these studies are the most cumbersome to conduct. The interrelations among the various 5-HT indicators are insufficiently known. [For a review of 5-HT and depression, see van Praag (1982), Goodwin and Post (1983), and Chapter 5 of this volume.]

Initially, depressed patients with and without demonstrable disturbances in central 5-HT seemed indistinguishable in psychopathological terms. In 1971, interpreting the available data at that time, we introduced the concept of biochemical heterogeneity of depression (van Praag & Korf, 1971b). We postulated that some forms of depression are linked to disturbances in 5-HT functions, while others are not so linked, or are linked to a lesser extent only. The same syndrome, then, could be the ultimate outcome of various pathophysiological processes. As an analogy, we discussed the syndrome of anemia. Anemic patients present with, by and large, the same symptoms, but the pathogenesis, and so the treatment of the syndrome, is heterogeneous in nature.

Subsequent studies, however, made the postulate of a separate category of 5-HT depression untenable (van Praag & Lemus, 1986). Data indicated that increasing 5-HT availability *alone* is not a sufficient antidepressant measure. This argues against the concept of a type of depression that is generated predominantly by central 5-HT disturbances, leading to decreased 5-HT availability.

Whither 5-HT depression

First we demonstrated in a double-blind, placebo-controlled, comparative study that 5-HTP is an active antidepressant in hospitalized patients with rather severe forms of melancholic depression, whereas tryptophan turned out to be no better than placebo (van Praag, 1984). Both 5-HT precursors increase central 5-HT metabolism to an equal extent, as reflected in the probenecid-induced accumulation of 5-HIAA in CSF. They appeared to differ, however, in their effect on CA metabolites in CSF (reflecting intracerebral metabolism of the mother amines). 5-HTP increases the metabolism of DA as well as of NE, while tryptophan does not (van Praag, 1983). In high doses (> 5 g intravenously), tryptophan even lowers DA and NE metabolism, possibly by interfering with the influx of tyrosine, the precursor substance of the CAs, in the CNS (van Praag et al., 1987a).

5-HTP's ability to stimulate CA metabolism is thought to be due to the presence of aromatic amino-acid decarboxylase in CAergic nerve cells. Hence, 5-HTP is converted to 5-HT not only in 5-HTergic, but also in CAergic, neurons. In the latter, 5-HT functions as a false transmitter, as a consequence of which the synthesis rate of CAs increases. The net functional effect of the two opposing processes—that is, false transmitter formation leading to decreased function and increased CA production leading to augmented function—is probably heightened CAergic activity.

If 5-HTP's therapeutic superiority to tryptophan is related to its combined effects on the 5-HT and CA systems, one would expect tryptophan's antidepressant efficacy to be raised above the significance level by combining it with a compound capable of increasing CA availability. We showed in humans that tyrosine is presumably such a compound, and combining tryptophan with tyrosine indeed led to significant antidepressant activity (van Praag, 1986b).

A second observation supports the hypothesis that 5-HTP derives its therapeutic efficacy from its dual influence on the 5-HTergic and CAergic systems. In about 25% of patients initially treated successfully with 5-HTP, the response subsided in the second month of treatment (van Praag, 1983). This phenomenon is paralleled by normalization of CA metabolism (again, as reflected by the CSF concentration of CA metabolites), while the metabolism of 5-HT remained increased (Figure 13-5). We thus hypothesized that clinical relapse and normalization of CA metabolism are related. If so, reactivating CA metabolism should restore clinical remission—and, indeed, it did. Adding tyrosine to the 5-HTP regime in the group of relapsers once again led to subsidence of the depression and to a rise in CA metabolism (van Praag & Lemus, 1986) (Figure 13-6).

These data suggest that *combined* augmentation of 5-HT and CA availability in the CNS provides the best conditions for antidepressant activity, and they argue against the existence of a separate diagnostic entity called "5-HT depression." 5-HTP's behavioral effects in monkeys have also been demonstrated to be a function of its influence on 5-HT and CA systems (Raleigh, 1987).

If 5-HT disturbances are not linked to a particular syndromal subtype of depression, could it be that they relate to particular psychopathological dimensions that may or may not occur in depression, explaining the occurrence of 5-HT disturbances in some, but not other, depressions (van Praag et al., 1987c)?

This hypothesis seems plausible in the light of recent observations, the relevant psychopathological dimensions being dysregulation of aggression and heightened anxiety. Supportive evidence is briefly summarized in the following.

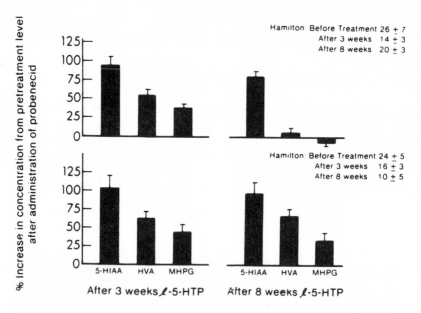

Figure 13-5. In the first month of treatment with L-5-HTP (200 mg/day in combination with carbidopa 150 mg/day) there is a substantial increase of HVA and MHPG in CSF after a probenecid load. In the second treatment month, the levels of the CA metabolites have returned to normal in patients who relapsed. The 5-HIAA response remains increased over time. In patients in whom the therapeutic response to 5-HTP continued, the effect on CA metabolites in CSF did not subside nor did the 5-HIAA level (van Praag, 1983).

5-HT and Disturbed Aggression Regulation

In 1976, Asberg et al. confirmed our findings of a subgroup of depressed individuals with low CSF 5-HIAA, and added the important observation that suicide attempters seemed to accumulate in this subgroup. This finding was confirmed by many, though not by all, investigators. Subsequent studies revealed, moreover, that low CSF 5-HIAA not only was observed in depressed suicide attempters, but also in nondepressed, nonpsychotic (e.g., personality-disturbed) suicide attempters and in schizophrenic patients who had made suicide attempts because "voices" had ordered them to do so, but who were not suffering from depression as defined by DSM-III (van Praag, 1986a).

Lowered concentrations of CSF 5-HIAA have also been reported in individuals with increased outwardly directed aggression, but belonging to different diagnostic categories (Brown et al., 1979, 1982; Bioulac et al., 1980; Linnoila et al., 1983; Lidberg et al., 1984, 1985; Virkkunen et al., 1987). The biological study of aggression in humans is known to be fraught with

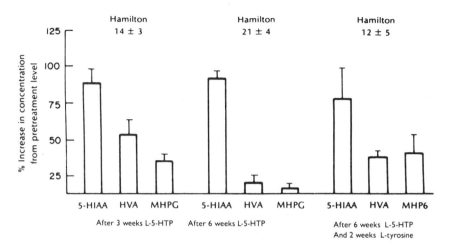

Figure 13-6. In the patients referred to in the top section of Figure 13-5, L-tyrosine (100 mg/kg/day) was added to the 5-HTP regimen. This led to significant clinical improvement and to a significant rise of the CSF HVA and MHPG concentrations after probenecid (van Praag, 1983).

methodological difficulties, such as the usually short duration of aggressive outbursts and the fact that these explosions are, more often than not, intertwined with a host of factors, social or toxicological in nature (e.g., drugs, alcohol), for which it is hard to control. The fact that all seven studies published so far on the subject have reported low CSF 5-HIAA seems to indicate that the finding is a robust one.

Dysregulation of aggression can be a major feature of depression, as evidenced by the greatly increased incidence of both suicidal behavior and signs of outwardly directed aggressiveness seen in depressed individuals. We have shown that depressed patients with low CSF 5-HIAA not only have an increased rate of suicide attempts, but also show an increased frequency of signs of outwardly directed aggression (van Praag et al., 1986) (Table 13-1).

The facts, then, seem sufficiently robust to carry the hypothesis that signs of diminished 5-HT metabolism in the CNS, as originally observed in depression, are related to dysregulated aggression, irrespective of the direction it takes and of the nosological context in which it occurs.

5-HT and Heightened Anxiety

Anxiety is a second psychopathological dimension occurring in depression, but by no means specific for that disorder, that also seems to be 5-HT related. Several pieces of evidence point in this direction.

TABLE 13-1
Low 5-HIAA Depressives Compared with Normal 5-HIAA Depressives Present:

Finding	P
More suicide attempts	< 0.01
Greater number of contacts with police	< 0.05
Increased arguments with	
relatives	< 0.05
spouse	< 0.01
colleagues	< 0.05
friends	< 0.05
More hostility at interview	< 0.05
Impaired employment history (arguments)	< 0.05

5-HT potentiating drugs (in particular, 5-HTP, increasing 5-HT synthesis) and the 5-HT uptake inhibitors (e.g., clomipramine, trazodone, fluvoxamine, and fluoxetine) have been reported as showing therapeutic efficacy in panic disorder (Evans & Moore, 1981; Koczkas et al., 1981; Kahn et al., 1984, 1987; Evans et al., 1986; Den Boer et al., 1987). Even more interesting, the effect of these indirect 5-HT agonists seems to be biphasic, at least in some patients (Kahn & Westenberg, 1985). These patients show an initial phase of increased anxiety, lasting two to three weeks, followed by a phase of amelioration in which anxiety and panic attacks diminish. We explained this biphasic effect by postulating (1) hypersensitivity of postsynaptic 5-HT receptors, and (2) a direct relation between this phenomenon and the anxiety attacks. Under these circumstances, increasing 5-HT availability would first lead to additional stimulation of an already hyperactive 5-HT system and, hence, to clinical deterioration. Downregulation of the receptor system as a result of increased 5-HT availability would eventually lead to amelioration of the anxiety disorder (Kahn et al., 1988c).

Additional evidence favoring this hypothesis recently was acquired. Panic disorder patients were challenged with m-chlorophenylpiperazine (mCPP), a relatively selective $5-HT_1$ receptor agonist. Normals and patients suffering from major depression served as controls. The major findings were twofold. Patients with panic disorder showed a substantial increase in anxiety during the mCPP test, in comparison with placebo. In the control groups, no significant response occurred on either mCPP or placebo (Kahn et al., 1988a). Moreover, the cortisol response to mCPP was augmented in panic disorder patients as compared with their response to placebo and with the mCPP response in the two control groups (Kahn et al., 1988b).

Another piece of confirmatory evidence is found in the development of two new anxiolytics that diminish central 5-HT activity—ritanserin, a selective $5-HT_2$ antagonist (Ceulemans et al., 1985), and buspirone, a substance with a high affinity for $5-HT_{1A}$ receptors that probably decreases 5-HTergic activity (Taylor et al., 1985). These drugs seem to be effective in generalized anxiety disorder; their effect in panic disorder has not yet been well studied. Also, Jones et al. (1988) recently reported animal data indicating that GR38032F, a selective $5-HT_3$ antagonist, appears to be a potential anxiolytic agent.

If, indeed, in (certain) states of increased anxiety, postsynaptic 5-HT receptors are hypersensitive, one would expect, as a consequence, a diminution of central 5-HT synthesis and a lowering of CSF 5-HIAA. No data are available on CSF 5-HIAA in anxiety-disordered patients. In depressed patients, a negative correlation between CSF 5-HIAA and anxiety levels has been observed (Banki, 1977b; Rydin et al., 1982; van Praag, unpublished).

The present data do not permit extending the 5-HT hypersensitivity hypothesis beyond panic disorder, but some preliminary evidence indicates that 5-HT receptor hypersensitivity may be related to increased anxiety in general, rather than to panic disorder alone. We have found a correlation between cortisol response to mCPP and anxiety level as measured one week before the mCPP challenge test in both panic disorder and major depression, suggesting a relationship between the general state of anxiety and 5-HT receptor hypersensitivity. The relation between CSF 5-HIAA and anxiety in depression points in the same direction, and so does the finding that suppressors of 5-HT activity, such as ritanserin and buspirone, are effective in generalized anxiety disorder.

A Dimensional 5-HT Hypothesis

Signs of decreased central 5-HT metabolism, then, seem to correlate not with a particular syndromal depression subtype, but with particular affective disturbances, such as increased (auto) aggression and augmented anxiety.

We define affects here as discrete, strong, transient emotions. The concept of "affect" is not identical to that of "mood." "Mood" refers to the degree of well-being one experiences, more or less habitually. Mood lowering, then, indicates a state in which one feels less than usually disposed. Mood is influenced by affects, but the two concepts are by no means synonymous. By way of analogy, mood refers to climate and affect more to the actual weather. "Mood" can also be used to indicate the entire gamut of affects and emotions. This usage creates confusion, however, and should be avoided. Functional psychopathology requires scrupulous definition of psychopathological dimensions.

If the psychopathological dimensions of increased aggression and heightened anxiety are both related to disordered 5-HT metabolism, one would expect them to intercorrelate, and indeed they do. In a recent series of studies on predictors of suicide and violence in groups of psychiatric patients with a diversity of diagnoses, we found trait anxiety to be strongly correlated with both suicide risk and violence risk (Apter et al., 1989; Apter et al., 1990).

The data favoring a dimensional 5-HT hypothesis, linking 5-HT disturbances to disordered aggression and anxiety regulation across diagnoses, seem fairly convincing.

THE ROLE OF NORADRENALINE IN ABNORMAL BEHAVIOR

Pleasure and Displeasure

So far, we have discussed MAergic involvement in drive and affect regulation. Both domains are frequently disturbed in depression, particularly in major depression, melancholic type. Those disturbances, however, are by no means specific for that disorder.

Another major sphere of dysfunction in melancholic depression pertains to the ability to experience pleasure. Normally, much of what we do, perceive, or think is not emotionally neutral, but is provided with a charge—globally speaking, either positive or negative. It generates pleasure or displeasure, in whatever way that may be defined. Anhedonia, the inability to experience pleasure, is a typical symptom of melancholic depression. It is one of the few almost pathognomonic symptoms in psychiatry.

Anhedonia is unlike flat affect or emotional blunting as seen in schizophrenia. Flat affect pertains to a global inability to experience, or at least to express, emotions; anhedonia indicates the inability to link a particular mental or motor activity with the experiential quality of gratification, a quality that was "stamped in" when similar activities were carried out in the past. In melancholic depression, the emotional defect is "localized" and there is no global defect in experiencing or expressing emotions. On the contrary, particularly negative emotions such as sadness, guilt, and shame are felt with profound intensity. In very severe cases of melancholic depression, the ability to experience discomfort is also impaired. Mental and physical activities that usually would be considered aversive are less likely to produce this effect. ("Someone close to me died recently, doctor, but it didn't have much effect on me. That is frightening.")

Behavior is strongly motivated by the attainment of pleasure and the avoidance of discomfort. The decreased ability to experience such modalities will reinforce the state of drive reduction characteristic of melancholic depression.

Inside the Pleasure Principle

In animals, brain systems that code for naturally occurring rewarding and aversive experiences have been demonstrated. The existence of the so-called reward and punishment systems was deduced from the observation that rats with chronically implanted electrodes will work to obtain electric stimulation at specific sites in the brain and to avoid stimulation at other specific sites (Olds & Milner, 1954). The highest self-stimulation rates are obtained when electrodes are located in the medial forebrain bundle of the lateral hypothalamus.

Reward and punishment systems are, at least in part, MAergically innervated, the former by CAs and the latter by 5-HT. DA is thought to be particularly involved in mobilizing and directing goal-directed behaviors. DA neurons constitute a "go-system" or "incentive system," guiding the organism to areas in the environment associated with reward (Crow, 1973). Though a role for NA in self-stimulation is less well supported than a role for DA, NAergic neurons seem to play a role in what we have called "emotional memory" (van Praag et al., 1988); that is, in the consolidation and retrieval of the emotional arousal induced by particular behaviors. Alternatively, NAergic tracts constitute the connections between the neural representation of rewards anticipated to be associated with particular behaviors and the DAergic incentive system (Crow, 1973, 1977). NAergic mechanisms have also been implicated in selecting among a choice of possible behaviors to attain a particular goal, based upon experiences of reward or punishment that those behaviors elicited on previous occasions (Ashton, 1987). A reward-related role of NAergic mechanisms in self-stimulation is supported by experiments with clonidine, an alpha$_2$-adrenergic agonist. This substance disrupts the rewarding component of brain stimulation in a selective manner, probably via activation of presynaptic alpha$_2$-receptors, and by doing so, curtails NAergic impulse flow (Hunt et al., 1976; Franklin, 1978). The CA synthesis inhibitor alpha-methyl-para-tyrosine magnifies this effect (Hunt et al., 1976).

A Noradrenalin Hypothesis of Anhedonia

NAergic mechanisms seem to enable the animal to couple the experience of reward or anticipated reward to a particular activity. The hedonic component of the melancholic syndrome can be conceived of as a dysfunction of exactly that coupling mechanism. "I used to love to go with my kids to a baseball game, doctor, but somehow it does not please me anymore." Situations that used to create pleasure are perceived as usual, but are now devoid of an emotional charge. Stein (1978) was the first to suggest that depression was "a disorder of positive reinforcement or reward function." We do not subscribe to this generalization, but would suggest a more focused version of the hypothesis. We propose that the hedonic disturbance in depression is related to NAergic insufficiency, a transmission defect resulting in the inability to couple the reward component with mental or physical activities that used to carry such a charge.

Stein (1978) also suggested that in depression the reward system might be primarily hypoactive, or secondarily hypoactive, namely overridden by the excessive activity of an anxiety-punishment system. On clinical grounds, the latter alternative is less plausible. There are many psychiatric states in which the anxiety-punishment system could be postulated to be hyperactive (e.g., the anxiety disorders). None of them, however, is accompanied by the hedonic disturbances so typical in melancholic depression.

The NA hypothesis of anhedonia fits into the general framework of the classic information-processing theory of human cognition, in which two sets of structures are being postulated—one for storing information and the other for information transfer from one structure to another. Following Kihlstrom's (1987) description, in this model information from the environment is transduced into a pattern of neural impulses by the sensory receptors. This pattern is briefly held in the sensory registers, one for each modality, where it is then analyzed by processes known as feature detection and pattern recognition. Information that has been identified as meaningful and relevant to current goals is then transferred to a structure known as primary or short-term memory, a process in which attention plays an important role. In short-term memory the information is subject to further analysis, whereby the perceptual information is combined with information retrieved from secondary or long-term memory. In the primary memory, processes such as judgment, inference, and problem solving take, place. On the basis of an analysis of the meaning of the stimulus input, a response is generated. Finally, a trace of the event is permanently encoded in the secondary memory.

It is in the primary memory, one might assume, that the percepts (i.e., the perceptual information) are linked with the appropriate emotion (i.e., the emotion that was aroused in similar circumstances on previous occasions).

The concept of the NAergic nature of hedonic disturbances has not been systematically studied, and hence is largely hypothetical. Some scattered data, however, although admittedly tentative at best, are sufficiently intriguing to prompt further investigation.

Preliminary Studies of the Noradrenaline Hypothesis of Anhedonia

Experiments with Clozapine

Anhedonia is a typical symptom of melancholic depression, but can also be pharmacologically induced (i.e., by antipsychotics). Apart from anticholinergic phenomena, the most common side effects of antipsychotics are

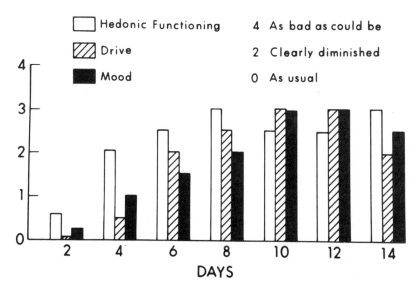

Figure 13-7. Clozapine (100 mg/day for two weeks) was administered to six normal individuals. After two to three days, listlessness was reported; after five to six days, lack of energy was reported; and in the second week, mood lowering was described. The "clozapine syndrome" resembled mild melancholic depression. Placebo was ineffectual (van Praag et al., unpublished observation).

extrapyramidal symptoms and anhedonia. The motor symptoms are thought to be related to nigro-striatal DAergic blockage. Most antipsychotics also variably block NAergic transmission. Conceivably, this effect could underlie the hedonic disturbances.

Clozapine is a so-called "atypical antipsychotic," one of a group of compounds with more selective effects on mesolimbic and mesocortical DA systems than their "typical" counterparts. This could explain why their propensity to elicit motor side effects is lower and their therapeutic potential is probably greater. In addition, clozapine has a profound blocking effect on NA receptors, particularly after acute administration (Bartholini et al., 1972, 1973; Burki et al., 1974; Buus Lassen, 1974).

We studied the psychological effects of 100 mg clozapine administered daily for two weeks to six normal volunteers in a placebo-controlled, double-blind, two-group design. We were particularly interested in clozapine's impact on mood, drive, and hedonic functions, which were assessed every other day in a structured interview and by a (blind) interviewer according to a five-point scale (Figure 13-7). Effects occurred more or less sequentially. After two to three days, listlessness, was reported; by the end of the first week, lack of energy became more prominent; finally, in the second week, lowering of mood was described. The "clozapine-syndrome" resembled that of mild melancholic (vital) depression, and was reported by all probands. In the control group, the placebo elicited, if anything, an energizing rather than a depressing effect. The hedonic deficit elicited by clozapine was pronounced, and in the first few days was "pure" (that is, not combined with other psychological disturbances).

This experiment does not provide information about a possible relationship between anhedonia and NAergic inhibition. However, a second experiment seemed to suggest such a relationship (van Praag et al., 1976). We compared perphenazine (average daily dose 21 mg) and clozapine (average daily dose 300 mg) in two groups, each made up of 12 patients suffering from different forms of acute psychoses. During perphenazine treatment, the postprobenecid concentration of HVA in CSF increased 70%, whereas clozapine failed to produce a significant rise. Conversely, clozapine caused a significant increase in the CSF concentration of MHPG, the major metabolite of NA in the CNS, while perphenazine did not. In contrast to perphenazine, clozapine apparently has a pronounced blocking effect on postsynaptic NA receptors. After 10 days of treatment, anhedonia was significantly more frequent in the clozapine group (eight of 12) than in the perphenazine group (two of 12).

Experiments with Tyrosine

In depressed patients, tyrosine, the precursor of DA and NA, increased the CSF concentration of HVA and MHPG (van Praag & Lemus, 1986). From these data, it was inferred that tyrosine furthers CA synthesis and metabolism (Figure 13-3). The effect on NA is much more pronounced than that on DA. As stated above, the reverse is true after administration of L-dopa (Figure 13-1).

In a double-blind study, we compared the effects of tyrosine (100 mg/kg/day) in 10 patients with major depression, melancholic type, with the effect of placebo in 10 comparable patients (van Praag, 1986b). We were particularly interested in tyrosine's effects on drive, mood, anxiety, and hedonic functions. These domains were explored weekly, using a structured interview, and results were recorded on a 10-point scale, ranging from "as good as could be" (10) to "as bad as could be" (1).

Tyrosine did not change the overall ratings on the Hamilton Depression Scale over a four-week period. Discrete components of the syndrome, however, did change significantly (Figure 13-4). This was particularly true for hedonic functioning and anxiety. In the first week, significant improvement occurred in the former domain, an effect that persisted during the four weeks the study lasted. Eight patients in the tyrosine group and one in the placebo group reported that they were less "deemotionalized." Anxiety was reported to be increased in nine patients on tyrosine and two on placebo. Mood and drive ratings improved slightly, but not significantly. Thus, tyrosine seems to exert an increasing effect on NA availability, while also significantly reducing anhedonia.

Clonidine Studies

In low doses, clonidine stimulates presynaptic alpha$_2$-adrenergic receptors, leading to diminished NA release. Administered to normal individuals, it has been shown to induce sedation impairment of paired-associated learning, particulary when the pairs to be learned are unrelated (Firth et al., 1985). Sedation is an unlikely explanation because clonidine did not affect other memory functions. It decreased blood pressure, suggesting diminished NAergic impulse flow, but this effect could, of course, be totally peripheral.

This finding suggests that NA neurons are involved in the coupling of the neural representation of associated stimuli. This is as far as one can go; it does not imply that these neurons are involved in linking an emotional memory trace ("pleasure") with a particular behavior.

Hormonal Studies

The growth hormone response to clonidine (supposedly mediated by postsynaptic alpha$_2$-adrenergic receptors in the hypothalamus) has been shown to be blunted in endogenous depression as compared with neurotic depression (Checkley et al., 1984) (Figure 13-8). The most important symptomatological distinction between the two syndromes is the presence or absence of anhedonia (van Praag, 1962). Conceivably, the NAergic deficit and the hedonic disturbances correlate, but data to this effect are not available.

Another hormonal disturbance observed in major depression is blunting of the plasma cortisol response to desmethylimipramine (DMI), a tricyclic antidepressant and a selective inhibitor of NA uptake (Asnis et al., 1985) (Figure 13-9). In correlating blunted DMI response with items of the SADS (Schedule for Affective Disorders and Schizophrenia—Endicott & Spitzer, 1978) related to anhedonia, we found a significant correlation with "lack of reactivity," but not with "loss of interest" and "social withdrawal" (Table 13-2). This study was a retrospective one, and no attempts had been made specifically to delineate the symptom of anhedonia and differentiate it from symptoms that show a certain similarity but which we consider basically different.

Conclusions

While the evidence in favor of an NAergic deficit underlying anhedonia is scanty and tentative, we believe it is of sufficient interest to warrant further investigation.

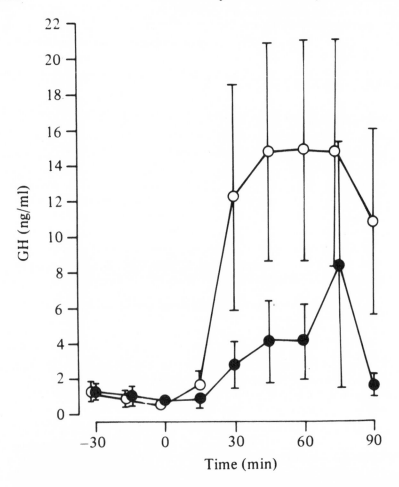

Figure 13-8. Mean plasma growth hormone concentrations (± SEM) before and after the infusion of clonidine (1.3 mg/kg) between 0 and 10 minutes in 10 patients with endogenous depression (0-0) and in 10 patients with reactive depression (0-0) (Checkley et al., 1984).

A DIMENSIONAL MONOAMINE HYPOTHESIS

Let us now amalgamate the biobehavioral relations we have suggested (Figure 13-10). First, we pointed out what we consider to be the major domains of psychological dysfunctioning in melancholic depression: drive, mood, and hedonic functioning. Next, we discussed evidence of MAergic dysfunctions underlying these psychological dysfunctions. Sufficient evidence seems available to implicate DA in drive reduction and 5-HT in dis-

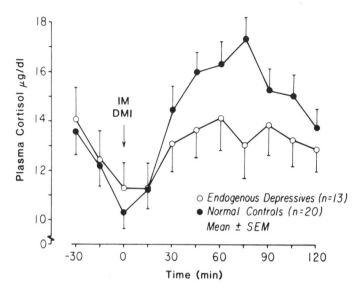

Figure 13-9. Cortisol response after 75 mg desipramine given intravenously in patients with major depressive disorder, endogenous subtype (RDC criteria) as compared with normal controls (Asnis et al., 1985).

turbed aggression regulation and heightened anxiety. Tentatively, a link has been proposed between NAergic dysfunction and anhedonia.

5-HTergic and DAergic systems (Green & Deakin, 1980; Williams & Davies, 1983; Curzon et al., 1985; Fuenmayor & Bermudez, 1985) and 5-HTergic and NAergic systems (Ferron et al., 1982; Reinhard et al., 1983; Manier et al., 1984; Feuerstein & Hertting, 1986; Heal et al., 1986; Asakura et al., 1987; Devau et al., 1987) are strongly and mutually intertwined. If

TABLE 13-2
**SADS Items Relating to Anhedonia and the Cortisol Response
to Desipramine in Major Depressives (Asnis et al., unpublished)**

	Zero-Order Correlation with Delta* 75 Cortisol	*Correlation with 75 Minutes Cortisol (Baseline Partialled Out)*	*Correlation with 75 Minutes Cortisol (Age and Baseline Partialled Out)*
Loss of interest	−0.109	−0.171	−0.171
Social withdrawal	0.152	0.060	0.076
Lack of reactivity	−0.066	−0.273†	−0.289†

* = Delta cortisol, 75 minutes after 75 mg desipramine IM.
† = $p < 0.05$ one-tailed test.

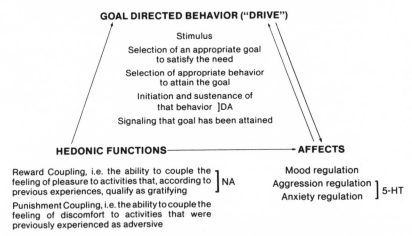

MAJOR AREAS OF DYSFUNCTION IN MAJOR DEPRESSION, MELANCHOLIC TYPE (ENDOGENOUS OR VITAL DEPRESSION)

GOAL DIRECTED BEHAVIOR ("DRIVE")

Stimulus

Selection of an appropriate goal to satisfy the need

Selection of appropriate behavior to attain the goal

Initiation and sustenance of that behavior]DA

Signaling that goal has been attained

HEDONIC FUNCTIONS —————————————→ AFFECTS

Reward Coupling, i.e. the ability to couple the feeling of pleasure to activities that, according to] NA previous experiences, qualify as gratifying

Punishment Coupling, i.e. the ability to couple the feeling of discomfort to activities that were previously experienced as adversive

Mood regulation
Aggression regulation] 5-HT
Anxiety regulation

Figure 13-10. Depiction of the major domains of psychological dysfunctioning in major depression, melancholic type, and the hypothesized MAergic dysfunctions underlying these psychological dysfunctions.

the psychological dysfunctions under discussion were linked to MAergic dysfunctions, one would expect the psychological dysfunctions to (1) often go in concert, and (2) influence each other's severity. Disorders of drive, mood, and hedonic functioning meet in the melancholic syndrome, but no systematic data are available about their quantitative interactions. Clinical experience, however, suggests the likelihood that such interactions do occur. Anhedonia reinforces lack of drive and will tend to aggravate mood lowering. Mood lowering, in turn, will negatively affect drive, whereas, conversely, drive reduction can be perceived as a mood-lowering force.

Disturbances in drive, and in anxiety and aggression regulation, are by no means specific for melancholic depression, but also are seen in other behavioral and certain neurological disorders. This could explain the nosological nonspecificity of MA disturbances. Signs of deceased DA metabolism have, for example, been found in retarded depression and in Parkinson's disease; 5-HT disturbances have been reported in depressed suicide attempters, but also in suicide attempters with other diagnoses and in individuals with outwardly directed aggression irrespective of diagnosis. Moreover, 5-HT disturbances have been implicated in panic disorder. The odds are, however, that they relate to increased anxiety, across diagnoses. Anhedonia seems to be relatively characteristic for melancholic depression. One would expect the same to be true for the alleged signs of NAergic hypofunction, but no data are as yet available.

So far, no data implicate particular MAergic disturbances in the mood component in melancholic depression. One reason for this lack of data could be that this issue has hardly been studied, but it could also be explained by hypothesizing that mood disturbances are secondary to other depressive dysfunctions, possibly lack of drive and anhedonia—and some observations suggest that this could be the case. Katz et al. (1987) have demonstrated that the therapeutic effects of amitriptyline in depression appear as early as the first week of treatment. The first symptoms to decrease are anxiety and hostility, correlated with plasma amitriptyline levels. Mood improvement follows later, in the second and third weeks (Katz et al., in preparation). When we examined initial symptoms in 100 patients admitted for first or second episodes of melancholic depression, we found that anhedonia had been the most frequent initial symptom (42%), with drive reduction second in frequency (31%). Mood lowering was indicated as a first symptom by only 11% of the sample.

Recently, Cloninger (1986, 1987) advocated the dimensional approach for the biological study of personality disorders. He introduced a system of personality variants based on three dimensions—novelty seeking, harm avoidance, and reward dependence—and he additionally linked these traits to particular MAergic systems. The scheme has elegance but lacks empirical foundation, and will be hard to verify. It is hard enough to define and measure psychopathological dimensions such as anhedonia, mood lowering, drive, and anxiety; to do the same for delicate distinctions in personality makeup is infinitely more difficult. To view biological variables occurring in psychiatric disorders from the vantage point of psychopathological dimensions has been demonstrated to be feasible, as well as productive. Whether it will still be true when personality dimensions are substituted for psychopathological dimensions remains to be seen. Considering the present state of psychiatry's diagnostic methodology, we predict that Cloninger went one step too far.

FUNCTIONAL PSYCHOPATHOLOGY: A LOOK FORWARD

Mainstream biological psychiatry has always had an orthodox nosological orientation, positing as its major goal the discovery of markers, and eventually causes, of psychiatric disorders. We have advocated an alternative: a functional-dimensional standpoint (van Praag & Leÿnse, 1965; van Praag et al., 1975, 1987c). This orientation entails dissection of a given psychiatric syndrome into its component parts—the various psychological dysfunctions—and analyzing them for correlations with biological dysfunctions. Functional psychopathology is dimensional in orientation, viewing a given psychiatric disorder as a conglomerate of psychological dimensions, each of them nosologically nonspecific and occurring in different degrees of severity and in different combinations in the various psychiatric syndromes. The nosological approach is categorical, viewing psychiatric disorders as discrete entities, each with its own causation, symptomatology, and course.

The term "functional" is not identical with "symptomatological." Psychiatric symptoms are the behavioral expression of a psychological dysfunction, not the dysfunction itself. For example, a visual hallucination is a symptom, and a particular perceptual disturbance is the underlying dysfunction. The latter is the target of biological research within the functional framework.

As discussed above, the functional approach has been productive in biological psychiatric research. Its implications, however, transcend the boundaries of biological psychiatry in several important ways.

First, there are major implications in the realm of clinical psychopharmacology. A number of psychotropic drugs have proved to be diagnostically nonspecific. Tricyclic antidepressants are efficacious in certain forms of depression, and also in certain anxiety states. Clomipramine is an effective antidepressant, and is also a useful treatment in obsessive compulsive disorder. Carbamazepine is an established antiepileptic agent, as well as an asset in the prophylaxis of episodic mood disorders. These observations are puzzling from a nosological but not from a functional point of view. A particular drug may influence a specific functional system in the brain, and thus a particular set of psychological dysfunctions, irrespective of diagnosis.

The implications of the functional approach, however, reach farther than simply providing a possible explanation for the nosological nonspecificity of some psychotropic drugs. Once correlations between psychological and biological dysfunctions have been established, the next step inevitably will be the search for drugs that can selectively correct these biological dysfunctions. Such drugs would be expected to ameliorate the corresponding psychological dysfunctions, regardless of nosological diagnosis. Within a nosological frame of reference, treatment is directed toward a particular disorder, whereas within a functional framework, it is directed toward the underlying or resulting dysfunctions. In the former approach, treatment is preferably restricted to one drug; in the latter approach, combinations of drugs will be used, contingent on the existing spectrum of dysfunctions. Functional psychopathology will lead to functional psychopharmacology, and functional psychopharmacology will inevitably tend to use drugs in combination.

As an example of transnosological indication for psychotropic drugs, we summarize a recent hypothesis of ours (van Praag et al., 1986). In the late 1950s and early 1960s, animal experiments had clearly demonstrated that the classical antidepressants increase the availability of MAs (including 5-HT) in the brain. These data prompted clinical research into the relation between 5-HT and depression. Findings indicative of such a relationship initiated the search for, and eventually the development of, drugs that increase central 5-HT selectively (e.g., the selective 5-HT reuptake inhibitors). Continued explorations indicated the likelihood that 5-HT was involved not so much in depression per se, as in certain components of the syndrome (i.e., anxiety and dyscontrol of aggression). These data, in turn, generated the hypothesis that compounds capable of potentiating 5-HT are not true antidepressants, but rather are indicated in states of heightened anxiety/aggression across (nosological) diagnoses.

One could even argue that the greater the biochemical specificity of a drug, the greater is the chance it will be nosologically nonspecific but effective against certain (clusters of) psychological dysfunctions, across diagnoses. We predict that the development of biochemically specific drugs will decrease the range of action of such medications, but will enable the clinician to compose tailor-made therapeutic regimens and to titrate each drug individually, based on the spectrum of psychological dysfunctions. In principle, this is an inviting perspective. In practice, however, its practicability will depend on the compatibility of the component drugs and their propensity to induce side effects.

Goal-directed, dysfunction-oriented polypharmacy (or, if one dislikes that work, multidimensional pharmacy, or multipharmacy) is more than a chimera. Cardiology provides a useful analogy. For example, once a myocardial infarction has been diagnosed and the cardiac condition has been functionally analyzed, drugs will be administered to regulate discrete disturbances in, for instance, rhythm, conduction, frequency, and output. These drugs are often prescribed simultaneously, and thus provide a model of goal-directed, dysfunction-oriented multipharmacy. This is a conceivable prospect for psychiatry as well, and the direction in which we expect to see clinical psychopharmacology develop. It would mean profound scientific progress.

A second field that will benefit from a functionally oriented psychopathology is that of the measurement of abnormal human behavior. So far, the presence of a psychiatric syndrome or symptom is psychometrically expressed as a rough estimate; that is, as mildly, moderately, or severely present, or anywhere in between. Many psychological functions and dysfunctions, however, are measurable in real quantitative terms and with considerable precision and reliability. Functional psychopathology will lay the groundwork for a scientifically based psychopathology.

Finally, the field of the psychotherapies will benefit from a functionally oriented psychopathology, because it will allow, much more precisely than is possible today, exposure and delineation of mental domains that are dysfunctional and those that are still relatively normal. This will permit a rather precise definition of treatment goals and a more rational choice of treatment method—and will help treatment planning immeasurably.

Thus, functional psychopathology not only is a productive framework for biological research in psychiatry, but could evolve into a forceful catalyst for psychiatry's ongoing scientific orientation.

We introduced the functional/dimensional approach in psychopathology as a complement of, and not as an alternative to, the nosological/categorical approach. We still fully subscribe to this standpoint, as much as we do to the view that the exclusive adherence to nosology has not served biological psychiatry well. In fact, we believe that it has been a factor stunting its growth (van Praag, 1990).

SUMMARY

Classical nosology has been the major cornerstone of biological psychiatric research; finding biological markers and eventually causes of disease entities has been the major goal. We have advocated another approach, one we have designated as "functional," that attempts to correlate biological variables with psychological dysfunctions, which are considered the basic units of classification in psychopathology. We have pursued this route for many years, and on the basis of the resulting data, we have formulated the following hypothesis. Signs of diminished DA, 5-HT, and NA metabolism have been found in a number of psychiatric disorders. We believe that these are not disorder specific, but rather are related to psychopathological dimensions (i.e., hypoactivity/inertia, increased aggression/anxiety, and anhedonia) independently of the nosological framework in which these dysfunctions occur. We have discussed implications of the functional approach for psychiatry, including a shift from nosological to functional application of psychotropic drugs. Functional psychopharmacology will be dysfunction oriented and, therefore, inevitably geared toward using drug combinations. We hail this prospect as progress, both practically and scientifically.

REFERENCES

American Psychiatric Association. (1988). Diagnostic and statistical manual of mental disorders. Third edition.
Apter, A., Plutchik, R., Sevy, S., Korn, M. L., Brown, S. L., & van Praag, H. M.

(1989). Suicide and violence in psychiatric patients. Presented at the American Psychiatric Association, San Francisco, Calif.

Apter, A., van Praag, H. M., Plutchik, R., Sevy, S., Korn, M., & Brown, S. L. (1990). The relationship between a serotonergically linked series of psycho-pathological dimensions. *Psych. Res.*, *32*, 191-192.

Asakura, M., Tsukamoto, T., Kubota, H., Imafuku, Ino, M., Nishizaki, J., Sata, A., Shinbo, K., & Hasegawa, K. (1987). Role of serotonin in the regulation of alpha-adrenoceptors by antidepressants. *Eur. J. Pharmacol.*, *141*, 95-100.

Asberg, M., Traskman, L., & Thoren, P. (1976). 5-HIAA in the cerebrospinal fluid: A biochemical suicide predictor? *Arch. Gen. Psychiatry*, *33*, 1193-1197.

Ashton, H. (1987). *Brain or systems disorders and psychotropic drugs.* Oxford: Oxford University Press.

Asnis, G. M., Halbreich, U., Rabinovich, H., Ryan, N. D., Sachar, E. J., Nelson, B., Puig-Antich, J., & Novacenko, H. (1985). The cortisol response to desipramine in endogenous depressives and normal controls: preliminary findings. *Psychiatr. Res.*, *14*, 225-233.

Banki, C. M. (1977a). Correlation between CSF metabolites and psychomotor activity in affective disorders. *J. Neurochem.*, *28*, 255-257.

Banki, C. M. (1977b). Correlation of anxiety and related symptoms with cerebrospinal fluid 5-hydroxyindoleacetic acid in depressed women. *J. Neural Transm.*, *41*, 135-143.

Banki, C. M., Molnar, G., & Vojnik, M. (1981). Cerebrospinal fluid amine metabolites, tryptophan and clinical parameters in depression. *J. Affect. Dis.*, *3*, 91-99.

Bartholini, G., Haefely, W., Jalfre, M., Keller, H. H., & Pletscher, A. (1972). Effects of clozapine on cerebral catecholaminergic neurone systems. *Br. J. Pharmacol.*, *46*, 736-740.

Bartholini, G., Keller, H. H., Pletscher, A. (1973). Effect of neuroleptics on endogenous norepinephrine in rat brain. *Neuropharmacol.*, *12*, 751-756.

Bioulac, B., Benezich, M., Renaud, B., Noel, B., & Roche, D. (1980). Serotonergic functions in the 47, XYZ syndrome. *Biol. Psychiat.*, *15*, 917-923.

Brown, G. L., Goodwin, F. K., Ballenger, J. C., Goyer, P. F., & Major, L. F. (1979). Aggression in humans correlates with cerebrospinal fluid metabolites. *Psychiatr. Res.*, *1*, 131-139.

Brown, G. L., Ebert, M. E., Goyer, P. F., Jimerson, D. C., Klein, W. J., Bunney, W. E., & Goodwin, F. K. (1982). Aggression, suicide and serotonin. Relationships to CSF amine metabolites. *Am. J. Psychiatr.*, *139*, 741-746.

Burki, H. R., Ruch, W., Asper, H., Baggiolini, M., & Stille, G. (1974). Effect of single and repeated administration of clozapine on the metabolism of dopamine and noradrenaline in the brain of the rat. *Eur. J. Pharmacol.*, *27*, 180-190.

Buus Lassen, J. (1974). Evidence of noradrenaline (NA)- and dopamine (DA)-receptor blockade by clozapine. *J. Pharmacol.*, *5*, 14.

Ceulemans, D. L. S., Hoppenbrouwers, M. I. J. A., Gelders, Y., & Reyntjens, A. J. M. (1985). The influence of ritanserin, a serotonin antagonist, in anxiety disorders: A double-blind placebo-controlled study versus lorazepam. *Pharmakopsychiat.*, *18*, 303-305.

Checkley, S. A., Glass, I. B., Thompson, C., Corn, T., & Robinson, P. (1984). The GH response to clonidine in endogenous as compared with reactive depression. *Psychol. Med.*, *14*, 773–777.

Cloninger, C. R. (1986). A unified biosocial theory of personality and its role in the development of anxiety states. *Psych. Dev.*, *3*, 167–226.

Cloninger, C. R. (1987). A systematic method for clinical description and classification of personality variants. *Arch. Gen. Psychiatry*, *44*, 573–588.

Crow, T. J. (1973). Catecholamine-containing neurones and electrical self-stimulation: 2. A theoretical interpretation and some psychiatric implications. *Psychol. Med.*, *3*, 66–73.

Crow, T. J. (1977). A general catecholamine hypothesis. *Neurosci. Res. Prog. Bull.*, *15*, 195–205.

Crow, T. J., & Deakin, J. F. W. (1985). Neurohormonal transmission, behaviour and mental disorder. In M. Shepherd (Ed.), *Handbook of psychiatry. part 5.* Cambridge, England: Cambridge University Press.

Curzon, G., Hutson, P. H., Kantamaneni, B. D., Sahakian, B. J., & Sarna, G. S. (1985). 3,4-Dihydroxphenylethylamine and 5-hydroxytryptamine metabolism in the rat: Acidic metabolites in cisternal cerebrospinal fluid before and after giving probenecid. *J. Neurochem.*, *45*, 508–513.

Den Boer, J. A., Westenberg, H. G. M., Kamerbeek, W. D. J., Verhoeven, W. M. A., & Kahn, R. S. (1987). Effect of serotonin uptake inhibitors in anxiety disorders: A double-blind comparison of clomipramine and fluvoxamine. *Int. Clin. Psychopharmacol.*, *2*, 21–32.

Devau, G., Multon, M. F., Pujol, J. F., & Buda, M. (1987). Inhibition of tyrosine hydroxylase activity by serotonin in explants of newborn rat locus ceruleus. *J. Neurochem.*, *49*, 665–670.

Endicott, J., & Spitzer, R. L. (1978). A diagnostic interview: The schedule for affective disorders and schizophrenia (SADS). *Arch. Gen. Psychiatry*, *35*, 837–844.

Evans, L., & Moore, G. (1981). The treatment of phobic anxiety by zimelidine. *Acta Psychiatr. Scan.*, *63*(Suppl 290), 342–345.

Evans, L., Kenardy, J., Schneider, P., & Hoey, H. (1986). Effect of a selective serotonin uptake inhibitor in agoraphobia with panic attacks. *Acta Psychiatr. Scand.*, *73*, 49–53.

Ferron, A., Descarries, L., & Reader, T. A. (1982). Altered neuronal responsiveness to biogenic amines in rat cerebral cortex after serotonin denervation or depletion. *Brain Res.*, *231*, 93–108.

Feuerstein, T. J., & Hertting, G. (1986). Serotonin (5-HT) enhances hippocampal noradrenaline (NA) release: Evidence for facilitatory 5-HT receptors within the CNS. *Naunyn-Schmiedeberg's Arch. Pharmacol.*, *333*, 191–197.

Firth, C. K., Dowdy, J., Ferrier, I. N., & Crow, T. J. (1985). Selective impairment of paired associate learning after administration of a centrally-acting adrenergic agonist (clonidine). *Psychopharmacol.*, *87*, 490–493.

Franklin, K. B. J. (1978). Catecholamines and self-stimulation: Reward and performance effects dissociated. *Pharmac. Biochem. Behav.*, *9*, 813–820.

Freed, C. R., & Yamamoto, B. K. (1985). Regional brain dopamine metabolism: A marker for the speed, direction and posture of moving animals. *Science, 229,* 62.

Fuenmayor, L. D., & Bermudez, M. (1985). Effect of the cerebral tryptaminergic system on the turnover of dopamine in the striatum of the rat. *J. Neurochem., 44,* 670–674.

Goodwin, F. V., & Post, R. M. (1983). 5-Hydroxytryptamine and depression: A model for the interaction of normal variances and pathology. *Br. J. Clin. Pharmacol., 15,* 393–405.

Green, A. R., & Deakin, J. F. W. (1980). Brain noradrenaline depletion prevents ECS-induced enhancement of serotonin- and dopamine-mediated behaviour. *Nature, 285,* 232–233.

Heal, D. J., Philpot, K. M., O'Shaughnessy, K. M., & Davies, C. L. (1986). The influence of central noradrenergic function on 5-HT2-mediated head-twitch responses in mice: Possible implications for the actions of antidepressant drugs. *Psychopharmacol., 89,* 414–420.

Hunt, G. E., Atrens, D. M., Chesher, G. B., & Becker, F. T. (1976). Alpha-noradrenergic modulation of hypothalamic self-stimulation: Studies employing clonidine, 1-phenylephrine and alpha-methyl-para-tyrosine. *Eur. J. Pharmacol., 37,* 105–111.

Jones, B. J., Costall, B., Domeney, A. M., Kelly, M. E., Naylor, R. J., Oakley, N. R., & Tyers, M. B. (1988). The potential anxiolytic activity of GR38032F, a 5-HT3-receptor antagonist. *Br. J. Pharmacol., 93,* 985–993.

Kahn, R. S., & Westenberg, H. G. M. (1985). l-5-Hydroxytryptophan in the treatment of anxiety disorders. *J. Affect. Dis., 8,* 197–200.

Kahn, R. S., Westenberg, H. G. M., & Jolles, J. (1984). Zimelidine treatment of obsessive-compulsive disorder. *Acta Psychiatr. Scand., 69,* 259–261.

Kahn, R. S., Westenberg, H. G. M., Verhoeven, W. M. A., Gispen-de Wied, C. C., & Kamerbeek, W. D. J. (1987). Effect of a serotonin precursor and uptake inhibitor in anxiety disorders: A double-blind comparison of 5-hydroxytryptophan, clomipramine and placebo. *Int. Clin. Psychopharmacol., 2,* 33–45.

Kahn. R. S., Wetzler, S., van Praag, H. M., & Asnis, G. M. (1988a). Behavioral indications of serotonergic supersensitivity in patients with panic disorder. *Psychiatr. Res., 25,* 101–104.

Kahn, R. S., Asnis, G. M., Wetzler, S., & van Praag, H. M. (1988b). Neuroendocrine evidence for 5-HT receptor hypersensitivity in panic disorder. *Psychopharmacol. (Berlin), 96,* 360–369.

Kahn, R. S., van Praag, H. M., Wetzler, S., Asnis, G. M., & Barr, G. (1988c). Serotonin and anxiety revisited. *Biol. Psychiat., 23,* 189–208.

Katz, M. M., Koslow, S., Maas, J. W., Frazer, A., Rowden, C., Casper, R. C., Croughan, J., Kocsis, J., & Redmond, E. (1987). The timing and specificity and clinical prediction of tricyclic drug effects in depression. *Psychol. Med., 17,* 297–309.

Katz, M. M., Koslow, S. H., Maas, J. W., Frazer, A., Kocsis, J., Secunda, S., Bowden, C. L., & Casper, R. C. (1990). Identifying the specific clinical actions of amitriptyline: Interrelationships of behavior, affect and plasma levels in depression. (Submitted).

Kihlstrom, J. F. (1987). The cognitive unconscious. *Science, 237,* 1445–1452.

Koczkas, S., Holmberg, G., & Wedin, L. (1981). A pilot study of the effect of the 5-HT uptake inhibitor, zimelidine, on phobic anxiety. *Acta Psychiatr. Scand.*, *63*(Suppl 290), 328–341.

Lakke, J. P. W. F., Korf, J., van Praag, H. M., & Schut, T. (1972). Predictive value of the probenecid test for the effect of L-DOPA therapy in Parkinson's disease. *Nature, 236*, 208–209.

Lidberg, L., Asberg, M., & Sundquist-Stensman, U. B. (1984). 5-Hydroxyindoleacetic acid in attempted suicides who have killed their children. *Lancet, ii*, 928.

Lidberg, L., Tuck, J. R., Asberg, M., Scalia-Tomba, G. P., & Bertilsson, L. (1985). Homicide, suicide and CSF 5-HIAA. *Acta Psychiatr. Scand., 71*, 230–236.

Lindstrom, L. H. (1985). Low HVA and normal 5-HIAA CSF levels in drug free schizophrenia patients, compared to healthy volunteers: Correlations to symptomatology and heredity. *Psychiatr. Res., 14*, 265–274.

Linnoila, M., Virkkunen, M., Scheinin, M., Nuutila, A., Rimon, R., & Goodwin, F. K. (1983). Low cerebrospinal fluid 5-hydroxyindoleacetic acid concentration differentiates impulsive from nonimpulsive violent behavior. *Life Sci., 33*, 2609–2614.

Manier, D. H., Gillespie, D. D., Steranka, L. R., & Sulser, F. (1984). A pivotal role for serotonin (5-HT) in the regulation of beta-adrenoceptors by antidepressants: Reversibility of the action of parachlorophenylalanine by 5-hydroxytryptophan. *Experientia, 40*, 1223–1226.

Olds, J., & Milner, P. (1954). Positive reinforcement produced by electrical stimulation of the septal area and other regions of the rat brain. *J. Comp. Phys. Psychiatr., 47*, 419–427.

Papeschi, R., & McClure, D. J. (1971). Homovanillic and 5-hydroxyindoleacetic acid in cerebrospinal fluid in depressed patients. *Arch. Gen. Psychiatr., 25*, 354–358.

Raleigh, M. J. (1987). Differential behavioral effects of tryptophan and 5-hydroxytryptophan in vervet monkeys: Influence of catecholaminergic systems. *Psychopharmacol., 93*, 44–50.

Reinhard, J. F., Jr., Galloway, M. P., & Roth, R. H. (1983). Noradrenergic modulation of serotonin synthesis and metabolism. II. Stimulation by 3-isobutyl-a-methylxanthine. *J. Pharm. Exp. Ther., 226*, 764–769.

Rydin, E., Schalling, D., & Asberg, M. (1982). Rorschach ratings in depressed and suicidal patients with low CSF 5-HIAA. *Psychiatr. Res., 7*, 229–243.

Stein, L. (1978). Reward transmitters: Catecholamines and opioid peptides. In M. A. Lipton, A. DiMascio, & K. F. Killam (Eds.), *Psychopharmacology: A generation of progress* (pp. 569–581). New York: Raven Press.

Taylor, D. P., Eison, M. S., Riblet, L. A., & Vandermaelen, C. P. (1985). Pharmacological and clinical effects of buspirone. *Pharmacol. Biochem. Behav., 23*, 687–694.

van Praag, H. M. (1962). A critical investigation of the importance of monoamine oxidase inhibition as a therapeutic principle in the treatment of depression. Thesis, Utrecht.

van Praag, H. M. (1982). Neurotransmitters and CNS disease: Depression. *Lancet, II*, 1259–1264.

van Praag, H. M. (1983). In search of the mode of action of antidepressants: 5-HT-tyrosine mixtures in depressions. *Neuropharmacol.*, *22*, 433–440.

van Praag, H. M. (1984). Studies in the mechanism of action of serotonin precursors in depression. *Psychopharmacol. Bull.*, *20*, 599–602.

van Praag, H. M. (1986a). Biological suicide research. Outcome and limitations. *Biol. Psychiat.*, *21*, 1305–1323.

van Praag, H. M. (1986b). Serotonin precursors with and without tyrosine in the treatment of depression. In C. Shagrass, R. Josias, W. Bridger, K. Weiss, D. Stoff, & J. Simpson (Eds.), *Biological psychiatry*. New York: Elsevier Science Publishers.

van Praag, H. M., & Korf, J. (1971a). Retarded depression and the dopamine metabolism. *Psychopharmacol.*, *19*, 199–203.

van Praag, H. M., & Korf, J. (1971b). Endogenous depressions with and without disturbances in the 5-hydroxytryptamine metabolism: A biochemical classification? *Psychopharmacol.*, *19*, 148–152.

van Praag, H. M., & Korf, J. (1975). Central monoamine deficiency in depression: Causative or secondary phenomenon? *Pharmakopsychiatr.*, *8*, 321–326.

van Praag, H. M., Korf, J., & Puite, J. (1970). 5-Hydroxyindoleacetic acid levels in the cerebrospinal fluid of depressive patients treated with probenecid. *Nature*, *225*, 1259–1260.

van Praag, H. M., Korf, J., Lakke, J. P. W. F., & Schut, T. (1975). Dopamine metabolism in depression, psychoses and Parkinson's disease: The problem of the specificity of biological variables in behaviour disorders. *Psychol. Med.*, *5*, 138–146.

van Praag, H. M., Korf, J., & Dols, L. C. W. (1976). Clozapine versus perphenazine: The value of the biochemical mode of action of neuroleptics in predicting their therapeutic activity. *Br. J. Psychiatr.*, *129*, 547–555.

van Praag, H. M., & Leijnse, B. (1965). Neubewertung des syndroms. Skizze einer funktionellen Pathologie. *Psychiatr. Neurol. Neurochir.*, *68*, 50–66.

van Praag, H. M., & Lemus, C. (1986). Monamine precursors in the treatment of psychiatric disorders. In R. J. Wurtman & J. J. Wurtman (Eds.), *Nutrition and the brain* (pp. 89–138). New York: Raven Press.

van Praag, H. M., Plutchik, R., & Conte, H. (1986). The serotonin-hypothesis of (auto) aggression. Critical appraisal of the evidence. *Ann. N.Y. Acad. Sci.*, *487*, 150–167.

van Praag, H. M., Lemus, C., & Kahn, R. (1987a). Hormonal probes of central serotonergic activity. Do they really exist? *Biol. Psychiatry*, *22*, 86–98.

van Praag, H. M., Kahn, R., Asnis, G. M., Lemus, C. Z., & Brown, S. L. (1987b). Therapeutic indications for serotonin potentiating compounds. A hypothesis. *Biol. Psychiatry*, *22*, 205–212.

van Praag, H. M., Kahn, R., Asnis, G. M., Wetzler, S., Brown, S., Bleich, A., & Korn, M. (1987c). Denosologization of biological psychiatry on the specificity of 5-HT disturbances in psychiatric disorders. *J. Affect. Dis.*, *13*, 1–8.

van Praag, H. M., Verhoeven, W. M. A., & Kahn. R. S. (1988). *Psychofarmaca* (3rd ed.). Assen/Maastricht: Van Gorcum.

van Praag, H. M. (1990).Two–tier diagnosing in psychiatry. *Psychiat. Res.* (in press).

Virkkunen, M., Nuutila, A., Goodwin, F. K., & Linnoila, M. (1987). Cerebrospinal fluid monoamine metabolite levels in male arsonists. *Arch. Gen. Psychiatry*, *44*, 241–247.

Williams, J., & Davies, J. A. (1983). The involvement of 5-hydroxytryptamine in the release of dendritic dopamine from slices of rat substantia nigra. *J. Pharm. Pharmacol.*, *35*, 734–737.

Name Index

333

Subject Index